内功推拿

（汉英对照）

Neigong Tuina

(Chinese-English)

主编译

林 勋 姚 斐

Chief Compilers/Translators Lin Xun Yao Fei

上海科学技术出版社

Shanghai Scientific & Technical Publishers

图书在版编目（CIP）数据

内功推拿：汉英对照 / 林勋，姚斐主编译. -- 上海：上海科学技术出版社，2024.3
ISBN 978-7-5478-6545-3

Ⅰ. ①内… Ⅱ. ①林… ②姚… Ⅲ. ①推拿－双语教学－高等学校－教材－汉、英 Ⅳ. ①R244.1

中国国家版本馆CIP数据核字(2024)第040449号

内功推拿(汉英对照)
主编译 林 勋 姚 斐

上海世纪出版(集团)有限公司
上海科学技术出版社 出版、发行
(上海市闵行区号景路159弄A座9F-10F)
邮政编码201101 www.sstp.cn
上海新华印刷有限公司印刷
开本 787×1092 1/16 印张 18
字数 300千字
2024年3月第1版 2024年3月第1次印刷
ISBN 978-7-5478-6545-3 / R·2968
定价：85.00元

内容提要　Abstract

> 《内功推拿》汉英双语对照教材包括绪论、源流、基本操作、特色疗法、练功法及临床应用六部分内容。

> 绪论部分，主要介绍内功推拿的定义与理念，内功推拿是中医推拿的一个重要分支，是在疾病的预防和治疗过程中，注重选择与少林内功有关的功法训练和接受推拿手法治疗相结合的一种推拿理论与技术，引导读者了解内功推拿的基本内涵和深厚底蕴。源流部分，简要阐述内功推拿的起源及发展过程。基本操作部分，详细阐述了内功推拿的各种手法、技巧及操作要领，同时结合丰富的图例，使读者能够迅速掌握内功推拿的要领。特色疗法部分，详细介绍了内功推拿在各类疾病中的应用及特色疗法，如棒击、膏摩、热敷、熏蒸等，充分展示了内功推拿在解决常见疾病、慢性病及疼痛性疾病等方面的独特优势。练功法部分，展示了少林内功的基本习练方法和技巧，帮助读者通过自身的锻炼，提高身体素质和抵抗力。临床应用部分，通过结合具体病例，详细阐述了内功推拿在临床上的应用及注意事项，帮助读者更好地掌握内功推拿的治疗原理和方法。

> 作为一部供外国留学生及中医爱好者使用的双语教材，本书集理论与实用技能于一体，以科学性、实用性和普适性为原则，全面展示了内功推拿的独特魅力与广泛应用，且图文并茂，以便读者理解内功推拿的治疗原理，能更直观地掌握手法操作技巧。

> The *Neigong Tuina* (Chinese-English) includes six parts: introduction, origin, basic operation, characteristic therapy, practice method and clinical application. The introduction part mainly introduces the definition and concept of Neigong Tuina. Neigong Tuina is an important branch of traditional Chinese medicine tuina. In the process of disease prevention and treatment,

it pays attention to the combination of exercise training related to Shaolin Neigong and tuina treatment, and guides readers to understand the basic connotation and deep inside information of Neigong Tuina. In the second part, the origin and development process of Neigong Tuina are briefly expounded. The basic operation section elaborates the various techniques, skills and operation essentials of the internal work massage, and combines rich legends to enable readers to quickly grasp the essentials of the Neigong Tuina. The special therapy chapter introduces the application and characteristic therapy of Neigong Tuina in various diseases in detail, which fully demonstrating the unique advantages of Neigong Tuina in solving common diseases, chronic diseases and painful diseases. The Shaolin Internal Exercise part shows the basic training methods and skills of Shaolin Internal Exercise, helping readers to improve their physical quality and resistance through their own exercises. Clinical application part, through the combination of specific cases, elaborated the clinical application of internal tuina and precautions, can help readers better grasp the principle and method of internal work massage treatment.

> As a bilingual textbook for foreign students and enthusiasts, this book integrates theory and practical skills, and fully demonstrates the unique charm and wide application of Neigong Tuina based on the principles of science, practicality and universality. This book is illustrated with so that readers can well understand the therapeutic principle of Neigong Tuina and master the manipulation skills more intuitively.

编委会 Compilation committee

主编译

林 勋 姚 斐

副主编译

肖 彬 陈 博 王尔亮

编委（以姓氏笔画为序）

朱静洲 任美玲 安光辉 李建华 沈永勤 沈慧萍
陈 晨 岳虹妤 袁恺文 高宁阳 郭光昕 谢芳芳
蓝涵皙 谭雁夫 薛玲玲

学术秘书

袁恺文

Chief Compilers/Translators

Lin Xun Yao Fei

Associate Compilers/Translators

Xiao Bin Chen Bo Wang Erliang

Contributors

Zhu Jingzhou Ren Meiling An Guanghui Li Jianhua
Shen Yongqin Shen Huiping Chen Chen Yue Hongyu
Yuan Kaiwen Gao Ningyang Guo Guangxin Xie Fangfang
Lan Hanxi Tan Yanfu Xue Lingling

Academic Secretary

Yuan Kaiwen

编写说明 Instructions

> 内功推拿是中医推拿特色流派，是文化和医学融合的产物，对推拿学科的发展影响很大，在中医推拿中占有举足轻重的地位。编写过程中，不仅突出内功推拿的源流、特色手法和功法，而且注重传授推拿名家独特的教学和训练方法，同时结合常见临床疾病治疗经验，现代研究进展等，力求展现内功推拿的功法魅力。全书文字简洁，图文并茂，论述精炼，深入浅出，通俗易懂。

> 本书在编译过程中，术语英译主要参考世界中医药学会联合会发布的《中医基本名词术语中英对照国际标准》、世界卫生组织总部发布的*WHO International Standard Terminologies on Traditional Chinese Medicine*两部术语标准，中药名采用音译及括号夹注中文及拉丁药名形式，古籍名采用英译，主要参考已出版书籍、教材中相关译法，力求译文语言表达的简洁性和准确性。

《内功推拿》编委会

2023.10

> Neigong Tuina is a characteristic school of Chinese medicine massage, is the product of the integration of culture and medicine, has a great impact on the development of the discipline of tuina, and occupies a pivotal position in Chinese medicine. In the process of writing, not only highlight the origin, characteristic techniques and exercises of Shaolin Internal Exercise, but also pay attention to the unique teaching and training methods of tuina masters, while combining the treatment experience of common clinical diseases, modern research progress, and so on, and strive

to show the charm of Shaolin Internal Exercise. The text is concise, illustrated, refined, simple and easy to understand.

> During the compilation of this textbook, The English translation of terms mainly refers to the *International Standards for Chinese-English Comparison of Basic Terms of Chinese Medicine* issued by the World Federation of Chinese Medicine Societies and *WHO International Standard Terminologies on Traditional Chinese* issued by the headquarters of the World Health Organization. The names of medicine are translated into Chinese and Latin medicine names. The ancient classics are translated mainly referring to the relevant translation methods in published books and textbooks, so as to strive for the simplicity and accuracy of the translation language expression.

Neigong Tuina Compilation Committee

Oct. 2023

目录 Contents

绪论

Introduction

释义

内功推拿是中医推拿的一个重要分支，是在疾病的预防和治疗过程中，注重选择与少林内功有关的功法训练和接受推拿手法治疗相结合的一种推拿理论与技术。曾名为擦法推拿、古法推拿等。

内功推拿起源于北方，形成于上海。经过几代人的发展和完善，形成了独特的学术思想、标志性的手法、明确的优势病种和有一定影响力的代表人物，逐渐发展为一支重要的推拿流派。

少林内功是内功推拿流派的标志性组成部分，除用于推拿医师自我锻炼强身外，还被用来指导患者练功治病，所有的推拿手法操作都是在患者锻炼少林内功的基础上进行的。

少林内功属于内功还是外功?

“内功”主要是“内练一口气”，也包括精神意念的修炼。练气讲究呼吸吐纳，多用腹式呼吸法，精神集中，循序渐进，从而达到锻炼身体内部器官的目的。包括佛家、道家和养生家的静功和各种调息功夫在内的内功，古代一般都在极少数人中私相授受，民国时期开始有人将其以“气功”之名用于治疗肺痨等慢性病。20世纪50年代以来，通过多地兴办气功疗养院而在辅助医疗方面得到了普遍应用。

“外功”就是“外练筋骨皮”，

Paraphrase

Neigong Tuina, once called Rubbing Tuina and Antique Tuina, is one of the significant branches of Tuina. It represents a theory and technique of Tuina, which attaches great importance to the combination of Shaolin internal exercise and manipulations, with the purpose of preventing and treating diseases.

Neigong Tuina originated in Northern China and took shape in Shanghai. Developed and improved by several generations, Neigong Tuina has become an important school of Tuina with defined academic thoughts, typical manipulations, distinctively-targeted diseases and famous figures.

Shaolin internal exercise is a significant component of Neigong Tuina. Tuina practitioners can do workout with it. But most importantly, patients are guided to exercise Shaolin internal exercise to treat diseases. Patients do Shaolin internal exercise first and then receive Tuina manipulations.

Shaolin internal exercise: internal exercise or external exercise?

“Internal exercise” is aimed at strengthening qi, and developing mind and will. Strengthening qi focuses on breathing, mainly abdominal breathing. When doing it, you must concentrate the mind and move towards progressively to exercise internal organs. Quiet qigong in Buddhism and Taoism, and internal exercise for adjusting breath were always transmitted among few people in ancient China. However, since the Republic of China (1912–1949), some TCM practitioners had used it in the name of “qigong” to treat chronic diseases like pulmonary tuberculosis. Since 1950s, internal exercise has got wide application in complementary medicine with the establishment of qigong

是锻炼筋、骨、皮的功夫。武术中，外功指习武者经过专门的系统训练，使身体的筋骨具有比常人较强的抗击打能力，达到外壮的效果，有拍打、棒击等锻炼方法。养生功法中的外功，主要是以肢体导引、按摩为主的动功。

民国金倜生所著《嫡派真传少林内功秘传》序云："易筋经为少林武术祖师达摩禅师所传授，分内、外两经。内经主柔，以静坐运气为事；至于外经，则主刚，以强筋练力为事，法偏重于上肢，实为练力运气、舒展筋脉之妙法。每日勤行四五次，百日之后，则食量增加、筋骨舒畅、百病不生。"外经的描述与内功推拿之少林内功颇有几分相似。内功推拿之少林内功的姿势锻炼法实为上肢姿势锻炼法搭配基本裆式组合锻炼法，着重锻炼两下肢的"霸力"和上肢的"灵活性"。且少林内功亦有"棒击""练力"，其内功推拿流派传人马万起曾是名震上海滩的武术教练。因此，少林内功有外功属性。

但不论是养生家还是武术家的内功，在习练时对"气"的体悟和运用都是其重要的组成部分。因此，强调"练气不见气""以气导力""气贯四肢"的少林内功之所以被称为"内功"也有一定道理。当然，这也与清末和民国时期武术、养生界崇尚"内功"的风气有关。

nursing homes in many places in China.

External exercise is aimed at strengthening the muscles, bones, and skin. By exercising external exercise in a systematic manner, people will make their tendons and bones stronger with higher tolerance to hitting. There are training methods such as flapping and stick knocking. External exercise in health-preserving exercises are mainly general exercises based on Daoyin and massage.

Direct Branch of Shaolin Internal Exercise: Preface written by Jin Disheng in the Republic of China said: "The book *Yijinjing* was written by Damo, the original master of Shaolin internal exercise and has two volumes, Nei Jing and Wai Jing. Nei Jing focuses on sit-in meditation and qi movement which can be featured as softening, while Wai Jing on enhancing sinews and bones and strength which can be featured as toughening. Its methods concentrate on upper body, a useful way to boosting strength, adjusting qi movement and stretching muscles. It should be performed four or five times a day for over three months, he would have better appetite, relax his muscles and never develop illnesses." The description of Wai Jing is much pretty similar to Shaolin internal exercise of Neigong Tuina. The movement of Shaolin internal exercise is the combination of upper body exercise and basic lower body one, with a focus on strengthening legs' stability and arms' flexibility. And Shaolin internal exercise also has "thrashing" and "strength training", the heir of which is Ma Wanqi, a kung fu coach well-known in Shanghai. That's to say, Shaolin internal exercise carries the characteristics of external exercise.

The most important part in internal exercise is to experience and apply qi, for both health-preservers and martial artists. So it makes sense that it is called by internal exercise, which emphasizes "exercise qi without seeing it", "strength is driven by qi", "four extremities is flooded by qi". Of course, it's also related with advocate of internal exercise in the circles of health-preservers and martial artists in the late Qing Dynasty (1636–1921) and the Republic of China around.

学术特点 Academic Features

内功推拿有一整套独特理论和治疗方法，其注重用中医基础理论指导临床实践，治疗上强调整体观念，善从脾胃论治，从而达到健脾和胃、扶助正气、调和气血、疏通经络、扶正祛邪、平衡阴阳，增强人体自身的抗病能力，并以此作为临床治疗疾病的纲领。内功推拿方法种类多，有特色的手法和棒击法、热敷法、练功等。治疗范围广泛，有病可治，无病可防，尚有强身健体之功效。

内功推拿的学术特点，可概括为以下几点。

Neigong Tuina has its own specific theories and treatment methods. Its clinical practice is guided by the basic theories of Traditional Chinese Medicine (TCM). When it comes to treatment, it puts emphasis on holistic concept with a focus on spleen and stomach's patterns identification. This is how it can improve people's resistance to diseases by strengthening spleen and harmonizing stomach, strengthening healthy qi, harmonizing between qi and blood, unblocking meridians and collaterals, balancing yin and yang. There are various methods within Neigong Tuina, including special manipulations, stick knocking manipulation, hot compress and exercise and so on. It can cure a wide range of diseases and strengthen body to prevent diseases.

The academic features of Neigong Tuina can be summarized as following:

一、强调扶正祛邪，重视整体观念

Focus on Strengthening Healthy Qi and Dissipating Pathogenic Factors, and Holistic Concept

内功推拿流派强调扶正祛邪，要求患者练功，提高自身正气，所谓正气存内，则邪不可干。待患者身体经过一段时间锻炼，身体状态有所改善，再结合手法治疗则易取效。从治疗手法来看，内功推拿善

The school of Neigong Tuina lays emphasis on strengthening healthy qi and dissipating pathogenic factors. It asks patients to do Shaolin internal exercise to cultivate and enhance healthy qi. It is due to the fact that there is sufficient healthy qi inside the body, that is why pathogenic

于平推法，尽管平推法是一种刺激性手法，对人体补泻作用取决于机体状态和手法所施部位或穴位，但总以温热为佳，偏于温补。即使刺激性较强的击法，也是通过穴位的配伍和击打力量的调节，达到激发阳气、扶正祛邪的功效，用于强身健体和内、妇虚损性疾病的治疗。从治疗部位上看，内功推拿注重推上腹、推两胁，旨在健脾和胃。脾胃乃后天之本，脾胃功能健全，正气则转虚为实；推肾俞、命门、八髎壮肾益气，肾主一身之精，肾强则体自强。从指导思想上看，内功推拿非常重视整体思想，认为人体是一个有机的整体，无论内、妇、虚劳杂病，还是伤科疾病，均以一定步骤的常规操作法作为基本方法，在此基础上进行手法治疗、刺激穴位。常规操作的施术区域遍及全身，又以头面、躯干部为手法刺激的重点，根据不同的疾病有所增减。这样，全身各穴均可受到手法的刺激，并且能够辨证施治，若能持之以恒，对慢性疾病，特别是慢性疑难杂症的治疗，往往会产生令人满意的奇效。

factors cannot invade the body. After doing Shaolin internal exercise for a period of time, people will have better health conditions. And receiving tuina manipulations at this time will be more effective. Flat-pushing manipulation is the most useful manipulation of Neigong Tuina, which is irritating. The tonifying and purging effect of flat-pushing manipulation depends on the patient's physical condition and the area or the acupuncture point treated. It has the function of warming and tonification and works better with warm hands. Knocking manipulation, which is more irritating, also achieves the efficacy of activating yang qi and reinforcing healthy qi to eliminate pathogenic factors by acupoints combination and knocking power adjustment. This can be used to obtain a stronger body and treat diseases including internal and female ones and others caused by deficiency and impairment.

For treatment parts, Neigong Tuina attaches much importance to pushing the upper abdomen and subcostal regions, with the purpose of strengthening the spleen and harmonizing the stomach. Spleen and stomach are two most essential organs for human to keep healthy, sound functions of which can replenish healthy qi. Kidneys and kidney qi can be tonified by pushing Shenshu (BL 23), Mingmen (DU 4) and Baliao (BL 31–34) points. Kidneys govern the whole essence in the body, so good function of kidneys makes an even stronger body. For guiding principles, Neigong Tuina pays high attention to holistic concept and regards human body as an organic whole. All diseases are treated by the same regular manipulation at the beginning and then by specialized manipulation or acupoints' rubbing.

The regular manipulation covers the entire body with a focus on head, face and trunk, and it can be adjusted according to various diseases. In that case, all acupoints can be stimulated by manipulations and patients can get treatment based on patterns identification. If making it a habit, you can be rewarded with unexpected recovery for chronic diseases especially chronic intractable ones.

二、特色功法

少林内功是内功推拿流派的特有功法，与一般的气功不同，少林内功的特点是练习时呼吸自如，不屏气，不运气。而四肢，特别是手和足要用够力量，做到所谓“练气不见气，以力带气，气贯四肢”。如此，气血就会随力而行，注于经脉，荣贯四肢九窍、五脏六腑，使阴阳平和、气血充沛。少林内功的练习方法很多，常用的有三个裆势（站裆、马裆、弓箭裆）和四个动作（前推八匹马、倒拉九头牛、霸王举鼎、风摆荷叶）。这种锻炼方法是以关节拮抗肌同时做强制性静力收缩的运动方式，不仅是一种有特色的功疗方法，也是一种有效地提高肌肉力量和耐力的锻炼方法，对推拿手法的渗透性亦有帮助。

Distinctive Internal Exercise

Shaolin internal exercise is the exercise only used by Neigong Tuina. Different from common Qigong, Shaolin internal exercise requires people to breathe naturally and store up strength in four limbs, especially in hands and feet. The ultimate goal is to gather enough strength to achieve the so-called “exercise qi without seeing it”, “strength is drove by qi”, and “four extremities is flooded by qi”. Qi and blood will flow into the meridians and collaterals along with strength to nourish four extremities and nine orifices and five zang-organs and six fu-organs which help reach yin-yang harmony and make qi and blood abundant within the human body. There are many ways to do Shaolin internal exercise, but three gestures (standing stance, horse stance and bow stance) and four movements: Qian Tui Ba Pi Ma (Pushing Eight Horses Forward), Dao La Jiu Tou Niu (Pulling Nine Oxen Backward), Ba Wang Jun Ding (Hegemonic King Supporting Tripot) and Feng Bai He Ye (Wind Blowing Lotus Leaf) are usually seen. This forces antagonistic muscle to statically contract, recognizing a distinctive treatment methods, a way to boost muscles' strength and resistance effectively and a great help to more effective manipulation.

三、特色治疗手法

内功推拿在临床实践中形成了部分有特色治疗手法，如平推法、提拿法、推桥弓、扫散法、理法、劈法等。其中，平推法是内功推拿

Distinctive Manipulation

During clinical practice, Neigong Tuina forms some distinctive manipulations, such as Pingtui manipulation (flat-pushing manipulation), Tina manipulation (lifting-grasping manipulation), Tuiqiaogong manipulation (pushing

的基本手法，可分为掌推法、大鱼际推法、小鱼际推法、指推法等，可借用一定的介质直接在体表操作，旨在取得温热深透的效果。五指拿法也称为抓法，一般仅用于头部，五指所经之处为两侧胆经、膀胱经和督脉。推桥弓是指以拇指推法施于两侧胸锁乳突肌前缘，上起翳风穴下抵缺盆。扫散法是指拇指与四指分开，拇指置于角孙穴，其余四指置于约脑空至风池处，由前向后靠腕关节，做扫散动作。内功推拿对部分手法进行发挥，如叩击类手法在内功推拿中被应用于全身各部，包括掌击法、拳击和棒击等，除在风湿、瘘、痹等证应用外，也广泛用于内科其他疾病。

bridge archpinching), Saosan manipulation (sweeping manipulation), Li manipulation (regulating manipulation) and Pi manipulation (splitting manipulation). Among them, flat-pushing manipulation is the basic manipulation in Neigong Tuina, which also can be divided into palm-pushing manipulation, great thenar pushing manipulation, hypothenar-pushing manipulation and finger-pushing manipulation. Flat-pushing manipulation can be operated directly on the surface of the body by using certain stuffs to heat the interior. Five-finger manipulation can also be called as grabbing manipulation, which is only used on head. During this manipulation, five fingers scratch gallbladder meridian, bladder meridian and the Du meridian on the two sides. Pushing bridge arch is to use thumbs to push the front side of sternocleidomastoid from Yifeng (SJ 17) to Quepen (ST 12). Sweeping manipulation means that a thumb separates from other fingers with the thumb putting at Jiaosun (SJ 20) and others putting from Naokong (GB 19) to Fengchi (GB 20) then five fingers wiggle front and back by wrist joints. Neigong Tuina expands the application of some manipulations, like knocking, which can be used around the body, including palm-slapping, punching and stick knocking. Apart from the application in wind dampness, fistula, and Bi-impediment, knocking is also widely used in various other internal diseases.

四、棒击法

棒击法也是内功推拿的一大特色。医者握住棒体的一端运用腕力，轻巧灵活地棒击全身各特定部位。棒击时要求患者全身放松、呼吸顺畅，击打的刺激性很强，适用于在疾病恢复期，患者体质已能承受棒力时或某些手法达不到一定力量而

Stick Knocking Manipulation

Stick knocking manipulation is another distinctive manipulation of Neigong Tuina. The practitioner holds one end of the stick and thrashes the certain part of body lightly with wrist force. When thrashing, the patient should relax the whole body and breathe smoothly. Due to its strong irritation, it applies at patients in rehabilitation who can withstand the force of thrashing, or in situation that other

不能起治疗作用时使用。尤其是病程较长的关节痹痛、感觉迟钝、肢体麻木等症和内伤杂病。也可用于强壮筋骨、祛病延年。使用时需要严格掌握中医辨证施治原则，视疾病的轻重不同、患病的部位不一而施以轻重不等的棒力。临床常用囟门棒击法、大椎棒击法、背部棒击法、胸背部棒击法、髋关节、大腿棒击法、小腿部棒击法等。

manipulations failing to cure, especially for patients having arthralgia, numbness of sensation and limbs, internal and miscellaneous diseases with long course. Stick knocking manipulation can also strengthen the tendons and bones, ward off diseases and prolong life. Based on the principle of TCM pattern identification and treatment, the stick knocking force depends on the severity and different parts of the disease. Clinically, stick knocking manipulation is often applied on fontanel, Dazhui (CV 14), back, thoracic and dorsal parts, hip joints, thighs and shanks.

五、全身推拿常规操作法

Routine Manipulation for Whole Body

内功推拿不仅可以治疗内、妇、杂症，还广泛应用于伤骨科疾病。内功推拿治疗内、妇疾病有一定的程序，这套手法习惯上被称为“常规手法”或“内功推拿常规操作”。一般顺序为头面部→颈项部→胸腹部→肩背腰部→肋胁部→上肢部→下肢部→头面部。常规操作从头面到腰骶，涉及十二经和奇经八脉，有疏通经络、调和气血、荣灌脏腑之功效。手法轻重因人而异，体弱者手法轻柔，体壮者手法可略重。临床应用时根据不同疾病适当加减变化。这套手法扶正祛邪、辨证论治，较好地反映了内功推拿流派的特点。内功推拿在治疗骨伤疾病时也有明确的步骤，并有盘、运、扳、提等各类手法。

Apart from miscellaneous internal and gynecological diseases, Neigong Tuina is also widely used in traumatological diseases treatment. There are certain processes for Neigong Tuina to treat internal and gynecological diseases, which are called the routine manipulation or the routine manipulations in Neigong Tuina. Generally routine manipulation is practiced in the order of head and face, neck, chest and abdomen, lateral thorax, upper limbs, lower limbs, and head and face. The routine manipulation covers head, face, waist to sacra, including twelve meridians and eight extra meridians, which can unblock meridians and collaterals, harmonize qi and blood and nourish internal organs. The manipulation on weak patients should be soft and light and on strong patients be a little harder. The force of manipulation should also be changed in accordance with different people and diseases. The routine manipulation is guided by the principle of pattern identification and treatment and can reinforce healthy qi to eliminate pathogenic factors, which reflects the characteristics of Neigong Tuina school. There are also clear processes of Neigong Tuina to treat orthopedic diseases with kneading, arc-pushing, pulling, lifting and other manipulations.

六、先练后推，功法手法有机结合

内功推拿在治疗时要求“先练后推”，功法锻炼和手法治疗有机结合，内功推拿在治疗内科虚损性疾病时，有“先练后推”的说法，即先指导患者练习少林内功。练习少林内功是为了扶助正气，正强则邪自去，通过功法的良性刺激激发人体经络系统的自身整体调节功能，使人体的生命活动恢复到正常状态。对于虚损明显的患者，更需要坚持练功，待脏腑和气血功能增强后再增加手法治疗。手法治疗具有疏通经络、行气活血的作用，刺激性手法在祛邪的同时会有消耗气机的副作用。因此，有时手法治疗后患者在感觉身体轻松的同时，会伴有轻度疲劳感，手法治疗如能结合功法锻炼则可以减缓单纯手法刺激产生的副作用。

Exercise Neigong First then Get Tuina Treatment

In treatment, Neigong Tuina requires patients to exercise before Tuina manipulations, which means integrating internal exercise with manipulation treatment. Doing Shaolin internal exercise can reinforce healthy qi to eliminate pathogenic factors. Shaolin internal exercise can also stimulate meridian system to arouse its self-adjustment function to enhance efficacy after the function of internal organs and qi and blood being strengthened. Manipulations can unblock meridian and activate qi and blood but some irritating manipulation can not only eliminate pathogenic factors but also curb qi activity. Therefore, after manipulation treatment, patients can feel relax with a little fatigue. Manipulation with exercising Neigong can release the side effects of only manipulation treatment.

七、擅长热敷和膏摩

湿热敷是内功推拿中不可分割的重要组成部分，在内功推拿中又称为“上水”。湿热敷是选用具有祛风散寒、疏经通络、理气、止痛、活血祛瘀的中草药配伍组方，放于布袋中在锅中煮沸，而后将毛巾浸湿后拧干，敷于病变部位，将热敷及药物外治相结合，其疗效明显，主要用于治疗关节风湿痹痛。湿热

Do Well in Hot Compress and Ointment Rubbing

Moist hot compress is an indispensable part of Neigong Tuina, which is called “Shangshui”. Moist hot compress is that put herbal formula which can dispel wind and dissipate cold, unblock meridians and collaterals, regulate qi, alleviate pain, circulate blood and eliminate stasis into a bag then throw the bag into a pot filled with water. Squeeze the towel which drowned in the boiling water and apply it to the area to be treated. It

敷能增强透热作用，提高手法治疗效果。一般在手法操作后应用，在不同部位使用具有不同的疗效。

内功推拿的另一特色是膏摩。膏摩是将手法与药物配合运用的一种方法，是用药物涂抹于施术部位，再施以手法，从而达到防治疾病的目的。擦法是内功推拿的主要代表手法，操作时多用冬青油膏或其他的油性介质，一是利于手法的操作，二可防止破皮，三可提高手法的效应。

gets greater efficacy when combing drugs with moist hot compress, which is often treated rheumatoid arthritis. Moist hot compress which applies after manipulation can increase penetration of heat and enhance the efficacy of manipulation. And moist hot compress in different part has different effects.

Another distinctive treatment method of Neigong Tuina is Gao Mo (Tuina combined with herbal ointment). Gao Mo is to apply herbal ointment on the surface of the area to be treated, following tuina manipulations, which aims to prevent and control diseases. Linear rubbing manipulation is the characteristic manipulation of Neigong Tuina. Practitioners may apply Chinese ilex ointment and other ointments first and then manipulate. The ointment can make manipulation easier, prevent broken skin and promote efficacy.

八、擅长治疗内妇科疾病，兼及伤科

内功推拿治疗手段丰富，手法多样，具有疏通经络、调和气血、调整脏腑的功效，治疗疾病范围广。在临床上善于治疗内科虚劳杂病、妇科经带胎产和伤骨科疾病。尤其擅长治疗劳倦内伤、胸胁屏伤、头痛失眠、高血压、神经衰弱以及部分呼吸道、消化道系统疾病。临床应用时功法强度和手法力度当结合具体疾病和体质灵活运用。

Specializes in the Treatment of Gynecological and Traumatological Diseases

Neigong Tuina can unblock meridians and collaterals, harmonize qi and blood and regulate internal organs to treat a wide array of diseases with various methods and manipulation. Clinically, Neigong Tuina is more effective in treating internal diseases, deficiency and miscellaneous diseases, menstruation, leukorrhea, pregnancy, childbirth and other gynecological diseases and orthopedic diseases, especially internal injury caused by fatigue, chest and hypochondrium injury, headache and insomnia, hypertension, neurasthenia and some respiratory and digestive system diseases. In clinical application, the force of the Neigong and the strength of the manipulation should be flexibly applied in light of specific diseases and constitutions.

学习方法 Learning Methods

一、根据自身生理特点训练

每个人的生理条件不尽相同，操作者性别年龄、高低胖瘦、形态体质等对手法效果有一定的影响。尤其是手指形状的差异对部分手法有较大的影响。可根据自己体质、生理特点去钻研训练，形成适合自己的推拿风格。不必完全模仿一个授课教师的手法，也不能要求学习者的手法都整齐划一。功法训练时间和强度也需要因人而异，不过分强求一致，要使学习者既能日有所进，又留有余兴。

Based on Your Physical Condition

Different physical conditions, such as ages, heights, shapes and constitutions result in different effects of manipulations. Particularly, the shapes of fingers have a great influence on some manipulations. In line with your constitutions and physical conditions, you can explore your own style of Tuina. It's unnecessary to copy teacher's manipulations or be identical with your counterparts. The training time and intensity also vary from person to person, which are the best that learners can make progress day by day and still have passion to learn it.

二、配合推拿功法训练

功法训练，尤其是少林内功，可以增强臂力、指力和下肢力量，更能从整体上提升专项耐力、灵敏性、柔韧性、协调性等身体素质。少林内功锻炼时要注意形体、呼吸和意念的配合，做到形松、气平、心定。

Together with Neigong Tuina

Exercising Shaolin internal exercise can enhance arms, fingers and legs' strength and boost your endurance, agility, flexibility, coordination etc. And during the process, pay attention to the coordination among gestures, breath and will to keep body relaxed, breath calm and mind stable.

三、循序渐进、持之以恒

手法是推拿取效的关键因素。因此，推拿手法训练和实践至关重要。但推拿手法的基本功训练不能

Be Progressive and Persistent

Manipulations are the essence to the effective treatment. That's why the training and practice of manipulations are important. However, do not expect to make achievement

急于求成，要一步一步地按计划循序渐进地进行。先米袋练习，后人体操作；先训练动作的准确性，再调整力量、耐力和频率；先单手练习，再双手训练；先训练功法、训练身形姿势的协调能力和平衡能力，再训练手法；先学习简单手法，再训练复杂手法；先形似，后神似；先继承，后创新。有机会多临床实践，不断摸索适合医患双方的治疗方法和手法。学习和训练一定要扎扎实实地坚持每天训练、持之以恒。绝不能采用那种“三天打鱼，两天晒网”式的训练方法。功法训练也应遵循“百日一小成，千日一大成”，不可操之过急。

immediately but practise step by step as scheduled. Practise on a bag of rice then on human body; focus on the correctness of manipulation gestures then adjusting strength, endurance and frequency; do one-hand practice then two-hand practice; exercise internal exercise and body posture coordination and balance then practise manipulations; practise simple manipulations then complicate ones; grasp the similar gestures of manipulations then comprehend their essences; learn then innovate. Conduct more clinical practice if possible to figure out the best treatment methods and manipulations suitable for both practitioners and patients. Tuina manipulations should be learned and practised every day, so should internal exercise.

四、利用一切条件配合手法训练

（1）要利用手法力学测定仪，实时检测手法指标。在观察手法的力量、频率、均匀性、运动轨迹等物理指标方面，现有的手法力学测定仪完全可以满足辅助教学的需要。当然，在其他很多方面，手法力学测定仪的智能还有待提高。

（2）要充分利用现代多媒体手段辅助学习推拿手法。要注意收集和利用DVD、网络等视频媒介，了解、学习和研究推拿手法。这是学习传统推拿手法的重要途径。“取法乎上，得乎其中”，不要仅仅满足于书本和老师授课。

Use All Conditions to Comply with Manipulation Practice

(1) Make use of measuring instrument of manipulation mechanics to detect of manipulation indicators in time. This instrument can aid teaching to observe strength, frequency, uniformity, movement trajectory and other physical indicators. But in other aspects, the functions of instrument need to be improved.

(2) Make full use of modern multimedia to learn Tuina manipulations. Collect and utilize DVD, Internet and other video media to learn about Tuina manipulations, which is an important channel to learn traditional Tuina manipulations. As a saying goes, “one sets the highest goals but may attain medium result”. So do not limit in your learning in textbooks and classes.

五、牢记身心放松，科学合理地训练技能

推拿不是单纯的体力劳动，手法学习和功法训练时要多动脑筋。要从人体解剖特点、生理学、生物力学、手法动力学等方面去认识理解手法和功法，理解掌握推拿技能的基本规律。需要明确某一手法运动的主动肌群是什么，如何使应该用力的肌肉紧张，而不应该用力的肌肉放松；要了解肌肉的紧张与放松如何交替进行，如何在保证完成手法动作的前提下，尽可能地放松肌肉以保证血液的持续供应；如何利用大肌肉群操作，以减少或延缓肌肉疲劳；如何在所有手法操作时尽可能保持身心放松、自然呼吸，避免屏气现象。这些都是在推拿手法训练的初始阶段应该学会的。

Relax Your Body and Mind, Practise Technique Scientifically

Tuina is not simply manual labor. It's important to keep brain ticking over when learning manipulations and exercising internal exercise. It is necessary to know and understand Tuina manipulations and master their basic laws from the human anatomy characteristics, physiology, biomechanics and manipulation dynamics. Learners should make it clear that each manipulation acts on which agonistic muscles group and how to tense the muscles that should tense, and relax the others; how to make muscle alternate between tension and relaxation and how to ensure the completion of manipulations, as much as possible to relax the muscle to ensure the continuous supply of blood; how to manipulate large muscle groups to decrease or delay muscle fatigue; how to remain body and mind relaxed and breathe naturally to avoid holding breath. Those all should be learned at the primary stage of practice.

六、掌握与推拿有关的医学基础知识

推拿不仅用于临床医学、预防保健，还可用于康复医学，治疗与应用领域广泛。学习内功推拿必须掌握相关疾病的基础知识才能更好地发挥推拿作用。要立足临床疗效，秉承“杂合而治”的理念，融合有效方法和技术。要能够综合运用相关基础知识和中西医诊疗知识来逐步加深对推拿治疗作用的理解，如与推拿密切相关的肌肉、骨骼、关

Master the Tuina-related Basic Medical Knowledge

Tuina can be used in a wide range of fields, including clinical medicine, disease prevention and rehabilitation medicine. When only master basic knowledge of relative diseases, Neigong Tuina can give its full play to treat. Based on clinical efficacy, Tuina practitioners should embrace the idea of “various methods to treatment together” to integrate effective methods and techniques. To get deeper understanding of Tuina treatment, use relevant basic knowledge and traditional Chinese and western medicine diagnosis and treatment knowledge,

节、神经、生理、经络、腧穴等知识，这是学习和提升内功推拿的必备基础和内在要求。

including knowledge about muscles, bones, joints, nerves, physiology, meridians, acupoints. It's the indispensable foundation and prerequisite to learn and promote theories and practice of Neigong Tuina.

第一章

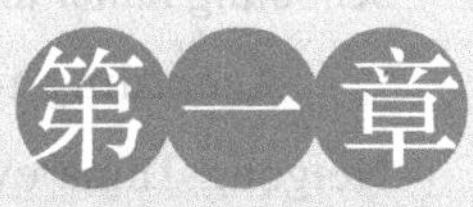

源流

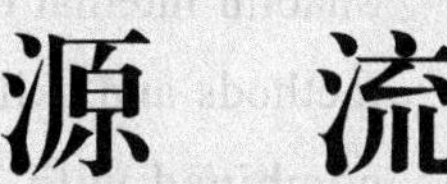

Chapter One
Origin

内功推拿具体源于何时尚有待于考证。一般认为内功推拿流派起源于北方，形成于上海，传播于全中国。内功推拿的师承脉络，可追溯到清末山东济宁的李嘉树，传马万起，后经马万龙和李锡九通过师带徒或学校教育进一步发扬光大。1956年10月10日，上海创办了第一期“推拿医师训练班”，后改为推拿学校，马万龙、李锡九等参与内功推拿理论或临床带教。至此，内功推拿教学打破了流派的壁垒，从过去单纯的师带徒形式走上了正规的学校教育途径，内功推拿的流传更为广泛。

根据目前现有资料的分析，内功推拿是在少林内功基础上逐步发展演化而形成的一种推拿流派。在长期的医疗实践过程中，由单纯的功法锻炼，逐渐融合了手法、膏摩、热敷和熏蒸等方法和技术，形成了内功推拿流派。经过几代人的发展和完善，形成了独特的学术思想、标志性手法、明确的优势病种和有一定影响力的代表人物，逐渐发展为一个重要的推拿流派。

It still remains to be proved when Neigong Tuina emerged. Generally speaking, Neigong Tuina had its origin in Northern China, took shape in Shanghai and then spread around China. The first Neigong Tuina master can be traced back to Li Jiashu who lived in Jining, Shandong province in the late Qing Dynasty. Ma Wanqi, the inheritor of Li Jiashu, and then Ma Wanlong and Li Xijiu enlarged their counterparts through apprenticeship and schooling. On October 10th, 1956, the first “Training Course for Tuina Practitioners” was held in Shanghai, which was renamed as Tuina College later. Ma Wanlong, Li Xijiu and other famous practitioners took part in teaching of Tuina theories and clinical practice. Therefore, the education for Neigong Tuina removed the barriers between different schools and distributed it even wider on the basis of formal schooling rather than apprenticeship.

According to current information, the school of Neigong Tuina evolved from Shaolin internal exercise. Shaolin internal exercise, an exercise absorbing medical methods and skills like manipulations, Gao Mo (Tuina combined with herbal ointment), hot compress and fumigation, leading its complete transformation into school of Neigong Tuina. Developed by several generations, Neigong Tuina has become an important school of Tuina with defined academic thoughts, typical manipulations, distinctively-targeted diseases and famous figures.

第一节 起源

Section One Origin

一、源于武

Derive from Kung Fu

推拿自诞生之日起，就与导引

From the very first day of its creation, Tuina has a

功法结下了不解之缘。导引疗法起源于古代的“舞蹈”。据《吕氏春秋·古乐》记载，“昔陶唐氏之始，阴多滞伏而湛积，水道壅塞，不行其原，民气郁阏而滞著，筋骨瑟缩不达，故作为舞以宣导之。”上古尧时洪水为患，造成“筋骨瑟缩”。当时的“舞”是导引的最早雏形。《庄子·刻意》谓：“吹呴呼吸，吐故纳新，熊经鸟伸，为寿而已矣。此道（导）引之士，养形之人，彭祖寿考者之所好也。”《引书》比较全面地反映了春秋战国时期的导引养生学成就，包括“导气令和，引体令柔”。

早期文献中导引与按摩并列，常常作为两种独立的疗法。中医经典著作《黄帝内经》把导引和按摩作为防治疾病的重要手段纳入医学体系之中，并指出了导引按摩的发源地是以河南为中心的中原地区。《素问·异法方宜论》记载：“中央者，其地平以湿，天地所生万物也众。其民食杂而不劳，故其病多痿厥寒热，其治宜导引按蹻。故导引按蹻者，亦从中央出也。”《素问·奇病论》《灵枢·病传》等也有导引按摩及其适应证的记载。医圣张仲景在《金匮要略》中将导引、膏摩与针灸等法并列，用于防治疾病。历史上也有医家将按摩与导引合并命名。如宋代张从正（子和）提出“按导”一词即为此意。民国以后出现《按导一得录》《袁氏按导学》等诸多以“按导”命名的文献，并出现了以“按导”为名从事推拿（按摩）开业者。

close bearing on Daoyin. Daoyin therapy is derived from ancient “dance”. According to *The Collection of Thoughts: Ancient Music chapter*, “When Yinkang came to the throne, excess yin qi deposited and blocked waterway. Everything in the world run in the opposed way. All people bottled themselves up with negative moods and hunched bodies. So the dance was created to release their emotions and free their bodies.” In the remote ages, when Yao was the leader of the Chinese nation, the flood caused tremendous havoc, contributing to people’s “cowering of tendons and bones”. At that time, “dance” was the earliest prototype of Daoyin. *Zhuangzi: One an Iron Will* said: “Breathe out waste and breathe in fresh air. It’s just like bears climbing trees and birds flying. All these lead to greater longevity. It’s the pursuit of people who exercise Daoyin and stay in shape like Pengzu, who lived 800 years.” The accomplishments of nourishing life by Daoyin in the Spring and Autumn Period and the Warring States Period (770 B.C.–221 B.C.) can be seen in the *Classic of Daoyin*. “Daoyin is to guide qi to adjust breath and stay calm, and to stretch body to enhance body flexibility and agility” is the famous sentence in the *Classic of Daoyin*.

Daoyin and massage were paid equal importance in the early literatures as two independent therapies. In *Yellow Emperor’s Canon of Medicine*, Daoyin and Anqiao (one of traditional Chinese massage) has been included in the medical system as two key methods to prevent and control diseases. And it has pointed that Daoyin and massage were originated in Henan province. It is recorded in *Plain Question: Discussion on Different Therapeutic Methods for Different Diseases*: “The central region, plain and humid, is the place rich in a variety of products. People living in the central region eat various kinds of food and do not need to do much work. So they tend to suffer from Weijue (flaccidity and coldness of limbs) and Hanre (Cold-Heat Syndrome) which can be treated by Anqiao.

内功推拿是在少林内功的基础上发展而形成的一种推拿流派，因此，推拿功法少林内功为内功推拿标志性组成部分。少林内功可使周身筋骨强健，气血充实，脏腑调和，阴阳平衡，力量陡增。少林内功起初是一种武术和功法锻炼，最初主要流传于我国北方山东、河南一带的农村。由于相关文献记载较少，少林内功精确的起源地仍需要进一步考证。目前主要有三种传说。

1. 少林说

天下功夫出少林，少林寺作为禅宗祖庭，在海内外享有极高的社会声誉。当前流传的少林内功有两种含义，广义的少林内功是少林寺僧人所练的内功，包括易筋经、洗髓经等。而特指的少林内功是内功推拿之少林内功，不仅用于针灸推拿学专业学生及推拿临床工作者自我锻炼以提高其身体素质和专业素质能力，亦被用于体弱病患者治病

So Daoyin and Anqiao were developed in the central region." There are also records about Daoyin and massage in *Plain Question: Discussion on Special Diseases* and *Miraculous Pivot: Diseases* have record of Daoyin and massage and their treatable diseases. Zhang Zhongjing regarded Daoyin and Gao Mo as methods to prevent and control diseases like acupuncture and moxibustion in his book *Synopsis of Prescriptions of the Golden Chamber*. In history, some doctors combined massage and Daoyin into one-word name, for example, Zhang Congzheng in the Song Dynasty put forward the word "Daoyin and Anqiao". In the Republic of China, many books were published in the name of "Daoyin and Anqiao", such as *Catalogue of Mass-Dao* and *Yuan's Mass- Dao*. And many massage practitioners emerged in the name of "Daoyin and Anqiao".

Neigong Tuina is a school of Tuina developed on the basis of Shaolin Neigong, which is the symbol of Neigong Tuina. Shaolin internal exercise can strengthen sinews and bones, replenish qi and blood, obtain harmony between internal organs, between yin and yang and increase power in short time. Shaolin internal exercise was a kind of kung fu, which spread mainly in villages of Shandong and Henan provinces. Due to few literatures, the accurate cradle of Shaolin internal exercise remains to be proved. At present, there are three folklores.

1. Derived from Shaolin

All kung fu come from Shaolin temple. Shaolin temple is the cradle of Chan School of Buddhism, which enjoys high reputation at home and abroad. The current Shaolin internal exercise has two meanings. Widely, it means the Neigong exercised by Shaolin monks, including Yijinjing, Xisuijing and so on; narrowly, it means Shaolin internal exercise of Neigong Tuina, which is exercised by students majoring in acupuncture and moxibustion and clinical practitioners as well as the infirm patients to strengthen the body and treat diseases. Shaolin internal

强身。内功推拿之少林内功为上肢姿势锻炼法搭配基本裆式组合锻炼法，着重锻炼两下肢的“霸力”和上肢的“灵活性”。1991年德虔所编《少林武术大全》及2007年冯永臣、王跃进、释永信等编著的《少林功夫》，都未发现与内功推拿之少林内功相同的内容。目前尚无足够证据表明，推拿功法之少林内功是河南少林寺之功夫，是否为托名，仍待进一步考证。

2. 达摩说

有人认为易筋经即为少林内功，为达摩所创。民国时期的倜庵识所著的《嫡派真传少林内功秘传》序中描述，“易筋经为少林武术祖师达摩禅师所传授，分内、外两经。内经主柔，以静坐运气为事；至于外经，则主刚，以强筋练力为事；其中外经法偏重于上肢，实为练力运气、舒展筋脉之妙法。每日勤行四五次，百日之后，则食量增加、筋骨舒畅、百病不生。”其中对易筋经外经“法偏重于上肢，实为练力运气、舒展筋脉之妙法”的描述与内功推拿之少林内功颇有几分相似。因此，认为少林内功实由易筋经演化而来，为达摩所创。但截至目前，易筋经是否即是少林内功，易筋经是否为达摩所创等，仍存争议。

3. 查拳说

相传在唐代，有一支东征的军队，路过冠县时，留下了一位身负战伤的青年将领，名叫滑宗歧。在当地百姓的精心照料下，滑宗歧恢复了健康。为了报答人们的调养

exercise of Neigong Tuina is the combination of the exercise of upper arms with basic stances, with the purpose of strengthening the stability of lower limbs and the flexibility of upper limbs. Both *Encyclopedia of Shaolin Kung Fu* compiled by De Qian in 1991 and *Shaolin Kung Fu* compiled in 2007 by Feng Yongchen, Wang Yuejin, Shi Yongxin and others didn't convey the same content as Shaolin internal exercise of Neigong Tuina. Now, it still needs more evidences to prove that Shaolin internal exercise of Neigong Tuina is the kung fu from Shaolin temple, Henan province, or it just borrowed the name.

2. Derived from Damo

Some think Yijinjing belongs to Shaolin internal exercise, which was created by Damo. *Direct Branch of Shaolin Internal Exercise · Preface* written by Ti Anshi in the Republic of China said: "The book *Yijinjing* was written by Damo, the original master of Shaolin kung fu and has two volumes, *Nei Jing* and *Wai Jing*. *Nei Jing* focuses on sit-in meditation and qi movement which can be featured as softening, while *Wai Jing* on enhancing sinews and bones and strength which can be featured as toughening. *Wai Jing* concentrates on upper body, a useful way to boosting strength, adjusting qi movement and stretching muscles. Men Should do Yijinjing four or five times a day for over three months, he would have better appetite, relax his muscles and never develop illnesses." In fact, the description of *Wai Jing* is much pretty similar to Shaolin internal exercise of Neigong Tuina. Therefore, some argues that Shaolin internal exercise is developed from Yijinjing. However, it is arguable that whether Yijinjing is Shaolin internal exercise and whether Yijinjing was created by Damo.

3. Derived from Zha boxing

It's said that one troop moved toward east in the Tang Dynasty (61–907). When they passed by Guan town, a young general called Hua Zongqi was left behind due to

之恩，他便把自己擅长的“架子拳”传授给了村民，后随其习武者日众，滑氏便将旅居长安的师兄查元义请来共同施教。当地人为纪念恩师，把查元义所传“身法势”称为“查拳”，滑宗岐所传“架子拳”称为“滑拳”。查拳在清代黄河流域盛传，清代乾隆年间在山东的冠县（今隶属聊城市）和任城（今隶属济宁市）逐渐形成了三个不同的流派，分别是冠县以张其维为代表的“张式”查拳；以杨鸿修为代表的“杨式”查拳；任城以李恩聚为代表的“李式”查拳，李氏家族祖辈习武，尤精查拳、弹腿。李恩聚的父辈李振基被尊为内功推拿流派的创始人。

heavy wound. Taken care of by local residents, Hua Zongqi recovered. In return, Hua taught villagers “Jiazi boxing” at which he was adept. As the number of students became larger and larger, Hua invited Zha Yuanyi, who had higher seniority to teach with him together. To memorize both of them, local people named the boxing they taught as “Zha boxing” and “Hua boxing” respectively. Zha boxing was popular at Yellow River basin in the Qing Dynasty. And from 1711 to 1799, Zha boxing had formed three schools in Guan town (belongs to Liaocheng city now) and Ren city (belongs to Jining city now) in Shandong province. “Zhang style” was represented by Zhang Qiwei, “Yang style” by Yang Hongxiu in Guan town and “Li style” by Li Enju in Ren city. Among them, Li family was a family of kung fu, who were especially skilled in Zha boxing and flipping leg. Li Enju’s father Li Zhenji was regarded as the founder of Neigong Tuina.

二、成于医

Take Shape in TCM

少林内功原为武林强身健体的基本功。主要用于提高习武者的身体素质和技击能力，经过几代人的调整，慢慢发展为同样适合于体弱病患者强身治病的一种武术运动。从武术发展史上看，练武的目的由技击转向健身，甚至是医疗，是随着社会的变迁逐渐呈现的。民国时期的上海就有许多以技击出名的推拿医家。

Shaolin internal exercise is the basic kung fu for fitness, which is mainly for improving exercisers’ healthy condition and their skills for hitting. And through the adjustment of several generations, it has developed into another kung fu that is suitable for infirm people to strengthen the body and treat diseases. Looking back to the history of kung fu, as society developed, the goal of exercising kung fu was transferred from hitting to fitness, even to medical care. In the Republic of China, there were many Tuina practitioners who were originally famous for their kung fu in Shanghai.

三、现代教育

Modern Education

在几代推拿人的不懈努力下，

The education cause for Tuina finally won the

推拿的教育事业获得了社会的认可和政府的支持，自20世纪50年代中期起，部分省市开始设立推拿科、按摩科。并以师带徒、开办培训班、建立学校等形式培养推拿专业人员，逐步开辟了推拿现代学校教育，出版推拿学教材，创立了推拿学历教育和人才培养模式。

1956年10月10日，上海创办了第一期“推拿医师训练班”，首批招收了60名学员，由当时著名的推拿老医生执教，马万龙、李锡九等均参与内功推拿理论或临床带教。至此，推拿教学从过去的师带徒形式走上了正规的学校教育途径。随后，训练班被改成“推拿医士学校”，并于1958年3月成立推拿联合诊所，继而又成立了推拿门诊部，解决了学生的临床实习问题，是推拿教育工作的一个重大改革和收获。同年11月25日成立了上海中医学院附属推拿医士学校（后改名为上海中医学院附属推拿学校）。该校自1956年至1965年招收了8届学员，培养了500多名推拿专业人才，并转送到全国各地，在推拿学的医教研工作中发挥了重要作用。在1960—1984年间，上海中医学院附属推拿门诊部受卫生部委托，承办了三期全国高等推拿师资训练班，为全国培养了高级推拿医学人才，构筑了现代推拿教育规划的蓝图。

中医推拿学的专科、教育和研究生教育逐步形成，为现代推拿的传承开辟了新的道路。1974年上海中医学院开设了针灸、推拿、骨伤

recognition and support from the public and government after constant efforts of several Tuina practitioners. Since the mid-1950s, some provinces has set up Tuina and massage departments in hospitals. Modern schooling for Tuina had been built step by step together with publication of related textbooks as Tuina professionals were trained in training courses, schools or as an apprentice. Thus, academic education and professional cultivation model for Tuina have been established.

On October 10th, 1956, the first “Training Course for Tuina Practitioners” received 60 students, taught by Tuina practitioners with high prestige including Ma Wanlong and Li Xijiu. From then on, the education of Tuina transferred from apprenticeship to formal school education. Then, the training course was transformed into Tuina Practitioner College. The United Tuina Clinic established in March, 1958, together with later-established outpatient clinic of Tuina became places for students to serve as an intern, which was a major reform and gains of Tuina education. On 25th November, Tuina Practitioner College affiliated to Shanghai College of Traditional Chinese Medicine (renamed as Tuina College affiliated to Shanghai College of Traditional Chinese Medicine) was established. From 1956 to 1965, the college had enrolled 8 classes of graduates, cultivating 500 Tuina professionals, who played major roles in clinical practice, education and research of Tuina around China. From 1960 to 1984, the Tuina outpatient clinic affiliated to Shanghai College of Traditional Chinese Medicine was entrusted by the Ministry of Health to undertake three national higher Tuina teachers’ training courses. The courses cultivated high-level Tuina professionals and laid the foundation for the modern Tuina education.

Gradually, vocation, graduate and postgraduate education of Tuina had been established and improved, which paved the new way for keeping modern Tuina

专业，1978年改为针灸、推拿专业，1979年改为针灸推拿系，1982年针灸推拿系分别设立针灸和推拿专科，1986年成立推拿系。推拿从业者越来越多，学习途径多样化，手法更加丰富，疾病谱顺应时代变化而调整。推拿现代教育的发展，培育了一批又一批的综合性推拿专业人才。而且推拿学的临床、现代教育和推拿科研逐步展开。

现代推拿教育改变了单纯的手把手教学的单一师承教育模式，逐步打破了门派交流的壁垒，一指禅推拿、内功推拿、㨰法等各种推拿学术流派开始交流和融合，内功推拿逐步成为推拿学的重要内容，为现代推拿学教育做出了重要贡献。随着疾病谱、就医形式和医疗管理等方面的变化，内功推拿目前在国内的应用情况不尽如人意。为了加强内功推拿流派的传承，一些省市开展了大量的研究和传承工作，如上海中医药大学于2013年6月成立了"内功推拿流派传承研究室"。2013年，上海中医药大学获得国家自然基金项目立项，题目为"少林内功防治慢性疲劳综合征的脑内信息响应特征研究"。这是第一个研究少林内功的国家自然基金项目，也是内功推拿研究迈入更高层次基础研究的标志。这些将有力地推动少林内功功法的研究，推广内功推拿的临床应用，促进内功推拿流派的传承。

alive. In 1974, Shanghai College of Traditional Chinese Medicine established acupuncture and moxibustion, Tuina and orthopedics specialties, which changed into acupuncture and moxibustion and Tuina specialties in 1978. In 1982, acupuncture and moxibustion, Tuina specialties set up under the school of Acupuncture and Moxibustion-Tuina which established in 1979. In 1986, the school of Tuina established. More and more people were devoted into Tuina cause with multiplie channels to learn. More manipulations were applied clinically for different diseases with the changing with time. The development of modern Tuina education has cultivated a batch of Tuina professionals with all-round Tuina knowledge. At the same time, the clinical and scientific research and modern education of Tuina all carried forward.

Modern Tuina education replaces the original apprenticeship which was the only form of learning before and breaks the barriers that impede communication and exchange between schools. Yi Zhi Chan pushing, Neigong Tuina, rolling manipulation and other schools began to integrate with each other and Neigong Tuina has become one of the important parts and contributors to modern Tuina education. With the change of the range of treatable diseases, form of medical treatment and medical management, the current application of Neigong Tuina in China is far from satisfying. In order to keep the school of Neigong Tuina alive, some provinces carried forward plenty of researches and inheritance works. For example, Shanghai University of Traditional Chinese Medicine established "Workroom for inheritance of Neigong Tuina" in June, 2013. At the same year, the university obtain a project about Shaolin Neiong, called "Research on the Brain Information Response Characteristics of Shaolin internal exercise in Prevention and Treatment of Chronic Fatigue Syndrome, sponsored by National Natural Science Foundation of China". This was the first Shaolin internal exercise research project sponsored by National Natural Science Foundation of China and also a sign of a higher level of basic research on Neigong Tuina. All researches can promote studies on the exercise of Shaolin internal exercise, expand clinical application of Neigong Tuina and keep it alive.

四、相关著作

目前尚无内功推拿或少林内功专著出版。大部分推拿教材和著作均单独列章、节编入了内功推拿或少林内功的内容。

上海推拿学校1959年1月整理编写的《中医推拿学》等教材，已将用内功推拿治疗肺痨和肺胀列入其中。1959年上海中医学院附属推拿医士学校编写的《中医推拿学》中推拿功法仅有易筋经，尚无少林内功。1960年上海中医学院附属推拿学校编写的《推拿学》和1961年上海中医学院编写的中医学院试用教材《中医推拿学讲义》已经纳入了少林内功锻炼方法。1963年上海中医学院附属推拿学校又编写了《少林内功》，作为推拿练功课程的专用教材。

1975年全国高等中医院校统编教材《推拿学》将内功推拿技术广泛应用于运动系统、消化系统、呼吸系统、心脑血管系统疾病和妇科疾病，治疗范围显著增加。1991年的《推拿大成》总结了虚劳、哮喘、便秘、失眠、痛经、胸胁屏伤等17种疾病的内功推拿治疗方法。推拿

Related Books

For now, no monograph about Neigong Tuina or Shaolin internal exercise has been published. But most of textbooks and masterpieces have set the context of Neigong Tuina in a sole chapter or part.

Shanghai Tuina College had been compiled *Tuina of Traditional Chinese Medicine* and other textbooks in January, 1959, which mentioned that Neigong Tuina can treat pulmonary tuberculosis and lung-distension. In the same year, *Tuina of Traditional Chinese Medicine* compiled by Tuina Practitioners College affiliated to Shanghai College of Traditional Chinese Medicine covered Yijinjing but no Shaolin internal exercise. *Tuina* compiled by Tuina College affiliated to Shanghai College of Traditional Chinese Medicine in 1960 and *The Handout for Tuina of Traditional Chinese Medicine* compiled by Shanghai College of Traditional Chinese Medicine as a textbook on trial had already contained the Shaolin internal exercise. In 1963, Tuina College affiliated with Shanghai College of Traditional Chinese Medicine compiled Shaolin internal exercise, as the specific textbook for exercise class.

Tuina complied by higher Traditional Chinese Medicine schools nationwide in 1975 expanded Neigong Tuina's range of treatment into motor, digestive, respiratory, cardiovascular and cerebrovascular system diseases and gynecological diseases. In 1991, *Tuina Collection* is

学教材建设取得了新成果，不仅有针对不同学历的教材，而且逐步分化为推拿手法、推拿功法等教材，教学内容随着推拿学科和推拿实践的发展逐步修改、补充，更加切合实用。

全国中医药行业高等教育“十二五”“十三五”规划教材《推拿手法学》《推拿功法学》，中华人民共和国国家卫生健康委员会“十二五”“十三五”规划教材《推拿手法学》《推拿功法学》，以及国家卫生健康委员会“十三五”研究生规划教材《推拿流派研究技术》都将内功推拿流派和少林内功纳入其中。此外，骆竞洪主编的《中华推拿医学志——手法源流》等著作也对内功推拿做了描述。

published which summarized how to use Neigong Tuina to treat deficiency, asthma, constipation, insomnia, dysmenorrhea, pain in the chest when breathing and other 17 kinds of diseases. New accomplishments had been made in developing textbooks of Tuina. People of different education phases have different textbooks, and the textbooks have gradually divided into smaller subjects, like tuina manipulations and Shaolin internal exercise. What's more, their contents became more practical thanks to continuous revisal and supplement in light of development of Tuina and its practice.

According to “the 12th Five-year Plan” and “the 13th Five-year Plan”, China TCM industry compiled textbooks *Tuina Manipulation* and *Tuina Exercise* for higher education and National Health Commission of the People's Republic of China also compiled *Tuina Manipulation* and *Tuina Exercise* of its own version. Besides, in light of “the 13th Five-year Plan”, National Health Commission of China compiled *Technique of Schools of Tuina* for postgraduate students. Neigong Tuina and Shaolin internal exercise are edited in all books above. In addition, books such as *Annals of Tuina: Source of Manipulation* edited by Luo Jinghong also added Neigong Tuina.

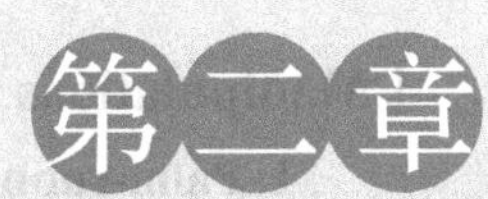

基本操作

Chapter Two
Basic Manipulations

第一节 特色手法

Section One Special Manipulations

一、擦法

擦法又称平推法，是内功推拿的主要手法，分为掌擦、大鱼际擦、小鱼际擦、指擦，不论哪一种擦法，都做直线来回的平推，故也称平推法。

Rubbing Manipulation

Rubbing manipulation, also known as horizontal pushing manipulation, is the main manipulation of Shaolin Internal Exercise and Tuina. It could be divided into palm-rubbing, thenar-rubbing, hypothenar-rubbing, and finger-rubbing. The patient is pushed back and forth in a straight line when using the above manipulations, so it is also called horizontal pushing manipulation.

【术式】

1. 掌擦法

嘱患者端坐方凳或站裆势（两手叉腰），穿单衣，术者立于一侧取站位，一手扶住患者（推胸腹扶背、推背扶胸），另一手成虚掌，再着力患者体表，做直线左右平推，由上而下慢慢移动，并由下而上反复3次。

前胸由锁骨下起，至上腹部中脘穴处，左右侧至腋中线。背部由大椎穴始至12胸椎，左右侧到腋后线。然后医者站于另一侧，重复平推胸腹及背部；再立于患者后面，两手同时平推两胁肋，由腋后上向前斜下方作直线来回推动2～3分钟。

术者一手拇指伸直，另一手扶患者肩背，四指并拢伸直，来回直线平推，称荡法，常用于胸背部。

【Manipulations】

1. Palm-rubbing manipulation

Ask the patient to sit upright on a stool or in a straight-standing posture (with hands on hips), and wear unlined clothes. The practitioner stands on one side to hold the patient with one hand (holding the back while pushing the chest and abdomen, and vice versa), concentrates his force on the patient's body surface with the other hand, and pushes the surface from the left to right horizontally, then slowly moves from top to bottom, and repeat the same manipulation from bottom to top for 3 times.

When pushing the chest, the manipulation should start from the subclavian region, to the Zhongwan (CV 12) in the upper abdomen, and from the left and right sides to the midaxillary line. When pushing the back, the manipulation should start from the Dazhui (GV 14) to 12 thoracic vertebrae, from left and right sides to the posterior axillary line. Then the practitioner stands on the other side, and repeatedly pushes the chest, abdomen, and back. After that, the practitioner turns to the rear side of the patient, pushes

2. 大鱼际擦法

使用时要求暴露治疗部位，常用于四肢部，术者一手握肢端，另一手以大鱼际由肢端向心方向直线来回平推，称之推三阴三阳。对四肢关节扭挫伤部位使用手法时可涂少许润滑剂，既可提高治疗效果，又能防止推破皮肤。

3. 小鱼际擦法

使用小鱼际擦法必须暴露治疗部位，常用于腰背部及臀部。患者端坐，身前屈两肘搁大腿上，术者一手扶转折肩，另一手小鱼际涂少许润滑剂，在治疗部位做直线来回平推。

4. 指擦法

指擦法常用拇指螺纹面平推。

both flanks simultaneously with both hands horizontally, and pushes back and forth in a straight line from the posterior to the anterior aspect of the axillary for 2 to 3 minutes.

The practitioner straightens the thumb with one hand, supports the patient's shoulder and back with the other hand, closes the four fingers and straightens them, and pushes back and forth in a straight line. This therapy is called oscillating manipulation and commonly applied on the chest and back.

2. Thenar-rubbing manipulation

It requires exposure of the treatment site, and commonly used on the extremities. The practitioner holds the extremities with one hand and pushes the thenar back and forth in a straight line from the extremities to the center with the other hand. This manipulation is called pushing along the Sanyin and Sanyang meridians. Applying a little lubricant to the torsion and contusion sites of the joints of the extremities can not only improve the therapeutic effect, but also prevent grazing the skin.

3. Hypothenar-rubbing manipulation

The hypothenar-rubbing manipulation necessitates exposure to the treatment site and is commonly applied to the lower back and buttocks.

The patient sits with both elbows flexed in the thigh, the practitioner turns the shoulder with one hand, applies a little lubricant to the hypothenar with the other hand, and makes a flat push back and forth on the treatment site.

4. Finger-rubbing manipulation

Horizontal pushing through the thumb ribbed surface is often used in finger-rubbing manipulation.

【要领】

（1）上肢放松，腕关节平伸，使前臂和手掌处于直线上。

（2）手掌、大鱼际或小鱼际、指面都需要紧贴治疗部位（但不能

【Essentials】

(1) Relax the upper limbs and extend the wrists so that the forearms and palms are in a straight line.

(2) The palm, thenar or hypothenar, and finger surfaces need to be close to the treatment site (but pressure

硬用压力，以免擦破皮肤），并可借助于介质（按摩膏、冬青膏等）进行平推。

should not be used hard to avoid abrading the skin) and can pushed flat with the help of media (massage ointment, holly ointment, etc.).

（3）以肩肘关节屈伸，带动手掌或大、小鱼际，指面做直线往返运动（上下或左右方向均可）。

(3) Flexion and extension of the shoulder and elbow joints, driving the palm, thenar, hypothenar, and finger surfaces to do a linear round-trip movement (up and down or left and right directions are acceptable).

（4）动作均匀连续，用力要稳，不能屏气，频率为每分钟100～120次。

(4) The manipulation should be uniform and continuous, the force and breath should be stable, with a frequency of 100 to 120 times per minute.

（5）掌擦法前胸部操作时男女有别。

(5) Men and women differ in chest manipulation.

（6）女性患者需要避开乳房。

(6) Breasts region need to be avoided when applied to female patients.

【应用】

擦法是一种柔和温热的刺激，具有温通经络、祛风散寒、活血祛瘀、消肿止痛和宽胸理气、健脾和胃的功效。

掌擦法温热量较低，多用于胸闷气急、胸胁屏伤、虚寒腹痛和消化不良等症。气喘胸闷可在掌擦过程中用中指螺纹面按揉膻中、中府、云门、华盖等穴，掌擦时间较长，见热为度；胃脘痛可在掌擦过程中按揉上脘、中脘等穴，两胁肋掌擦时间稍长，见热为度，有舒肝理气止痛的功效；若见胸胁屏伤，可在掌擦两胁肋时结合中指螺纹面按揉期门、章门、大包等穴；呼吸胁肋牵痛可拿胸大肌，嘱患者深呼吸，手法随呼吸慢慢移动。

荡法有宽胸理气之功用，适宜慢性病恢复期、体质强的肥胖者，或肺气肿、肺结核、哮喘等证，并可嘱患者在治疗期中结合少林内功

【Applications】

Rubbing is a mild and warm stimulation, which has the effects of warming meridians, dispelling wind and dissipating cold, activating blood and removing stasis, alleviating swelling and relieving pain, loosening the chest and regulating qi, invigorating spleen and harmonizing stomach. Palm-rubbing manipulation could only produce little heat and is mostly used for the treatment of chest tightness and shortness of breath, chest and rib-side injury, and abdominal pain caused by deficiency cold and indigestion. Asthma and chest tightness can be treated by rubbing at Danzhong (CV 17), Zhongfu (LU 1), Yunmen (LU 2), Huagai (CV 20) and other points with the ribbed surface of the middle finger during palm rubbing, and it should be rubbed for a long time until feeling the heat. Epigastric pain can be treated by kneading Shangwan (CV 13), Zhongwan (CV 12) and other points during palm rubbing. When applied to the two flanks, the manipulation time is slightly longer as long as the patient feel warm. It has the effects of soothing the liver and regulating qi and relieving pain. As for respiratory hypochondriac pain, the points such as Qimen (LR 14), Zhangmen (LR 13), and

锻炼，促使疾病早愈。

大鱼际擦法温热量中等，常用于四肢部，适用于四肢关节扭挫伤、劳损和类风湿关节炎等症。可结合拍法、按揉法等进行治疗，并可结合热敷。

小鱼际擦法温热量较高，常用于腰背部和臀部，适用于急慢性损伤、风湿痹证麻木不仁等症。可结合拍打法、点法、按揉法进行治疗，并可结合热敷。

指擦法常用于颈部两侧，适宜于肝阳头痛，能平肝熄风、清醒头目、安神定魄。对高血压、失眠患者，手法时间、次数适当延长。

Dabao (SP 21) can be kneaded in combination with the rubbing manipulation on the two flanks. Moreover, the chest muscle can be rubbed for respiratory flank traction pain. Instruct the patient to take deep breaths, while slowly moving the hands with the breath.

The oscillating manipulation plays a role in expanding the chest and regulating qi, which is suitable for obese patients in recovery period with chronic disease, and patients with strong constitution, emphysema, pulmonary tuberculosis, asthma, etc.. Patients can combine Shaolin internal exercise in the treatment to promote recovery of the disease.

Thenar-rubbing manipulation could produce moderate heat, which is commonly used in the extremities, and is suitable for limb joint torsion and contusion, strain, and rheumatoid arthritis. It can be combined with flapping manipulation, kneading manipulation, etc., and can be performed with hot compress simultaneously.

Hypothenar-rubbing manipulation could generate higher heat, which is commonly used in the lower back and buttocks. It is suitable for patients with acute and chronic injuries, rheumatism arthralgia, numbness, and other diseases. It can be combined with flapping manipulation, pressing manipulation, kneading manipulation for treatment, and can be performed with hot compress simultaneously.

The finger-rubbing manipulation is commonly used on both sides of the neck and is suitable for liver-yang headaches, which can calm the liver and extinguish the wind, clear the head and vision, and tranquilize the mind. For patients with hypertension and insomnia, they need more extension and higher frequency of manipulation.

二、提拿法

Lifting-grasping Manipulation

用拇指与其余手指螺纹面同时用力，进行一紧一松地拿住并提起，

Use the thumb and the ribbed surface of the other four fingers at the same time to grasp and lift skin tightly and

称为提拿法。

提拿法是内功推拿的特有手法，“捏而提起谓之拿”，使用时拿中带提，主要分为三指提拿法和五指提拿法，可用于全身各部。

loosely.

"Tina" is a unique technique in Shaolin Internal Exercise and Tuina, "The action that pinching and lifting at the same time is called lifting-grasping". This therapy is mainly divided into three-finger lifting-grasping manipulation and five-finger lifting-grasping manipulation, and both can be used in all parts of the body.

【术式】

1. 头部

患者正坐，术者立于患者的侧后方，一手扶住前额以固定头部，另一手五指分开，微曲，放于患者头顶部，指尖均在前发际处（五指的位置分别为：中指放在督脉，示指、环指放在膀胱经：拇指、小指放在胆经）。

五指螺纹面着力，指间关节屈伸，由前向后捏提拿移动至头顶，随后拇指与四指分开于颈项两侧（虎口对枕后）对称用力，提拿脑空、风池、风府等穴，由下至项部，操作3～5次。亦称拿五经法或抓五经。

2. 胸部

患者取坐位，术者站于侧面，一手托住患者上臂，一手四指紧贴其胸前（胸大肌处），拇指紧贴其腋下，四指由上而下移动，螺纹面用力，又称拿血浪，操作3～5次。

3. 颈肩部

患者取坐位，术者站于患者后侧，一手扶肩一手捏拿颈侧部（胸锁乳突肌处），左右两手交替，操作3～5次。提拿肩井部时，拇指伸直，四指并拢成鸭嘴形，拇指紧贴

【Manipulations】

1. Head

The patient sits upright, and the practitioner stands on the lateral posterior of the patient, holding the patient's forehead with one hand, and placed the other hand on the top of the patient's head with fingers separated and slightly curved at the front hairline (the positions of the five fingers are as follows, the middle finger is placed on the Governor Vessel, the index finger and the ring finger on the Bladder Meridian, the thumb and the little finger on the Gallbladder Meridian).

Focus force on the ribbed surface of the five fingers, flex and extend the interphalangeal joints, lift the skin from front to back and to the top of the head. Then separate the thumb and the other four fingers on both sides of the neck (hold patient's occiput on the area between the thumb and the index finger), exert symmetrical force to lift the Naokong (GB 19), Fengchi (GB 20), Fengfu (GV 16) etc., from bottom to top, and operate 3 to 5 times. It is also known as lifting-grasping the five meridians or grasping the five meridians.

2. Chest

Ask the patient to take a sitting position. The practitioner stands on the side, holds the patient's upper arm with one hand, put four fingers of the other hand on the patient's ectopectoralis and the thumb on the armpit, moves four fingers from top to bottom, and exerts force on the ribbed surface. This manipulation also known as

肩井穴，四指紧贴缺盆穴，对称用力提拿。

4. 背部

患者取坐位，术生站于一侧，患者将一上臂后伸屈曲贴住腰部，术者一手扶住患者肩部，另一手拇指与四指指端沿着患者肩胛骨内侧及脊柱之间，紧贴皮下摸到条索状肌腱，提拿3～5次。

5. 腹部

患者取坐位，术者位于患者前面，嘱患者放松腹肌，术者一手扶患者腰部，一手紧贴其肚脐旁（天枢穴），在腹壁下摸到条索状肌腱一提即放，又称拿肚筋。

6. 四肢部

上肢部：患者取坐位，术者站于一侧，一手托住患者前臂，另一手拇指与四指成鸭嘴形，提拿三角肌、肱三头肌、肱二头肌及极泉、曲池、手三里、少海、小海、合谷等穴，其中提拿极泉穴又称拿电门。

下肢部：患者俯卧，术者在患者侧面，提拿内收肌、股四头肌，向下提拿委中、承山（腓肠肌）、阳陵泉。

lifting-grasping blood waves and needs to be repeated 3 to 5 times.

3. Neck and shoulder

The patient is in a sitting position, and the practitioner stands on the back of the patient, pinches the lateral neck (at the sternocleidomastoid) with one hand and supports the shoulder with the other hand. The practitioner alternates the left and right hands, and operates this process 3 to 5 times. When operating the manipulation, straighten the thumb, close the four fingers into a duck mouth shape, press the thumb against the Jianjing (GB 21) and the four fingers against the Quepen (ST 12), and lift with symmetrical force.

4. Back

Ask the patient to take a sitting position, and the practitioner stands on his side. The patient flexes one upper arm against the waist. The practitioner supports the patient's shoulder with one hand, and lifts the cord-like tendon close to the subcutaneous tissue in the area between the inner side of scapula and the spine of the patient with the other hand for 3 to 5 times.

5. Abdomen

The patient is in a sitting position and relaxes the abdominal muscles. The practitioner stands in front of the patient, supports the patient's waist with one hand and abuts the Tianshu (ST 25) with the other hand. The cord-like tendon is felt under the abdominal wall and released quickly after being lifted up. This manipulation is also known as lifting-grasping abdominal sinew.

6. Limbs

Upper limb: The patient is seated, and the practitioner stands on one side, holds the patient's forearm with one hand, forms the other hand in the shape of a duck bill to lift the deltoid muscle, triceps brachii muscle, biceps brachii muscle and the Jiquan (HT 1), Quchi (LI 11), Shousanli (LI 10), Shaohai (HT 3), Xiaohai (SI 8), Hegu (LI 4) and other points. Among these, lifting the Jiquan (HT 1) is also known as lifting-grasping electric gate.

Lower limbs: The patient takes a prone position, and the practitioner lifts the adductor internus and quadriceps femoris on the side of the patient and lifts Weizhong (BL 40), Chengshan (BL 57) (gastrocnemius), and Yanglingquan (GB 34) downward.

【要领】

（1）肩肘关节放松，五指关节做屈伸，指面着力，不可指甲掐压及拖拉。

（2）手法轻快有力、柔和，动作协调有节律。

（3）作用力由轻而重，根据病情轻重而用力，但应在患者能忍受的范围内进行手法。

【Essentials】

(1) The practitioner should relax shoulder and elbow joints, and flexes and extends in five knuckles. The force must be focused on finger surfaces, and pinching and dragging with nails should be avoided.

(2) The maneuver should be nimble and powerful and the movements should be coordinated and rhythmic.

(3) The intensity of force is from light to heavy according to the severity of the disease, but the manipulation should be performed to the extent that is tolerated by the patient.

【应用】

提拿法有祛风散寒、疏通经络、调和气血、清利头目、安神定魄、宽胸理气等功效。

常用于头部，治疗头痛、失眠等症；用于胸部治疗胸胁屏伤、肺气肿、肺结核、哮喘等证；用于治疗高血压、肩周炎、颈椎病等证；用于背部，如捏拿背部大筋治疗背部牵痛、麻木不仁等症；用于腹部，如捏拿脐旁两侧（天枢穴）腹下肌腱，适用于腹痛、腹泻等证；用于四肢，如提拿极泉、少海、小海、曲池、委中、阳陵泉、承山等穴，治疗手足麻木，风湿痹痛等症。

【Applications】

Lifting-grasping manipulation has the effects of expelling wind and dispersing cold, dredging meridians, harmonizing qi and blood, clearing the head and vision, tranquilizing the mind, and expanding the chest and regulating qi. It is commonly used in the head to treat headache, insomnia and other diseases. It is used in the chest to treat chest and subcostal regions, emphysema, tuberculosis, asthma and other diseases. It is used in the treatment of hypertension, scapulohumeral periarthritis, cervical spondylosis and other diseases. It is used in the back, such as lifting-grasping the back tendons to treat back traction pain, numbness and other diseases. It is used in the abdomen, such as lifting-grasping the lower abdominal tendons on both sides of the umbilicus, Tianshu (ST 25) to treat abdominal pain, diarrhea and other diseases. It is used in the limbs, such as lifting-grasping Jiquan (HT 1), Shaohai (HT 3), Xiaohai (SI 8), Quchi (LI 11), Weizhong (BL 40), Yanglingquan (GB 34), Chengshan (BL 57) and other points to treat numbness of the hands and feet and wind-damp and impediment pain.

三、点法

Point-pressing Manipulation

用拇指指端或屈指第2关节（拇、示、中指均可）突起部点按一定部位，并深压揉动，称为点法。

Knead and apply pressure to the surface of the body with thumb tips or interphalangeal joints of thumb, index finger and middle finger.

【术式】

在人体选定部位，用拇指指端或屈指第2关节（拇、示、中指均可）突起部进行点按，刺激量由轻到重，由浅入深，以酸胀得气为度。

【Manipulations】

Knead and apply pressure to the surface of the body with thumb tips or interphalangeal joints of thumb, index finger and middle finger, with the intensity of stimulation ranges from light to heavy, shallow to deep as long as obtaining qi.

【要领】

（1）指端点，需手握空拳，前臂及腕用力下压。

（2）指关节点时握拳，前臂及腕用力下压。

（3）点时需紧贴穴位，用力由轻到重，由浅入深点压。

【Essentials】

(1) When applying point-pressing manipulation with the finger end, the practitioner should hold a hollow fist and press downward with forearm and wrist.

(2) When performing the manipulation with finger joints, the practitioner should press downward with forearm and wrist.

(3) When performing the manipulation, the practitioner should stick his fingers to acupoints and point-press them with growing force.

【应用】

点法是一种刺激量较强的手法，具有疏通经络、和气止痛、祛风散寒、开窍醒脑之功效。

适用于全身各部位，常用于骨

【Applications】

Point-pressing manipulation is a technique with strong stimulation, which has the effects of dredging meridians, harmonizing qi and relieving pain, expelling wind and dissipating cold, and opening the orifices and refreshing

缝间或循经选穴，在临诊时主要是根据不同疾病循经取穴。如点头维穴、风池穴可除头风；用拇指端点人中穴（又称掐人中）可使昏迷患者苏醒，达到开窍醒脑的目的；如点脾俞、胃俞、胆俞、胆囊穴可以对胃脘痛、胆绞痛患者立即止痛；点大肠俞和上髎、次髎可治外伤风湿引起的腰痛；点三阴交可治疗痛经；点阑尾穴可止腹痛；点天宗、肩贞，可治疗漏肩风；点居髎、环跳可治疗腰腿痛；点角孙、脑空可治疗头痛、头胀、鼻塞等。

the mind.

It is applicable to various parts of the body, and commonly used in bone seams or selected points on the affected channels. In the clinical diagnosis, selection of points on the affected area is performed according to diseases. For example, head-wind could be treated by point-pressing Touwei (ST 8) and Fengchi (GB 20). Point-pressing philtrum with fingertip (also known as pinching the philtrum) can make comatose patients wake up and open the orifices and refresh the mind. Point-pressing Pishu (BL 20), Weishu (BL 21), Danshu (BL 19), and Dannang (EX–LE 6) can relieve epigastric pain and biliary colic immediately; point-pressing Dachangshu (BL 25), Shangliao (BL 31) and Ciliao (BL 32) can treat low back pain caused by traumatic rheumatism; point-pressing Sanyinjiao (SP 6) can treat dysmenorrhea; point-pressing appendix acupoint can relieve abdominal pain; point-pressing Tianzong (SI 11) and Jianzhen (SI 9) can treat omalgia; Juliao (GB 29) and Huantiao (GB 30) can treat pain in lower extremities and waist; Jiaosun (SJ 20) and Naokong (GB 19) can treat headache, fullness in head, and nasal congestion.

四、分法

Separating Manipulation

用双手拇指螺纹面紧贴皮肤，向左右两侧直线推动，称为分法。

About the thumb ribbed surface of both hands to the skin and push linearly to the left and right sides.

【术式】

患者取坐位，术者站于患者前侧，两手拇指螺纹面紧贴皮肤，向左右两侧均匀推开。

如分前额印堂穴，四指扶住两颞或面部两侧，由中间向两侧分抹，由印堂推向两侧太阳；分眉弓，即

【Manipulations】

Ask the patient to take a sitting position. The practitioner stands on the front side of the patient, with the thumb ribbed surface of both hands abutting the skin and pushing skin evenly to the left and right sides.

Take forehead Yintang (EX–HN 3) for example, hold the two temporal or both sides of the face with four

由眉头推向两侧眉梢分；分迎香，即由迎香穴向地仓穴分推；分人中，即由人中穴向口角分推；分承浆，即由承浆向地仓分推。

fingers, wiping from the middle to both sides, from the Yintang (EX–HN 3) to the Taiyang (EX–HN 5) ; fork the superciliary arch, that is, push from the head to tip of the eyebrow; fork the Yingxiang (LI 20), that is, push from the Yingxiang (LI 20) to the Dicang (ST 4) ; fork the middle, that is, push from the Shuigou (DU 26) to the corner of mouth; fork the Chengjiang (CV 24), that is, push from the Chengjiang (CV 24) to the Dicang (ST 4).

【要领】

（1）指面紧贴皮肤做缓慢的直线移动，其余手指要协同助力。

（2）左右两手用力要相同，用力要缓和。

（3）用力重而不滞，轻而不浮。

【Essentials】

(1) Make a slow linear movement with the finger surface close to the skin, and the other fingers should assist synergistically.

(2) Two hands should exert the same moderate force on the skin.

(3) The force should be strong but not stagnant, light but not floating.

【应用】

分法具有镇静安神、醒脑开窍等功效。

适用于头面部印堂、眉棱骨、迎香、人中、承浆等部位或穴位，对感冒头痛、鼻塞、高血压、失眠等证均有疗效。

【Applications】

Separating manipulation has the effects of calming and tranquilizing the mind, refreshing the brain and opening the orifices.

It is applicable to Yintang (EX–HN 3), supra-orbital bone, Yingxiang (LI 20), Shuigou (DU 26), Chengjiang (CV 24) and other parts or acupoints in the head and face. It is also effective for cold, headaches, nasal congestion, high blood pressure and insomnia.

五、合法

Joining Manipulation

用双手拇指螺纹面或两手大、小鱼际在一定部位上合而用力，有两侧向中间推拢称为合法。合法是与分法相对而言。

Exert joint force at the treatment site with the thumb ribbed surface or the palmar thenar and hypothenar area, and perform the manipulation from two sides to the middle. Joining manipulation and Separating manipulation are practiced in the same way but of two opposite directions.

【术式】

患者取坐位，术者站于患者前侧，双手大鱼际紧贴患者两颞前部，四指微屈，由前额向后沿胆经缓慢用力移至枕部。或者医者两手掌朝上，小鱼际紧贴患者枕部，由上而下至风池沿胸锁乳突肌缓慢用力移至锁骨上区。

【Manipulations】

The patient is asked to take a sitting position. The practitioner stands in front of the patient, clings thenar region of both hands to the anterior part of temporal regions of the patient, slightly flexes four fingers, and slowly and forcefully moves fingers from the forehead backward along the to the gallbladder meridian to the occipital region. Alternatively, the manipulation could be performed with the practitioner's palms facing up, the hypothenar area abuts the patient's occipital region and moves slowly and forcefully from the top to Fenchi (GB 20), then along the sternocleidomastoid muscle to the supraclavicular region.

【要领】

（1）两手大鱼际及小鱼际分别紧贴皮肤，合掌用力缓慢移动。

（2）左右两手用力要相同，用力要缓和。

（3）用力要轻而不浮，重而不滞。

【Essentials】

(1) The practitioner's thenar and hypothenar areas of both hands need to cling to the skin, and the palms are pressed together and moved slowly.

(2) Both hands should exert the same force, and the force should be appropriate.

(3) The force should be strong but not stagnant, light but not floating.

【应用】

合法常用于两颞、枕部及项部，有祛风散寒、清头目、平肝阳、安心神之功效，适用于感冒头痛、头晕、失眠、高血压等证。

【Applications】

Combining manipulation is commonly used to treat diseases related to the two temporal regions, occipital rengions, and neck, and has the effects of expelling wind and dispersing cold, clearing the head and vision, calming the liver yang, and tranquilizing the mind. It is suitable for cold headache, dizziness, insomnia, and hypertension.

六、扫散法

Sweeping Manipulation

以拇指偏锋及其余四指指端在头侧做前后上下往返扫散动作，称

Push and scrub on the side of the head using the radial side of the thumb and tips of the other four fingers.

扫散法。

【术式】

患者取正坐位，术者立于前侧，一手扶患者头部一侧，另一手拇指和四指分开，拇指偏锋置于率谷穴，其余四指依次置于头部一侧，腕关节摆动，由前向后做扫散动作约15次，可向后扫散至枕后脑空、风池，换手操作头部另一侧。

【Manipulations】

The patient sits uprightly. The practitioner stands on the front side with one hand supports the patient's head, the lateral side of the thumb of the other hand places at the Shuaigu (GB 8), and the remaining four fingers successively places on one side of the head. Then, swing the wrist, make sweeping movements from front to back about 15 times, sweep backward to Naokong (GB 19) and Fengchi (GB 20) and alternate the other hand to operate the same manipulation on the other side of the head.

【要领】

（1）操作时术者腕关节放松，以前臂主动的屈伸运动带动腕关节来回摆动，来完成整个扫散动作。

（2）手法操作过程中，应保持患者头部固定，勿来回摇动，以免引起头晕等不适。

（3）手法力量不宜太轻或太重，推出时以拇指桡面接触到皮肤为度，勿过分加力或浮于头发之上；收回时微微离开皮肤。

（4）操作时，紧贴皮肤之拇指应顺发而动，头发较多者，可将拇指伸入发间进行操作，避免牵拉发根而致疼痛。

（5）注意动作连贯，快慢适度，轻重有致，一气呵成。

【Essentials】

(1) During the manipulation, the practitioner relaxes the wrist joint, and takes flexion and extension movements of the forearm to drive the wrist joint to swing back and forth.

(2) During the manipulation, the patient's head should be kept fixed to avoid causing dizziness and other discomfort.

(3) The force should remain moderate, that is to say, it should not be too great, nor should it float on the hair. The thumb radial surface should in contact with the skin when pushing out, and slightly away from skin when withdrawing.

(4) During the manipulation, the thumb should smoothly move along the hair. For those with more hair, the practitioner can extend the thumb into the hair for Manipulations to avoid pain caused by pulling the hair root.

(5) Pay attention to the coherence of the movement, keep moderate speed and apply appropriate force to complete consecutive actions.

【应用】

扫散法有明目醒脑、祛风散寒、平肝潜阳之功效。

【Applications】

The sweeping manipulation has the effects of brightening the eyes and refreshing the brain, dispelling

主要用于头部，对头痛、头昏、头晕、失眠、高血压及脑震荡后遗症均有治疗作用。

wind and dissipating cold, and pacifying the liver to subdue yang.

It is mainly used on the head and has therapeutic effects on headache, dizziness, insomnia, hypertension and sequelae of concussion.

七、理法

Regulating Manipulation

用单手或双手拇指螺纹面紧贴皮肤，或示、中两指指节夹紧指节做左右拨动或由上而下用力捋过，称为理法。

Applied with the ribbed surface of the thumb of one hand or both hands stick to the skin, or the knuckles of the index and middle fingers clamped and moved from left to right or pushed from top to bottom.

【术式】

患者取正坐或站立位，术者一手握掌，另一手拇指螺纹面紧按掌背肌腱，其余四指抵住掌心，随后一手握腕，另一手示、中两指屈曲，用第二指节夹住患者手指由上而下移动，依次对五指进行理顺，指节同时出现松动和响声为宜。

一般结合其他操作后再理掌背及五指。

【Manipulations】

The patient is asked to take a sitting or standing position. The practitioner holds the patient's palm with one hand, and presses the dorsal tendon of the palm tightly with the thumb ribbed surface of the other hand. Then, the other four fingers are held against the palm, and the thumb is slid to the side, or the ribbed side of the thumb of both hands is performed simultaneously. Moreover, hold the patient's wrist with one hand, flex the index finger and middle finger of the other, clamp the patient's fingers with the second knuckle and move from top to bottom, and perform this exercise sequentially on five fingers. The most appropriate condition is that the knuckles of patients have looseness and sound at the same time.

Generally, this manipulation is always applied after other manipulations are done.

【要领】

（1）用拇指螺纹面紧贴掌指皮肤，四指抵住另一侧，按住肌腱向左右拨动，两手拇指同时进行交互进行。

【Essentials】

(1) The practitioner needs to stick the ribbed surface of the thumb close to the skin, with four fingers against the palm, and press the tendon to the left or right side. This manipulation can be performed with the thumbs of both

（2）两指屈曲以第2指节夹住一指由上而下用力捋过，五指依次进行。

（3）用力重而不滞，轻而不浮。

hands at the same time.

(2) The practitioner needs to flex the index finger and middle finger of one hand, clamp the patient's fingers with the second knuckle and move from top to bottom, and perform this exercise sequentially on five fingers.

(3) The force should be strong but not stagnant, light but not floating.

【应用】

理法有疏通经络、活利指节之功效。

适用于手掌背、手五指及足背。对肢体麻木等症如类风湿关节炎、肢体伤筋均有治疗作用。

【Applications】

The regulating manipulation has the effect of dredging the meridians and activating the knuckles.

It is applicable to the back of the palm, fingers, and dorsum of the foot. It has a therapeutic effect on limb numbness such as rheumatoid arthritis and limb tendon injury.

八、劈法

Chopping Manipulation

以手掌侧劈击指缝，称为劈法。

Chop the area between the fingers with the ulnar side of the palm.

【术式】

患者取正坐或站立位，在理掌背及五指后，嘱患者上臂向前侧方平举，将五指用力分开，术者一手握住患者腕部，拇指抵住其掌腕部，另一手掌平直，四指并拢，用手掌尺侧面，劈击四指缝，依次逐个劈击。

【Manipulations】

The patient takes a sitting or standing position. After regulating the back of the palm and the five fingers, the patient is instructed to raise the upper arm to the anterolateral side, and the five fingers are separated by force. The practitioner holds the patient's wrist with one hand and the thumb is against the wrist, while the other palm is straightened with four fingers close together. Then, chop the area between the four figures with the ulnar side of the palm one by one.

【要领】

（1）手掌平直，四指并拢，手掌尺侧作力点。

【Essentials】

(1) The palm should be put flat with four figures closely hold together, and it is the ulnar side of the palm

（2）用力要稳，重而不滞，轻而不浮。

that is taken as the stress point.

(2) The force should be stable, strong but not stagnant, light but not floating.

【应用】

劈法有疏通经络之功效。

适用于两手四缝，肢体麻木、气血不和及内妇科杂证均可配合治疗。

【Applications】

Chopping manipulation has the effect of dredging the meridians.

It is applicable to the area between fingers and it can be used in combination with the treatment of limb numbness, disharmony between qi and blood and internal gynecological miscellaneous diseases.

九、运法

Arc-pushing Manipulation

握住上臂作缓和回旋或环转动作，称为运法。

Gripping the upper arm and performing gentle rotation or circular movements is called arc-pushing manipulation.

【术式】

患者取正坐或立位，嘱患者放松上臂，术者两手将患者一侧上臂握住托起由前而后运转。

以左臂为例，术者一手握住患肢的掌心腕部，另一手以掌背相抵，将患肢腕部徐徐向前向上、由前向后，当上臂上举至160°左右时，随即反转，托腕转为握腕，另一手（原握腕之手）随手腕沿前臂向下滑至肩部按住，此时握腕之手向上拉，按肩之手向下压，使患肢充分伸展，随即向后环转，往复3次，再转为由后向前，手势反之重复，往复3次结束。同法用于另一侧上臂。

【Manipulations】

The patient is seated or standing in an upright position. Instruct the patient to relax the upper arm. The practitioner uses both hands to grip and support the patient's upper arm from front to back.

Taking the left arm as an example, one hand of the practitioner grips the palm and wrist of the affected limb, while the other hand opposes with the back of the hand, gently moving the wrist of the affected limb forward and upward, and then backward. When the upper arm is raised to about 160°, the movement is reversed. The hand supporting the wrist changes to gripping the wrist, while the other hand (the original hand gripping the wrist) slides down the forearm to the shoulder and presses down. At this point, the hand gripping the wrist pulls upwards while the hand pressing the shoulder pushes downwards, fully stretching the affected limb. Then, it is rotated backward and repeated 3 times before switching to rotating forward. The same actions are repeated in reverse, and the process is repeated 3 times. The same technique is applied to the other arm.

【要领】

运法动作缓和，用力要稳，运动方向及幅度须在生理许可范围内或在患者能忍受的范围内进行

【Essentials】

The requirement of the rotating manipulation should be moderate, the force should be stable, and the direction and range of the movement should be based on physiology or within the range that the patient can tolerate.

【应用】

运法有滑利关节、舒筋通络、调和气血之功效。

适用于上肢，对上肢麻木、肩关节粘连，以及内妇科虚劳杂证均有治疗作用，可配合其他手法使用。

【Applications】

The rotating manipulation has the effect of smoothing joints, relaxing tendons and dredging collaterals, and harmonizing qi and blood.

It is applicable to the upper limbs, and has therapeutic effects on upper limb numbness, shoulder joint adhesion, and miscellaneous internal gynecological vacuity taxation diseases, and can be used in combination with other manipulations.

十、背法

Back-carrying Manipulation

术者用两肘套住患者肘弯部，弯腰将患者背起，并牵伸抖动患者腰部的方法，称为背法。

Carry the patient on the back and apply traction, shaking, vibration and instant extension to the affected lumbar area.

【术式】

术者和患者背靠背站立，嘱患者两肘微曲稍外展，术者将两肘套住患者肘弯部，弯腰将患者背起，两脚离地，术者臀部抵住患者腰部，同时屈膝挺臀，伸膝抖动背伸患者腰部，并令患者咳嗽配合，对症状

【Manipulations】

The practitioner and the patient stand back-to-back, and the patient is instructed to slightly bend and abduct elbows. The practitioner puts both arms over the patient's elbow, bends down to carry the patient on the back, and keeps the patient's feet off the ground. The practitioner's hip is pressed against the patient's waist, while bending

重者，可做左右摆动再做抖动，效果更佳。

the knees and lifting the hip, or extending the knees and shaking the back to stretch the patient's waist. For those with severe symptoms, the practitioner can do a side-to-side swing and then make shaking movements, which could achieve a better effect.

【要领】

（1）手挽手背起时，注意臀部顶住患者腰骶部。

（2）伸屈膝动作和臀部的抖动要协调。

（3）在做抖动动作时，让患者放松勿紧张，可做咳嗽动作配合。

【Essentials】

(1) When back-carrying the patient arm in arm, the practitioner should be aware of that the hip needs to against the patient's lumbosacral region.

(2) Knee extension and hip shaking should be coordinated.

(3) When making shaking movements, let the patient relax, and cough movements can be done in co-Manipulations.

【应用】

背法具有行气活血、滑利关节之功效。

常用于胸腰部损伤，促使扭挫的小关节复位，对胸胁屏伤、岔气、腰部扭伤及腰椎间盘突出症均有较好的治疗效果。

【Applications】

Back-carrying manipulation has the effects of moving qi and activating the blood, and disinhibiting the joints.

It is commonly used for thoracolumbar injury, promoting the reduction of twisted facet joints, and has a good therapeutic effect on the injury of chest and hypochondria, bifurcation, lumbar sprain, and lumbar disc herniation.

十一、拔伸法

Pulling-stretching Manipulation

拔伸即牵拉、牵引的意思，固定肢体或关节的一端，牵拉另一端的方法，称为拔伸法。

Immobilize one end of the affected joints or limbs and pull the other end. Pulling means traction and stretching.

【术式】

1. 颈椎拔伸法

患者正坐，术者站在患者背后，用双手拇指顶在患者枕骨下方，掌

【Manipulations】

1. Cervical vertebrae pulling-stretching manipulation

The patient sits upright. The practitioner stands behind the patient, with both thumbs behind the patient's

根托住其两侧下颌角的下方，并用两前臂压住患者两肩，双手用力向上牵拉，两前臂下压，同时往相反方向用力。

2. 肩关节拔伸法

患者坐势，术者用双手握住其腕或肘部，逐渐用力牵拉，嘱患者身体向另一侧倾斜（或有一助手帮助固定患者身体）与牵拉之力对抗。

3. 腕关节拔伸法

患者正坐，术者坐于患侧，两手握患者掌腕部，一足抵住腋下，做腕关节用力牵拉。

4. 指间关节拔伸法

用一手捏住被拔伸指间关节的近侧端，另一手捏住其远侧端，两手同时朝相反方向用力牵拉。

5. 踝关节拔伸法

患者取仰卧位，术者一手握住患者脚大趾处，一手托住足跟，嘱患者两手握住床边，用力牵拉踝关节。

occipital bone and palms hold the lower jaw bones. Then, the practitioner presses the patient's shoulders with both forearms, and forcefully pull upwards with both hands.

2. Shoulder pulling-stretching manipulation

The patient takes a sitting position. The practitioner holds the wrist or elbow of the patient with both hands, and gradually stretches with stronger force. The patient is asked to lean to the other side (or arrange an assistant to help fix the patient's body) to resist the pulling force.

3. Wrist pulling-stretching manipulation

The patient sits upright. The practitioner sits beside the patient, holds the patient's palm and wrist with both hands, and stretches the wrist joint with force.

4. Finger pulling-stretching manipulation

The practitioner holds two ends of fingers with both hands, and pulls in opposite directions at the same time.

5. Ankle pulling-stretching manipulation

The patient takes a supine position and is instructed to hold the bedside with both hands. The practitioner holds the thumb of the foot with one hand and the heel with the other, and pulls the ankle joint forcefully.

【要领】

（1）一手固定关节一端，另一手做对抗性用力，或以身体自重固定近端，两手握住关节远端，徐徐用力。

（2）用力要均匀而持续，动作要缓和。

【Essentials】

(1) Fix one end of the joint with one hand and use the other hand to exert resisting force, or fix the proximal end by body weight and hold the distal end of the joint with both hands applying force gradually.

(2) The force should be stable and continuous, and the movements should be moderate.

【应用】

拔伸法有理筋整复之功效，适用于项、肩、腕、指、踝关节的错位伤筋等。

【Applications】

Pulling-stretching manipulations has the effect of restoring soft tissues and restitution. It is applicable to dislocation and tendon injury of neck, shoulder, wrist, finger and ankle joints.

十二、击法

用拳、掌、桑枝棒等叩击体表，称为击法。

Knocking Manipulation

Knock the surface of the body with the fist, palms, fingers or mulberry sticks. Stick knocking manipulation is one of the special manipulations of Shaolin Internal Exercise and Tuina.

【术式】

1. 掌击法

手指自然松开，腕略背伸，用掌根部击打体表。如掌击囟门，患者取正坐位，嘱患者齿咬紧，舌抵上腭，目平视，术者立于前侧，一手托住患者枕后，另一手用掌根叩击其囟门穴，先轻轻叩击几下，再稍加力重击3次即可。

2. 拳击法

术者手握拳，腕背要挺直，以拳背着力于治疗部位，运用肘关节屈伸和前臂的力量，将拳背平击在治疗部位上。如拳击大椎、八髎穴，患者取正坐位，术者立于患者后侧，一手扶肩，另一手用拳背平击患者大椎，再击八髎穴，多在常规手法操作即将结束手法时使用。

3. 侧击法

手指并拢伸直，腕略背伸，用小指侧及小鱼际侧击打患者体表。

4. 指尖击法

手指半屈，腕关节放松，运用腕关节的屈伸，以指端轻轻击打患者体表，双手可交替操作。

【Manipulations】

1. Palm-knocking manipulation

The practitioner should naturally loose the fingers, slightly extend the wrist, and use the base of palm to knock the body surface. For example, when knocking the fontanelle with palm, the patient should sit upright, clench the teeth with the tongue touches against the upper palate, and look straight ahead. The practitioner stands on the front side, holds the patients' occiput with one hand, and knocks the Xinhui (DU 22) with the base of palm of the other hand. Gently tap the acupoint a few times first, and then knock 3 times with stronger force.

2. Fist-knocking manipulation

The practitioner should make a fist, straighten the wrist back, and use the fist back to concentrate the force on the treatment site. Hit the treatment site with the back of the fist through the flexion of the elbow and the strength of the forearm. Take fist-knocking Dazhui (GV 14) and Baliao (BL 31–34) as an example. The patient sits upright. And the practitioner stands behind the patient, holds the shoulder with one hand, knocks the Dazhui (GV 14) firstly and Baliao (BL 31–34) secondly. It is mostly used after the Manipulations of conventional manipulations.

3. Lateral-knocking manipulation

The practitioner should close and straighten fingers, extend the wrist slightly, and hit the patient's body surface with the lateral side of the little finger and the hypothenar.

4. Fingertip-knocking manipulation

The practitioner should half bend the fingers, relax the wrist joints, and tap the patient's body surface lightly with the fingertips through the flexion and extension of the wrist joints. The practitioner could alternate hands during manipulation.

【要领】

（1）动作要快速而短暂，垂直叩击体表，不能有拖拉动作。

（2）频率均匀有节奏，不要断断续续。

（3）用力要由轻到重，拳击法操作时，要轻轻引击，随后重击3次即可。

【Essentials】

(1) The movements should be quick and brief, knocking vertically on the body surface.

(2) The frequency should be even and rhythmic without intermittence.

(3) The strength of force should be from light to heavy. It should be performed gently at the beginning, then knocking harder for 3 times.

【应用】

击法有醒脑开窍、平肝潜阳、调和气血之功效。

常作为辅助手法，适用于头顶、肩背、腰臀及四肢部，如击囟门、大椎、八髎等穴，配合治疗头痛、失眠、风湿痹痛和肌肉麻木不仁等症。

【Applications】

Knocking manipulation has effects of refreshing the brain and opening the orifices, calming the liver and subduing the yang, and harmonizing the qi and blood.

It is suitable for treating the top of the head, shoulder and back, waist and hip and limbs, such as hitting fontanel, Dazhui (GV 14), Baliao (BL 31–34) and other points. This manipulation is often used as an auxiliary maneuver for the treatment of headache, insomnia, rheumatism and arthralgia and muscle numbness.

十三、啄法

Pecking Manipulation

五指端聚拢成梅花状，啄击治疗部位的手法，如鸡啄米状，故称为啄法，又称为餐法。

Place the five fingers together like a plum blossom and peck the area to be treated. This movement is similar to the behavior of the chicken pecking rice, so it is called pecking manipulation, or (chicken's) dining manipulation.

【术式】

术者五指屈曲，拇指与其余四指聚拢成梅花状，做腕关节伸屈运动，使指端垂直啄击治疗部位。

【Manipulations】

The practitioner flexes the five fingers, gathers fingers into a plum blossom shape, and performs the wrist joint extension and flexion movement, so that the fingertips vertically peck the treatment site.

【要领】

（1）腕关节放松，动作轻巧、灵活。

（2）头部、胸部操作，宜幅度小、频率快；背部操作，宜幅度大、频率慢。

（3）用力轻快，着力均匀。

【Essentials】

(1) Relax the wrist joint. The movement should be light and flexible.

(2) For the Manipulations on the head and chest, the range should be small and the frequency should be fast; for the Manipulations on the back, the range should be large and the frequency should be slow.

(3) The force should be light and evenly distributed.

【应用】

本法具有活血止痛、通经活络、开胸顺气、安神醒脑的功效，适用于头部及胸背部。

头顶前额部应用：与抹法、推拿、按法、揉法配合应用。常用于治疗头痛、头晕、失眠、神经衰弱、脑震荡后遗症以及脑栓塞后遗症等病症。

颈背部以及胸部的应用：常与滚法、摩法、揉法、按法等方法配合运用。

治疗颈背部肌肉酸痛、板滞以及胸胁胀痛等病症。

【Applications】

The manipulation has the effects of activating the blood and relieving pain, dredging the meridians and collaterals, relieving/regulating the chest and soothening the qi, soothing the nerves and refreshing the brain, and is applicable for the head, chest and back.

The application on the top of the head and forehead: It is used in combination with wiping manipulation, massage, pressing manipulation and kneading manipulation. It is commonly used to treat headache, dizziness, insomnia, neurasthenia, concussion sequelae, and cerebral embolism sequelae.

The application on the back of the neck and chest: It is often used in conjunction with rolling, rubbing, kneading, and pressing manipulations. It could be used to treat neck and back muscle soreness, stiffness, and chest and rib pain.

第二节 辅助手法

Section Two Auxiliary Manipulations

一、推法

Pushing Manipulation

术者用指、掌、拳、肘着力于人体的治疗部位作单方向直线移动的手法称为推法。

用拇指指面着力的称为拇指推法；用手掌或掌根着力的称为掌推法；手握拳，用拳面着力的称为拳推法；用肘尖着力的称为肘推法。

When using the pushing manipulation, the practitioner exerts force on the treatment site with fingers, palms, fists, and elbows and moves straightly in one direction.

Pushing with the thumb surface as the point of strength is called thumb-pushing manipulation; with the palm or the base of the palm is called palm-pushing manipulation; with the fist is called fist-pushing manipulation; and with the tip of the elbow is called elbow-pushing manipulation.

【术式】

1. 指推法

（1）拇指推法：术者用拇指指面着力于一定的治疗部位或穴位上，其余四指分开助力，做拇指内收运动，使指面在治疗部位或穴位上做直线推进（按经络循行或肌纤维平行方向推进）。

（2）屈拇指推法：用拇指指骨间关节背部着力于一定的治疗部位或穴位，做单方向直线推动。

（3）屈食指推法：用示指第1节指骨间关节背部着力于治疗部位或穴位，做单方向直线推动。

2. 掌推法

术者用手掌或掌根着力于一定的治疗部位或穴位上，以掌根为重点，运用前臂力量向一定方向推进。需要增大压力时，可用另一手掌重

【Manipulations】

1. Finger-pushing manipulation

(1) Thumb-pushing manipulation: The practitioner concentrates the force on certain treatment site or acupoint with the thumb surface, and the other four fingers are separated to assist, then, performs thumb adduction movement horizontally on the treatment site or acupoint. (Follow the meridians or advance in parallel to the muscle fibers).

(2) Flexed-thumb pushing manipulation: Exert force on the certain treatment site or acupoint with the back of the thumb joint, and move straightly in one direction.

(3) Flexed index finger pushing manipulation: Exert force on the certain treatment site or acupoint with the back of the first index finger joint, and move straightly in one direction.

2. Palm-pushing manipulation

The practitioner exerts force on the certain treatment site or acupoint with the palm or the base of palm, uses the

叠于掌背推进。

3. 拳推法

术者手握成拳，以示指、中指、环指、小指四指的指间关节背部突起处着力，向一定方向推进。

4. 肘推法

术者屈曲肘关节，用尺骨鹰嘴突起处（肘尖）着力于一定的治疗部位，向一定方向推进。

base of the palm as the focus, and applies the strength of the forearm to advance in a certain direction. When need to increase the force, push forward with both hands folded.

3. Fist-pushing manipulation

The practitioner makes a fist, and exerts force on the back protrusions of the four fingers' joints, and push them in a certain direction.

4. Elbow-pushing manipulation

The practitioner flexes the elbow joint, concentrates force on the protrusion of the olecranon (the tip of the elbow) and push forward in a certain direction.

【要领】

（1）着力面要紧贴体表的治疗部位。

（2）向下压力应均匀适中，过轻起不到治疗作用，过重易引起皮肤折叠而发生破损。

（3）用力深沉、平稳，呈直线移动，不可歪斜。

（4）推进的速度宜缓慢均匀，特别是肘推法。

（5）推法宜直接在体表操作，临床应用时，可在施治部位涂抹少许介质。

【Essentials】

(1) The surface of the force should stick to the treatment site.

(2) Downward pressure should be even and moderate, otherwise it is too light to play a therapeutic role or so strong that the skin is folded and injured.

(3) Move in a straight line with deep and steady force.

(4) The speed of movement should be slow and even, especially in the elbow pushing manipulation.

(5) The pushing manipulation should be performed directly on the body surface. In clinical application, a little Tuina medium can be applied on the treatment site.

【应用】

推法具有温经活络、解郁除闷、活血止痛、健脾和胃、调和气血的功效，在全身各部位均可使用。

一般拇指推法适用于肩背部、胸腹部、腰臀部及四肢部，如推桥弓，即用拇指从翳风穴由上而下推至锁骨上窝，具有平肝熄风、清脑明目、宁心安神的功效。常与五指抓头顶、扫散法、抹前额和一指禅

【Applications】

The pushing manipulation has the effects of warming meridians and activating collaterals, relieving depression and removing stuffiness, activating blood to relieve pain, invigorating the spleen and harmonizing the stomach, and harmonizing qi and blood. It can be applied in all parts of the body.

Generally, the thumb pushing manipulation is applicable to the shoulder-back area, chest-abdomen area, waist-buttock area and limbs. Take pushing the bridge

推法配合应用，治疗高血压、头痛、头晕、失眠等症。

掌推法适用于面积较大的部位，如腰背部、胸腹部及大腿部等。如掌推腰背及四肢，具有舒筋通络、理筋止痛的功效。治疗四肢关节软组织损伤、局部肿痛、活动不利等症时，常与擦法、按揉法、湿热敷配合使用。治疗背部肌肉酸痛、板滞时，常与丁氏㨰法、按揉法配合应用。

拳推法是平推法中刺激较强的一种手法，适用于腰背部及四肢部的劳损、宿伤及风湿痹痛等。

肘推法是推法中刺激最强的一种，适用于脊柱两侧华佗夹脊穴及大腿后侧，常用于体型壮实，肌肉丰厚，以及脊柱强直或感觉迟钝的患者。如治疗迁延日久的腰腿痛、腰背部僵直、感觉迟钝等病症，常与拍法、丁氏㨰法、肘压法等配合应用。

arch as an example, in this manipulation, the practitioner uses thumb to push downward from Yifeng (TE 17) to supraclavicular fossa. It has the effects of pacifying the liver and extinguishing the wind, clearing the brain and improving eyesight, quieting the spirit and tranquilizing the mind. It is often used in combination with the manipulation of five fingers grasping the top of the head, sweeping manipulation, wiping the forehead and pushing manipulation with one finger to treat hypertension, headache, dizziness, and insomnia.

The palm pushing manipulation is suitable for discomforts in larger areas, such as the lower back, chest and abdomen, and thighs. For example, the manipulation of pushing the waist, back and limbs with the palm has the effects of soothing tendons and dredging collaterals, regulating tendons and relieving pain. In the treatment of limb joint soft tissue injury, local swelling and pain, unfavorable movement and other symptoms, this manipulation is often used in combination with rubbing manipulation, kneading manipulation and hot compress. In the treatment of back muscle soreness and sluggishness, it is often used in combination with Ding's rolling manipulation and kneading manipulation.

Fist pushing is a manipulation with strong stimuli among pushing manipulations. It is suitable for strain, persistent injury and rheumatic arthralgia of the lower back and limbs.

Elbow pushing is one of the most stimulating pushing manipulations. It could be applied on the Huatuo Jiaji (EX–B 2) on both sides and the posterior side of the thigh. It is commonly used in strong patients with spinal rigidity or dysesthesia. For example, in the treatment of prolonged low back pain, low back stiffness, sluggishness and other symptoms, this manipulation is often used in combination with the patting manipulation, the Ding's rolling manipulation, and the elbow pressing manipulation.

二、拿法

Grasping Manipulation

用拇指与其余四指螺纹面对称用力内收提起并捏揉的手法称为拿法。

Pinch and knead the area to be treated with the thumb and the other four fingers..

【术式】

1. 二指拿法

拇指螺纹面和食指螺纹面相对用力夹住治疗部位的肌筋逐渐用力内收提起，并作轻重交替而连续的一紧一松的捏提和捏揉动作。

2. 三指拿法

拇指螺纹面和示、中指螺纹面相对用力夹住治疗部位的肌筋，逐渐用力内收提起，并做轻重交替且连续的一紧一松的捏提和捏揉动作。

3. 四指拿法

拇指螺纹面和示、中、环指螺纹面相对用力夹住治疗部位的肌筋，逐渐用力内收提起，并做轻重交替且连续的一紧一松的捏提和捏揉动作。

4. 五指拿法

拇指螺纹面与其余四指螺纹面相对用力夹住治疗部位的肌筋，逐渐用力内收提起，并做轻重交替而连续的一紧一松的捏提和捏揉动作。

【Manipulations】

1. Two-finger grasping manipulation

Clamp the muscle in the treatment site with the ribbed surfaces of the thumb and the index finger forcefully. Then lift the treatment site up with increasing force, and apply continuous pinching and kneading movements.

2. Three-finger grasping manipulation

Clamp the muscle in the treatment site with the ribbed surfaces of the thumb, the index finger and the middle finger forcefully. Then lift the treatment site up with increasing force, and apply continuous pinching and kneading movements.

3. Four-finger grasping manipulation

Clamp the muscle in the treatment site with the ribbed surfaces of the thumb, the index finger, the middle finger and the ring finger forcefully. Then lift the treatment site up with increasing force, and apply continuous pinching and kneading movements tightly and loosely.

4. Five-finger grasping manipulation

Clamp the muscle in the treatment site with the ribbed surfaces of the thumb and the other four fingers forcefully. Then lift the treatment site up with increasing force, and apply continuous pinching and kneading movements.

【要领】

（1）操作时腕关节要放松，动作灵活而柔和。

（2）着力面为螺纹面，不可用指端、爪甲内抠。

（3）操作时捏揉动作要连贯而

【Essentials】

(1) During the manipulations, the wrist joint should be relaxed and the movement should be flexible and gentle.

(2) The force should be focused on the ribbed surface but not fingertips or nails.

有节奏。

（4）拿法运劲要由轻到重，不可突然用力或使用暴力。

（5）拿法刺激较强，拿后常继以搓揉，以缓和刺激。

(3) The kneading movements should be consistent and rhythmic during manipulations.

(4) The strength should be from light to heavy, and sudden force or very hard force are not allowed during the grasping manipulation.

(5) Grasping manipulation has strong stimulation so it is often followed by rubbing manipulation to ease the stimulation.

【应用】

拿法临床应用相当广泛，常用于颈项部、肩背部、四肢部。

拿风池穴：具有发汗解表、开窍醒神的功效。常与按揉太阳、睛明穴以及扫散法等方法配合应用。用于治疗头痛、感冒、鼻塞、项强等症。

拿肩井：具有祛风散寒、调和气血的功效。用于治疗感冒、上肢痹痛等症。

拿颈项部：具有祛风散寒、开窍明目、疏通经络的功效。

拿上肢（内、外、后束）：具有疏经通络、松肌解痉的功效。用于上肢痹痛等。

【Applications】

Grasping manipulation is widely used in clinical practice and is commonly performed on the neck, shoulders, back, and extremities.

Grasping Fengchi (GB 20): It has the effects of inducing sweating to release the exterior and opening the orifices and refreshing the mind. It is often used in combination with kneading Taiyang (EX–HN 5), Jingming (BL 1) and sweeping manipulation for the treatment of headache, cold, nasal congestion, strong neck and other diseases.

Grasping Jianjing (GB 21): It has the effects of dispelling wind and dissipating cold, harmonizing qi and blood, and is used to treat colds and upper limb arthralgia.

Grasping neck: It has the effects of dispelling wind and dissipating cold, opening orifices and improving eyesight, and dredging meridians.

Grasping the upper limbs (inner, outer, posterior fasciculus): It has the effects of soothing meridians and dredging collaterals, relaxing muscle and releasing spasm. It could be used to treat upper limb arthralgia.

三、按法

Pressing Manipulation

用手指或手掌着力于治疗部位或穴位上，逐渐用力向下按压的方法，称为按法。

Exert the strength on the treatment site with the finger or the palm and press downward with increasing force.

When performed with the thumb, index, middle, or

其中以拇指或示、中、环指指面着力的，称为指按法；以掌根、鱼际、全掌或双掌重叠着力的，称为掌按法。

1. 指按法

（1）拇指按法：术者拇指伸直，用拇指指面着力于治疗部位（经络或穴位），垂直用力，向下按压，使刺激充分达到肌肉组织的深层，使患者产生酸、麻、重、胀和走窜等感觉，持续数秒后，渐渐放松，如此反复操作。其余四指握拳或张开，起支持作用，以协同助力。

（2）中指按法：术者中指指骨间关节、掌指关节伸直，示指搭于中指末节指骨间关节背侧，其余四指弯曲，用中指指端着力于治疗部位（经络或穴位），垂直用力，向下按压，使刺激充分达到肌肉组织的深层，使患者产生酸、麻、重、胀和走窜等感觉，持续数秒后，渐渐放松，如此反复操作。

（3）三指按法：术者示、中、环三指指间关节和掌指关节均伸直，用示、中、环三指指腹着力于治疗部位（经络或穴位），垂直用力向下按压，使刺激充分达到肌肉组织的深层，使患者产生酸、麻、重、胀和走窜等感觉，持续数秒后，渐渐放松，如此反复操作。

2. 掌按法

术者腕关节放松，用掌根、鱼际或全掌着力于治疗部位，而后做垂直用力向下按压。在按压时应稍停留3～5秒，松开后再重复按压，即“按而留之”。掌按法在操作时，

ring finger, it is called the finger-pressing manipulation; with the lower part of the palm, the thenar, the whole palm or the overlapping of the palms, it is called the palm-pressing manipulation.

1. Finger-pressing manipulation

(1) Thumb-pressing manipulation: The practitioner should straighten the thumb, put the thumb surface on the treatment site (meridians or acupoints), and press downward with perpendicular pressure, so that the force could be fully transmitted into the deep layer of muscle tissue. In so doing, the patient would have senses such as soreness, numbness, heaviness, distension and migratory pain. After a few seconds, the practitioner could gradually relax the finger, and repeat this progress several times. The remaining four fingers could make a fist or open up for support so as to assist in synergy.

(2) Middle Finger-pressing manipulation: The practitioner should straighten the interphalangeal joints and metacarpophalangeal joints of the middle finger, place the index finger on the back of the interphalangeal joint of the middle finger, and bent the remaining fingers. Apply vertical force on the treatment site (meridians or acupoints) with the tip of middle finger and press downward forcefully so that the force could be fully transmitted into the deep layer of muscle tissue. In so doing, the patient would have senses such as soreness, numbness, heaviness, distension and migratory pain. After a few seconds, the practitioner could gradually relax the finger, and repeat this progress several times.

(3) Three Fingers-pressing manipulation: The practitioner should straighten the interphalangeal joints and metacarpophalangeal joints of index finger, middle finger and ring finger. Apply vertical force on the treatment site (meridians or acupoints) with index finger, middle finger and ring finger and press downward forcefully, so that the force could be transmitted into the deep layers of the

根据疾病治疗的需要或者部位的不同，可采用单掌按法或双掌按法。

muscle tissue. In so doing, the patient would have senses such as soreness, numbness, heaviness, distension and migratory pain. After a few seconds, the practitioner could gradually relax the finger, and repeat this progress several times.

2. Palm-pressing manipulation

The practitioner should relax the wrist, apply vertical pressure on the treatment site (meridians or acupoints) with the lower part of the palm, the thenar, or the whole palm. When pressing, hold on for 3 to 5 seconds, then release and press the treatment site again. That is pressing andstaying for a while. When using palm-pressing manipulation, the practitioner can choose single-hand pressing manipulation or double hand-manipulation based on the demands of the treatment or the differences of the treatment areas.

【要领】

（1）按法操作时，按压的方向应垂直于治疗部位。

（2）用力要由轻到重，平稳而持续，力量逐渐增加，使刺激充分透达到机体组织深部。

（3）按而留之，不宜突然松手。

（4）忌粗暴施力。

（5）指按法时掌指关节以及指间关节均应伸直。

（6）若要增加按压力量，可用双指或双掌重叠按压（即叠指按法或叠掌按法），也可上身前倾伸肘，以借助身体的重力增加按压力量。

【Essentials】

(1) During pressing manipulation, the direction of pressing should be perpendicular to the treatment site.

(2) The strength should be from light to heavy and remain stable and sustaining. The force should be gradually increased, so that the stimulation can fully penetrate into the body tissue.

(3) The practitioner needs to remember to press downward and hold on for seconds. It's inappropriate to let hands go quickly.

(4) Don't exert force violently.

(5) The metacarpophalangeal joints and interphalangeal joints should be straightened when the pressing manipulation is performed.

(6) The pressure could be enhanced through overlapping two fingers or two palms or by leaning forward to rely on the body's weight.

【应用】

按是压抑的意思，指按法主要

【Applications】

To press is known as to force downward. It is mainly

用于经穴及阿是穴，适用于全身各部位或穴位。具有较好的行气活血、开通闭塞、缓急止痛的功效。

常用于治疗各种急、慢性疼痛。掌按法有接触面积大，压力重而刺激缓和的特点。适用于面积大而又较为平坦的腰背部、腹部、下肢等部位。具有疏经通络、开通闭塞、温中散寒的功效。

applied on acupoints and Ashi point, and is applicable to various parts or acupoints of the body. It has the effects of moving qi and activating the blood, releasing occlusion and relieving pain, relieving spasm and pain.

The palm-pressing manipulation featuring large contact area, heavy pressure and mild stimulation is suitable for treatment sites characterized by larger and flat area, such as lower back, abdomen, lower limbs and other parts. It has the effects of dredging meridians and collaterals, opening occlusion, warming the abdomen and dispelling cold.

四、摩法

Rubbing Manipulation

术者用手掌或指腹轻放于体表治疗部位，做环形、有节律摩动的手法。

用手指指面着力摩动的称为指摩法；用手掌面着力摩动的手法称为掌摩法。

The practitioner gently places the palm or the finger pulp on the treatment area, and performs a circular, rhythmic rubbing manipulation. The manipulation of rubbing with the finger surface is called the finger-rubbing manipulation, while the manipulation of rubbing with the palm is called the palm-rubbing manipulation.

【术式】

术者用手指指面或手掌面，轻放于患者体表的一定治疗部位或穴位，做环形的、有节律的摩动。

1. 指摩法

用手指着力做环形有节律的摩动。术者指掌部自然伸直，并拢，腕关节微屈，将示指、中指、环指、小指的末节指面附着于治疗部位上，沉肩、垂肘，以肘关节为支点，前臂作主动摆动，带动四指在体表作环转摩动（顺时针或逆时针方向）。

2. 掌摩法

用手掌着力做环形有节律的摩动。术者手掌自然伸直，腕关节微

【Manipulations】

The practitioner gently places the palm or the finger pulp on the treatment site or acupoints of the body surface, and performs a circular, rhythmic rubbing manipulation.

1. Finger-rubbing manipulation

Rub the treatment site or acupoints in a circular or rhythmic way with fingers. The practitioner should naturally straighten the fingers and the palm, slightly flex the wrist joint, and put the distal ends of the index finger, middle finger, ring finger, and little finger on the treatment site. Then sink the shoulders, drop the elbows, and take the elbow joint as the fulcrum to drive the four fingers to make a circular rubbing movement (clockwise or counterclockwise) on the body surface by swing forearm initiatively.

背伸，将手掌平放于体表治疗部位或穴位上，以掌心或掌根部作为着力点，腕关节放松，以肘关节为支点，前臂做主动摆动，带动手掌在体表做环转摩动（顺时针或逆时针方向）。

2. Palm-rubbing manipulation

Rub the treatment site or acupoints in a circular or rhythmic way with the palm. The practitioner should naturally straighten the palm, and put the palm flatly on treatment sites or acupoints, then focus the strength on the center or base of the palm and relax the elbow joint to make a circular rubbing movement (clockwise or counterclockwise) on the body surface by swinging forearm initiatively with the elbow joint as the fulcrum.

【要领】

（1）摩法操作时，肘关节微屈在120°～150°。

（2）腕关节放松，指掌关节自然伸直，手指并拢。

（3）操作时指面或掌面要紧贴体表治疗部位，可做顺时针或逆时针方向摩动。

（4）摩动时压力要均匀，动作要轻柔。指摩法操作时宜轻快，频率约120次/分钟；掌摩法操作时宜稍重缓，频率约100次/分钟。

【Essentials】

(1) In the process of rubbing, the elbow joint should be slightly flexed at the angle between 120° and 150°.

(2) Relax the wrist joint and the metacarpal joints should be naturally straightened with the fingers closed together.

(3) During the manipulations, the finger surface or palm surface should be clung to the treatment site, and the rubbing manipulation could be performed in a clockwise or counterclockwise direction.

(4) The pressure should be even and the movement should be gentle when rubbing. The finger-rubbing manipulation should be operated lightly with a frequency of about 120 times per minute, while the palm-rubbing manipulation should be performed slightly heavier and more slowly with a frequency of about 100 times per minute.

【应用】

摩法刺激柔和舒适，应用在全身各部位，以胸腹部以及胁肋部为常用。

（1）在腹部应用时，临床上常与推摩法、振法以及鱼际揉法配合应用，治疗脘腹部胀痛、泄泻、便秘、消化不良等胃肠道疾病。具有

【Applications】

Due to the comfort and gentle stimulation the rubbing manipulation could provide, it could be used all over the body, especially in the chest, abdomen and flanks.

(1) When applied on the abdomen, it is often used in combination with the pushing-rubbing manipulation, the vibrating manipulation and the thenar-kneading manipulation to treat gastrointestinal diseases such as abdominal distention,

和中理气、消食导滞、调节胃肠等功能。

（2）胸胁部应用时，常与指摩法、擦法等方法配合应用，治疗胸胁胀满、咳嗽、气喘以及胸胁屏伤，挫伤等症。具有宽胸理气，宣肺止咳的功效。

（3）在腰背、四肢部位应用时，常与㨰法配合应用，治疗四肢关节外伤肿痛以及风湿痹痛等症。具有行气活血，散瘀消肿之功效。

（4）在少腹部应用时，常与一指禅推法和擦法合用，治疗遗尿、女子不孕、痛经、闭经或男子阳痿、遗精等病症。

古人按照摩法操作的速度以及摩动的方向，将摩法分为补法和泻法。如《厘正按摩要术》云："急摩为泻，缓摩为补。"也有顺时针方向摩动为补，逆时针方向摩动为泻之论述。

diarrhea, constipation, and indigestion. It has the functions of harmonizing the middle energizer and rectifying qi, dispersing food and removing food stagnation, and regulating gastrointestinal and other functions.

(2) When applied on the chest and rib-side, it is often used in conjunction with finger-rubbing manipulation and rubbing manipulation to treat painful distention in the chest and rib-side, cough, asthma, and injury in chest and rib-side. It has the effects of loosening the chest and regulating qi, ventilating lung and relieving cough.

(3) When applied on the lower back and limbs, it is often used in conjunction with the rolling manipulation to treat impediment pain caused by wind dampness, and traumatic swelling and pain of joints. It has the effects of moving qi and promoting blood circulation, dissipating stasis and removing swelling.

(4) When applied on the lower abdomen, it is often used in combination with one-finger pushing manipulation and rubbing manipulation to treat enuresis, female infertility, dysmenorrhea, amenorrhea or male impotence, nocturnal emission and other diseases.

According to the speed and the direction of rubbing, the ancients divided rubbing manipulation into tonifying method and reduction method. For example, it is recorded in the *Revised Version of Massage Essentials* that "Quick rubbing is for reduction, and slow rubbing is for tonifying." There are also discussions that rubbing in a clockwise direction is for supplementation, and rubbing in a counter-clockwise direction is for drainage.

五、揉法

Kneading Manipulation

术者用手指的螺纹面或手掌面着力于治疗部位或穴位，做轻柔缓和的环旋运动并带动该处的皮肤及皮下

The practitioner places the ribbed surface of the fingers or the palm on the treatment site or acupoint, and makes a gentle and slow circular motion to transmit the

组织一起揉动的手法，称为揉法。

force into the skin and subcutaneous tissues.

【术式】

1. 指揉法

（1）拇指揉法：用拇指的螺纹面，轻按于一定的治疗部位或穴位，腕关节放松，前臂做主动摆动，带动腕关节的摆动，使拇指螺纹面在治疗部位上做小幅度轻柔的环旋运动，并带动该处的皮肤及皮下组织一起揉动。

（2）中指揉法：术者中指伸直，示指搭于中指远端指间关节背侧，腕关节微屈，用中指指腹着力于一定的治疗部位或穴位上，以肘关节为支点，前臂做主动摆动，带动腕关节的摆动，使中指指腹在治疗部位上做小幅度轻柔的环旋运动。

（3）双指揉法：术者示、中指伸直，腕关节微屈，用示、中指螺纹面着力于一定的治疗部位或穴位，以肘关节为节点，前臂做主动摆动，带动腕关节的摆动，使示、中指指腹在治疗部位上做小幅度轻柔的环旋运动。

（4）三指揉法：术者示、中、环指伸直，腕关节微屈，用示、中、环指螺纹面着力于一定的治疗部位或穴位，以肘关节为支点，前臂做主动摆动，带动腕关节的摆动，使三指的指腹在治疗部位上做小幅度轻柔的环旋运动。

（5）叠拇指揉法：双手拇指相叠做揉法称为叠拇指揉法，此法是为了加强揉法的强度。

【Manipulations】

1. Finger-kneading manipulation

(1) Thumb-kneading manipulation: Press gently on the treatment site or acupoint with the ribbed surface of the thumb. Relax the wrist joint and make active swing with forearm to drive the wrist joint. Then make a small and gentle circular motion on the treatment site with the ribbed surface of the thumb to drive the skin and subcutaneous tissue there to be kneaded together.

(2) Middle finger-kneading manipulation: The practitioner should straighten the middle finger, put the index finger on the back of the distal interphalangeal joint of the middle finger, slightly flex the wrist joint, and then exert force on the certain treatment site or acupoint with the pulp of the middle finger. Take the elbow joint as the fulcrum and make an active swing with forearm to drive the wrist joint, so that a small gentle whirling movement is made on the treatment site with the pulp of the middle fingers.

(3) Double finger-kneading manipulation: The practitioner should straighten the index and middle fingers, slightly flex the wrist joint, and then exert force on the certain treatment site or acupoint with the ribbed surface of the index and middle fingers. Take the elbow joint as the fulcrum and make an active swing with the forearm to drive the wrist joint. Then a small gentle whirling movement is made on the treatment site with the pulp of the index and middle fingers.

(4) Three finger-kneading manipulation: The practitioner should straighten the index, middle and ring fingers, slightly flex the wrist joint, and then exert force on the certain treatment site or acupoint with the ribbed surface of the index, middle and ring fingers. Take the elbow joint as the fulcrum and make an active swing with

2. 鱼际揉法

术者用鱼际吸定于治疗部位或穴位，沉肩、垂肘，腕关节放松呈微屈或水平状，拇指内收，四指自然伸直，以肘关节为支点，前臂作主动摆动，带动腕关节带动皮下组织一起揉动。

3. 掌揉法

术者用手掌根附着于治疗部位或穴位，稍用力下压，腕关节放松，运用前臂力量带动腕、掌、指在治疗部位上作小幅度轻柔缓和的环旋运动，并带动该处的皮肤及皮下组织一起揉动。为加强刺激强度可以双掌相叠揉动（称为叠掌揉法）。

the forearm to drive the wrist joint. Then a small gentle whirling movement is made on the treatment site with the pulp of the three fingers.

(5) Overlapped fingers-kneading manipulation: The manipulation that is operated through overlapping index fingers of both hands is called overlapped fingers-kneading manipulation. This is used to enhance the strength of kneading manipulation.

2. Thenar-kneading manipulation

The practitioner should stick thenar on the treatment site or acupoint, sink the shoulder, drop the elbow and then relax the wrist joint to make it stay slightly flexed or horizontal. The thumb is flexed and the other four fingers are naturally straightened. Take the elbow joint as the fulcrum and make an active swing with the forearm to drive the wrist joint and subcutaneous tissue.

3. Palm-kneading manipulation

The practitioner should stick the lower part of the palm to the treatment site or acupoint and press downward. Relax the wrist joint, make small gentle whirling movement on the treatment site with the wrist joint, palm and fingers and drive the skin and subcutaneous tissue through the force of forearm. Both palms could be overlapped to knead for promoting the stimulation (which is called overlapped palm-kneading manipulation).

【要领】

（1）揉法着力点要吸附，不可有摩擦与移动。

（2）揉法动作灵活、协调而有节律性。

（3）指揉法揉动时幅度要小，频率要适中；中指揉时，指骨间关节、掌指关节均要伸直；拇指揉法时，仅靠拇指掌指关节作环旋运动。

（4）鱼际揉法术者不可耸肩，

【Essentials】

(1) During the kneading manipulation, the point of strength should be fixed to avoid friction or movement.

(2) The manipulation should be flexible, coordinated and rhythmic.

(3) When performing finger-kneading manipulation, the range of the motion should be small and the frequency should be moderate. When kneading with middle finger, the interphalangeal joints and metacarpophalangeal joints should be straightened; when kneading with thumb, only

腕关节不可背伸。

（5）掌揉法操作时，腕关节放松，压力轻柔，动作灵活，吸定，既不能有体表的摩擦，也不能有向下按压的动作。

（6）频率120～160次/分钟。

the metacarpophalangeal joints of thumb should be used for cyclic movement.

(4) The practitioner shall not shrug shoulders or extend wrist joint backwards while practicing thenar-kneading manipulation.

(5) During the palm-kneading manipulation, the wrist joint should be relaxed, the pressure should be gentle, and the movement should be flexible. There should be neither friction on the body surface nor downward compression.

(6) The frequency should be about 120 to 160 times per minute.

【应用】

指揉法：施术面积较小，动力集中，动作柔和而深沉，适用于全身各部位或穴位，其治疗作用取决于所取穴位的特异性。

双指揉法：临床上常用于同时分揉二穴，多用于小儿。

三指揉法：临床常用于同时分揉三穴，如三指揉神阙与两侧天枢，治疗脘腹胀痛、便秘等症，以及三指同时揉胸锁乳突肌治疗小儿斜颈。

鱼际揉法：主要用于头面、胸腹和四肢部。鱼际揉头面部具有祛风通络，安神醒脑明目功效，用于治疗头痛、头晕、失眠、面瘫等。鱼际揉胸胁部具有宽胸理气，行气活血功效，用于治疗咳嗽、胸闷、气喘、胸胁屏挫伤。鱼际揉脘腹部具有健脾和胃，消积导滞功效，用于治疗脘腹胀痛、泄泻、便秘等。鱼际揉四肢关节具有舒筋活血，消肿止痛功效，用于治疗软组织急性扭挫伤，局部肿痛，运动障碍等。

掌揉法：着力面积大，刺激柔

【Applications】

The finger-kneading manipulation is performed on small area so the strength is focused, and the movement is gentle and deep. Therefore, it is suitable for various parts or acupoints of the body, and its therapeutic effect depends on the specificity of the acupoints.

Double finger-kneading manipulation is commonly used to knead two points at the same time in clinical practice and is mostly used to treat children.

Three Finger-kneading manipulation is commonly used in clinical practice to knead three points at the same time, such as kneading Shenque (CV 8) and Tianshu (ST 25) on both sides to treat abdominal pain and constipation, as well as kneading sternocleidomastoid muscle at the same time to treat torticollis in children.

Thenar-kneading manipulation is mainly performed on the head, face, chest and abdomen, and extremities. Thenar kneading could be performed on the head and face to produce the effects of expelling wind and dredging collaterals, tranquilizing the mind and refreshing the eyes, and is used to treat headache, dizziness, insomnia, and facial paralysis.

Thenar kneading manipulation performed on the chest and rib-side could produce the effects of soothing

和舒适，适用于面积大又较为平坦的部位，如腰背部、腹部以及四肢。

（1）掌揉腹部：具有温中散寒的功效，常用于治疗脘腹疼痛，与按揉足三里，背部的脾俞、肝俞（18）、胆俞、阿是穴等配合应用。

（2）掌揉腰背部：掌根揉腰背部两侧肾俞、命门、腰阳关、八髎穴，用于治疗肾虚腰痛、腰三横突综合征，常与按法、擦法等配合应用。

（3）掌揉膝部：常由于治疗膝关节酸痛、屈伸不利等症。操作时患者取仰卧位，两下肢伸直，术者用手掌轻放于髌上，作环转揉动并带动髌骨一起揉动。

（4）掌揉腰背部以及四肢肌肉，有较好的放松肌肉，松解痉挛的作用，常用于治疗腰背部以及四肢肌肉的酸痛及强刺激手法作用后引起的不适感。

the chest and regulating qi, moving qi and activating blood circulation. It is used to treat cough, chest tightness, asthma, and chest and flank injury. Thenar kneading manipulation performed on the abdomen produce the effects of invigorating spleen and harmonizing stomach, promoting digestion and removing food stagnation. It could be used to treat abdominal pain, diarrhea, and constipation. Thenar kneading manipulation performed on the extremities could produce the effects of relaxing tendons and activating blood circulation, dispersing swelling and relieving pain. It could be used to treat acute torsion and contusion of soft tissues, local swelling and pain, and dyskinesia.

Palm-kneading manipulation is performed on the larger area. It could produce soft and comfortable stimulation, and is suitable for large and relatively flat areas including the lower back, abdomen and limbs.

(1) Kneading the abdomen with the palm: It has the effects of warming the middle and dispelling cold. It is often used to treat abdominal pain. It is used in conjunction with the massage and rubbing of Zusanli (ST 36), Pishu (BL 20), Ganshu (BL 18), Danshu (BL 19) and Ashi point on the back.

(2) Kneading the lower back with the palm: Rubbing the Shenshu (BL 23), Mingmen (GV 4), Yaoyangguan (GV 3), and Baliao (BL 31–34) with the lower part of the palm on both sides of the waist and back. It is used to treat low back pain due to kidney deficiency, and third lumbar transverse process syndrome. It is often used in conjunction with pressing and rubbing manipulations.

(3) Kneading the knees with the palm: It is often used to treat soreness of the knee joints, unfavorable flexion and extension, etc. During the manipulations, the patient should take a supine position, and straighten the lower limbs. The practitioner should gently place the palm on the patella of the patient and make a circular motion on the treatment area.

(4) Kneading the muscles of the lower back and

limbs with the palm: It can relax the muscles and relieve spasm. It is often used to treat the soreness of the muscles and the discomfort caused by manipulations with strong stimulation.

六、搓法

Palm-twisting Manipulation

用手掌面着力于治疗部位或夹住肢体做交替搓动的方法，称为搓法。

Hold the limb or treatment areas with both hands/palms and apply alternating or back-and-forth twisting.

【术式】

患者肢体放松，术者用双手掌面夹住肢体的治疗部位，然后相对用力，做方向相反的快速搓揉、搓转或搓摩运动，并同时做上下往返移动。

双手掌对称用力，作前后环转搓摩运动的，称搓摩法；用双手掌对称用力，搓揉肩部，称为搓揉法。

【Manipulations】

The patient should be relaxed. The practitioner holds the patient's limb with both palms, and then performs rapid kneading, twisting and rubbing manipulations in opposite directions and moves up and down simultaneously.

Manipulation that characterized by applying symmetrical force with both palms on the body to rub and twist the skin back and forth is called twisting-rubbing manipulation; manipulation that characterized by applying symmetrical force with both palms on the body to knead and twist shoulder is called twisting-kneading manipulation.

【要领】

（1）操作时，双手用力要对称。

（2）搓揉、搓摩动作要快，但移动要慢。

（3）术者腕关节放松，动作要灵活，治疗部位不宜夹得太紧。

（4）操作时动作要连贯。

【Essentials】

(1) During manipulation, the force of both hands should be symmetrical.

(2) The practitioner should twist, rub, and knead quickly but move from up to down slowly.

(3) The practitioner should relax the wrist joint and manipulate flexibly. It's inappropriate to clamp the treatment site too tightly.

(4) Please operate in a consistent manner.

【应用】

《医宗金鉴·正骨心法要旨》谓："以手轻轻搓揉，令其骨合筋舒。"其

【Applications】

It is said in *Golden Mirror of the Medical Tradition: Essentials for Bone Orthopedics* that "(The doctor should)

治疗作用根据治疗部位而论，操作方法亦随不同部位而变化。临床上常作为辅助性结束手法应用，适用于四肢、腰背及胁肋部，以上肢为常用。

肩及上肢部应用：常用于治疗肩及上肢部酸痛，活动不利。具有调和气血、疏通经络以及放松肌肉的功效。操作时患者取坐位，患侧上肢部放松，并自然下垂。术者站于患者侧方，上身略前倾，用双手分别夹住患者肩部前后部，然后由上而下，由肩部→上臂→前臂→腕部。在搓肩关节时，双手呈顺时针方向的环形搓揉法，然后顺势向下搓上臂、前臂部，双手呈一前一后的交替搓转动作，并向下移动至腕部，再由腕部向上搓至腋下，如此反复3～5遍。

搓法常与抖法合用，作为治疗的结束手法，以缓解因刺激手法可能引起的不良反应。

腰背部应用：常用于治疗腰背部肌肉酸痛、板滞等症。具有行气活血、疏经通络的功效。操作时，患者取卧位或坐位（上身前倾），术者双掌夹扶住患者腰背部肌肉，然后双手同时用力做快速的搓摩运动，同时做上下来回往返移动。

胁肋部应用：临床上常用于治疗胸闷、气喘腹胀以及因肝气郁结引起的头痛、头晕、失眠等症。具有疏肝理气、平喘降逆的功效。操作时，患者取坐位，术者站于患者身后，用双手夹住其腋下，然后双手同时用力做快速的搓揉动作，沿胁肋部搓至平脐处。一般自上而下

twist, rub and knead with hands gently to relax bones and tendons". Clinically, it is often used as an auxiliary ending manipulation which is suitable for the four limbs, lower back and flank. The uppers limbs are commonly used in the clinics.

Twisting the shoulder and upper limbs: It is commonly used for the treatment of the soreness pain in shoulders and upper limbs, and other unfavorable symptoms. It has the effects of harmonizing qi and blood, dredging meridians, and relaxing muscles. During the treatment, the patient should take a sitting position, and naturally relax and drop the upper limbs. The practitioner stands on the side of the patient, leans his upper body slightly forward, and clamps the patient's shoulder with both hands, and then performs the treatment from top to bottom according to the order of shoulder→ upper arm→ forearm→wrist. When twisting the shoulder joints, twisting-kneading manipulation should be operated in a clockwise circular motion. Next, rub the upper arm and forearm downwards, and alternately make twisting actions with both hands, and move down to the wrist, and then rub upwards from the wrist to the armpit. Repeat the manipulation 3 to 5 times.

Palm-twisting manipulation is often used in combination with the shaking manipulation as the finishing touch to alleviate the adverse reactions caused by the stimulation.

Twisting the lower back: It is commonly used for the treatment of lower back muscle soreness and stagnation. It has the functions of moving qi and activating blood, and dredging meridians and collaterals. During the Manipulations, the patient should take a supine or sitting position (upper body leans forward), the practitioner holds the patient's waist and back muscles with both palms, and then forcefully performs the twisting-rubbing manipulation at the same time.

Twisting the rib side: Clinically, it is commonly used to treat chest tightness, asthma and abdominal distension,

单方向移动，以免引起气机上逆。

下肢部应用：用于治疗腰腿痛、下肢部肌肉痉挛。如腰椎间盘突出症、股内收肌综合征、小腿腓肠肌痉挛等病症。具有调和气血、疏经通络的功效。操作时，患者取仰卧位，下肢部自然放松，微屈膝屈髋。术者双手夹住患者下肢部，双手同时用力做快速的搓转动作，由髋部搓至踝部，往返数遍后，然后重点搓病变部位，并配合下肢抖法作为结束手法。

膝部应用：常用于治疗膝关节酸痛、活动不利等症，如慢性骨关节炎、膝关节软组织损伤、软骨炎等。具有活血祛瘀、消肿止痛的功效。治疗时，患者侧卧，微屈膝屈髋。术者用双手夹住患者膝关节部，同时用力做顺时针方向的环形的快速搓揉或搓摩运动，常与擦膝关节、揉膝关节等方法配合应用。

as well as headache, dizziness and insomnia caused by liver qi stagnation. It has the effects of soothing the liver and regulating qi, relieving asthma and descending the adverse qi. During the treatment, the patient should take a sitting position, and the practitioner stands behind the patient, clamps the patient's armpit with both hands, and then does a quick twisting-rubbing action from the rib side to the umbilicus. Generally, this manipulation moves in one direction from top to bottom, so as to avoid the counterflow of qi.

Twisting the lower limbs: It is used for the treatment of low back pain, lower extremity muscle spasm including lumbar disc herniation, adductor femoris syndrome, calf gastrocnemius spasm and other diseases. It has the effects of harmonizing qi and blood, and dredging meridians and collaterals. During the treatment, the patient should take a supine position, and naturally relax the lower limbs with the knees and hips slightly flexed. The practitioner clamps the patient's lower limbs with both hands, and performs rapid twisting-rubbing movements from the hip to the ankle. After several times, take the lesion site as the focus, and combined with the lower limb-shaking manipulation in the end.

Twisting the knees: It is commonly used to treat knee soreness and other unfavorable symptoms such as chronic osteoarthritis, knee soft tissue injury, and chondritis. It has the effects of activating blood and removing blood stasis, reducing swelling and relieving pain. During the treatment, the patient lies on the side with the hips flexed slightly. The practitioner clamps the knee of the patient with both hands, and vigorously performs a circular rapid twisting-rubbing or twisting-kneading movement in a clockwise direction simultaneously. It is often used in conjunction with manipulations such as rubbing the knee and kneading the knee.

七、抖法

Shaking Manipulation

用单手或双手握住患肢远端，做连续的、小幅度的、频率较高的上下抖动的手法，称为抖法。

Holding the distal end of the affected limb with one or both hands and shaking the limb up and down continuously in a small-amplitude, high-frequency way.

【术式】

1. 抖上肢法

术者用双手或单手握住患者的手腕部或手掌部，将其上肢慢慢地向前外侧抬起约60°，然后稍用力做连续的、小幅度的、频率较高的上下抖动，并将抖动波由腕关节逐渐传递到肩部，使肩关节和上肢产生舒适的感觉。

2. 抖下肢法

患者取仰卧位，下肢放松伸直，术者站于其脚后方，用单手或双手分别握患者的两踝部，使其下肢呈内旋状，并提起离开床面，然后做连续的、小幅度的上下抖动，使髋部和大腿部有舒适放松的感觉。

3. 抖腕部法

患者取坐位，腕关节放松，术者用双手拇指按放于腕背部，两示指相对，横置于患者腕关节掌侧横纹，双手拇指和示指相对用力捏住患者腕关节上下横纹并做相反方向的快速搓动，带动腕关节做频率较快的、连续的、小幅度的上下抖动。或者术者用示指桡侧抵住腕关节掌侧，拇指按住其前臂近腕关节处将其前臂上下快速运动，使腕关节产生小幅度的、连续的、频率较快的上下抖动。

【Manipulations】

1. Shaking upper limbs

The practitioner holds the patient's wrist or palm with hands, slowly lifts the upper limbs anteriorly and laterally at an angel of 60°, and then makes continuous, small-amplitude, high-frequency up-and-down shaking manipulation with slight force. The shaking wave is gradually transmitted from the wrist joint to the shoulder to relax the shoulder joint and upper limbs.

2. Shaking lower limbs

The patient should take a supine position and straighten the lower limbs. The practitioner stands behind the patient's feet, holds the patient's two ankles with one or two hands, makes the patient's lower limbs rotate inwards, and lifts them off the bed. Then do continuous, small-amplitude up and down shaking to relax the hips and thighs.

3. Shaking wrist

The patient should take a sitting position, and relax the wrist joint. The practitioner presses on the back of the patient's wrist with the thumbs of both hands, and places both index fingers transversely on the patient's wrist joint. Then squeeze the horizontal lines of the patient's wrist joints and do quick twisting-rubbing movements in the opposite direction, driving the wrist joints to do frequent, continuous, small-amplitude up and down shaking movements. Alternatively, the practitioner presses the radial side of the index finger against the volar side of the wrist joint, and presses on the forearm near the wrist joint with the thumb to move the forearm up and down rapidly, so that the wrist joint could make a small, continuous and high-frequency up and down shaking.

【要领】

（1）被抖动的肢体要自然伸直、放松，使患肢的肌肉处于最佳的松弛状态，否则抖动的力量不易发挥。

（2）操作时动作要连续。

（3）抖动幅度要小、频率要快。

（4）术者操作时呼吸自然，不可屏气。

【Essentials】

(1) The shaken limbs should be naturally straightened and relaxed, so that the muscles of the affected limb are in the best state, otherwise it would be difficult to exert force.

(2) The movements should be continuous during manipulations.

(3) Shaking manipulation should be small-amplitude and high-frequency.

(4) The practitioner should breathe naturally without holding his/her breathe during manipulation.

【应用】

抖法是一种和缓、放松的手法，具有疏松经脉、通利关节、松解粘连、消除疲劳的功效，适用于四肢，以上肢为常用。

上肢的应用：治疗时常配合搓法，作为上肢或者肩部治疗的结束手法。治疗肩关节周围炎，肩部伤筋以及肩、肘关节酸痛、活动不利等病症。

下肢的应用：治疗时常配合搓法、叩法以及牵引等方法，用于治疗腰部扭伤、腰椎间盘突出症和腰椎退行性病症。

【Applications】

Shaking manipulation is a gentle and relaxing technique which has the effects of relaxing meridians, unblocking joints, loosening adhesions, and eliminating fatigue. It is suitable for the limbs, especially the upper limbs.

Shaking the upper limbs: It is often combined with palm-twisting manipulation and be the ending manipulation for the treatment of upper limbs or shoulders. It could be used to treat shoulder periarthritis, shoulder tendon injury, shoulder and elbow joint pain, and other inhibited movements.

Shaking the lower limbs: It is often combined with palm-twisting, tapping and pulling-stretching manipulations for the treatment of lumbar sprains, lumbar disc herniation and lumbar degenerative diseases.

八、拨法

Plucking Manipulation

用指、拳、肘着力于治疗部位，按而拨动的手法称为拨法，又称为弹拨法。

Press the area to be treated with fingers, fists, or elbows and then apply perpendicular plucking force to the subcutaneous tissue.

【术式】

1. 拇指拨法

用拇指指端着力于治疗部位（肌筋施治部位），适当用力下压至一定深度，待有酸胀感时，再做与肌纤维方向（或肌腱、韧带）成垂直方向的来回拨动。

2. 三指拨法

用示指、中指和环指的螺纹面着力于治疗部位（肌筋施治部位），适当用力下压至一定深度，待有酸胀感时，再做与肌纤维方向（或肌腱、韧带）成垂直方向的来回拨动。

3. 肘拨法

用肘尖着力于治疗部位（肌筋施治部位），适当用力下压至一定深度，待有酸胀感时，再做与肌纤维方向（或肌腱、韧带）成垂直方向的来回拨动。

【Manipulations】

1. Thumb-plucking manipulation

Apply force to the treatment site with thumb tip, press downward to a certain depth, and when the patient feels soreness, apply perpendicular plucking force to the subcutaneous tissue.

2. Three fingers-plucking manipulation

Apply force to the treatment site with the ribbed surfaces of index finger, middle finger and ring finger, press with appropriate force to a certain depth until feel soreness, and apply perpendicular plucking force to the subcutaneous tissue.

3. Elbow-plucking manipulation

Concentrate force to the treatment site with the tip of the elbow, press to a certain depth with appropriate force, and when feel soreness, apply perpendicular plucking force to the subcutaneous tissue.

【要领】

（1）施力的大小，应根据部位及病症性质而定。

（2）拨动的方向应与肌纤维方向垂直。

（3）施术时，向下的压力不宜过重，以患者能忍受为度。

（4）拨动时，指下应有弹动感，不能在皮肤表面有摩擦移动。

【Essentials】

(1) The intensity of force depends on the location and the nature of the symptoms.

(2) The direction of plucking manipulation should be perpendicular to the direction of muscle fiber.

(3) During the manipulation, the downward pressure should be within the extent that the patient can tolerate.

(4) When plucking, there should be a sense of bouncing under the fingers, and there should be no frictional movements on the surface of the skin.

【应用】

拨法是较强刺激的手法之一，常在阿是穴，或在指下有“筋结”感的部位应用。具有解痉止痛、分

【Applications】

Plucking manipulation is one of the strongest stimulating manipulations, and it is often applied at the Ashi point, or in the sites where there is a sense of “muscle knot” under

解粘连、疏理肌筋的功效。常用于治疗落枕、漏肩风、腰腿痛等软组织损伤引起的肌肉痉挛、疼痛。

（1）落枕：治疗落枕时，先嘱患者缓缓转动颈部，至疼痛最明显时，即保持在此体位，然后术者在颈背部最高带、疼痛最敏感点施以弹拨法，并配合颈部的被动前俯、后仰活动。当疼痛减轻后，疼痛明显缓解为止。

（2）肩关节粘连：治疗肩关节粘连、活动功能障碍时，可用拇指指端着力于肩穴处或阿是穴处弹拨、拨动，并配合做肩关节的被动运动。

（3）第3腰椎横突综合征：治疗第3腰椎横突综合征，可用双拇指重叠着力于阿是穴处，而后进行轻重交替的弹拨、拨动。

（4）肱二头肌长头肌腱腱鞘炎：对肱二头肌长头肌腱腱鞘炎，可用拇指指端着力于结节间沟处，做垂直肌腱方向来回的拨动。

the fingers. It has the effects of relieving spasm and pain, decomposing adhesions, and relaxing muscles and tendons. It is often used to treat muscle spasm and pain caused by soft tissue injuries such as stiff neck, frozen shoulder (omalgia), low back and lumbago and leg pain.

(1) Neck stiffness: In the treatment of neck stiffness, the patient needs to slowly turn the neck until he/she cannot bear the pain, then keeps in this posture. The practitioner performs the plucking manipulation on the area where the pain is the most acute, and in conjunction with passive flexion and retroversion of the neck until the pain is significantly relieved.

(2) Shoulder joints adhesion: In the treatment of shoulder joints adhesion and motor dysfunction, the practitioner could perform plucking manipulation on the meridian points of shoulder or the Ashi point with the thumb end, and it can be combined with passive movements of the shoulder joints.

(3) Third lumbar transverse process syndrome: In the treatment of third lumbar transverse process syndrome, the practitioner could overlap both thumbs to apply force on the Ashi point and then conduct plucking manipulation.

(4) Tenosynovitis of the long head of the biceps brachii muscle: In the treatment of tenosynovitis of the long head of the biceps brachii muscle, the practitioner could make back and forth plucking manipulation which is perpendicular to the tendon at the intertubercular groove.

九、捻法

Finger-twisting Manipulation

用拇指与示指相对捏住治疗部位，稍用力，作对称的快速捻搓动作称为捻法。

Hold the treatment site with the thumb and the index finger with slight force, and make a back-and-forth twisting.

【术式】

术者用拇指和示指的螺纹面（或

【Manipulations】

The practitioner grasps the treatment site with the

示指桡侧面），夹住患者的治疗部位，稍用力，做对称的快速捻搓。

ribbed surface of the thumb and index finger (or radial surface of the index finger), applies slight force and performs rapid twirling movements like twisting the thread back and forth in a symmetrical way.

【要领】

（1）操作时，腕关节放松，动作要灵活而连贯。

（2）用力轻快柔和，做到捻而不滞，转而不浮。

（3）捻搓动作要快，移动要慢，做到紧捻慢移。

（4）局部撕脱、骨折血肿初期，禁用捻法。

（5）施术时可用介质，以保护皮肤，提高疗效。

【Essentials】

(1) When practicing the manipulation, the wrist joint should be relaxed and the movement should be flexible and coherent.

(2) The force should be light and tender to achieve the effects of twisting without stagnation, and turning without floating.

(3) Twist quickly but move hands slowly.

(4) Finger-twisting manipulation is prohibited at the early stage of local tearing and fracture hematoma.

(5) Tuina mediums can be applied during manipulation to protect the skin and improve efficacy.

【应用】

捻法具有疏通关节、理筋通络之功效，适用于指（趾）小关节及浅表肌肤。常用于治疗指（趾）小关节疼痛、肿胀、屈伸不利等症，如类风湿关节炎、指骨关节损伤、指深浅屈肌腱腱鞘炎等病症。

本法也常用于咽喉部，用拇指与示指指面夹住患者喉结两旁，两指相对用力，做快速、柔和的捻搓动作。常与缠法、抖法配合治疗声门闭合功能不全引起的声音嘶哑、失音等症。

【Applications】

Finger-twisting manipulation has the effects of dredging joints, regulating tendons and collaterals, and is suitable for small joints of fingers (toes) and superficial skin. It is often used to treat pain, swelling, and unfavorable flexion and extension of the small joints of the fingers (toes), such as rheumatoid arthritis, phalangeal joint injuries, and superficial and superficial flexor tendons and tenosynovitis.

This manipulation is also commonly used in the sore throat. Clamp both sides of the patient's laryngeal knot with the thumb and the index finger. Apply force with the two fingers facing each other and perform rapid and tender twisting and rubbing movements. It is often used in combination with the pushing manipulation and shaking manipulation to treat hoarseness and aphonia caused by glottic closure insufficiency.

十、勒法

Tweezering Manipulation

用手指夹住患指，相对用力，做急速滑拉动作的手法，称为勒法。

Clamp the affected fingers or toes with the fingers and apply rapid pulling.

【术式】

术者用拇指与示指第2节或者屈示、中指分开成钳状，夹住患指，从指根部至指端，做急速的滑拉动作，或用寸劲抖动。每勒一指，均以有响声为宜。

【Manipulations】

The practitioner uses the thumb and the second segment of the index finger or flexes the index finger and the middle finger, separates these two fingers into a forceps shape, clamps the affected finger, and performs a rapid pulling movement from the base of the finger to the end of the finger, or shakes with strength. When applying this manipulation, it is advisable to make a sound with each movement.

【要领】

（1）手法要轻快柔和。

（2）施术前各指均放松，避免滞而不滑，滑而不实。

（3）必须急速拉滑。

【Essentials】

(1) The manipulation should be light and gentle.

(2) Relax fingers to avoid stagnation.

(3) Pull fingers down rapidly.

【应用】

勒法具有通经活络、滑利关节的功效，适用于手指部。常与捻法、抹法等方法配合应用，治疗肢体麻木、酸痛、屈伸不利等症。

【Applications】

Tightening manipulation has the effects of dredging meridians and activating collaterals, smoothing joints, and is suitable for treating discomforts in fingers. It is often used in conjunction with finger-twisting and wiping manipulations to treat limb numbness, soreness, and unfavorable flexion and extension of limbs.

十一、摇法

Rotating Manipulation

以患肢关节为轴心，使肢体、关节做被动环转运动的手法，称为摇法。

Take the joint of the affected limb as the axis to conduct passive rotation of limbs and joints.

【术式】

术者用一手握住或扶住被摇关节的近端（固定肢体），另一手握住远端，然后做缓和的环转运动，使被摇的关节做顺时针或逆时针方向的摇动。

1. 颈部摇法

（1）坐位颈部摇法：患者取坐位，颈项部放松。术者站于其背后侧方，一手扶住其头顶稍后部，另一手托住其下颌部，双手做相反方向用力，使患者头部向左或向右缓缓转动。

（2）卧位颈部摇法：患者仰卧，头部放松。术者站于其头一侧，以一手上肢前臂背侧托住患者头部，并扶住其对侧肩部，另一手扶住其头顶部，然后利用前臂的摆动，带动患者头部做顺时针环转摇动。再交换左右手，用另一前臂托住患者头部，做头部逆时针方向的环转摇动，每侧 3 ～ 5 周。

2. 肩部摇法

（1）托肘摇肩法：患者取坐位，肩部放松，患肢自然屈肘，术者站于其患侧，上身略前倾，一手扶住患者肩关节上部（用拇指按于结节间沟处），同时用另一手托起患者肘部（使患肢前臂搭于术者的前臂部），然后做缓慢的顺时针或逆时针方向的转动。

（2）扶肘摇肩法：患者取坐位，肩关节放松，患肢自然屈肘。术者站于患者侧后方，一手扶住患者肩上部，另一手扶住患者肘部，而后

【Manipulations】

The practitioner holds or supports the proximal end of the affected joint (fixed limb) with one hand, and the distal end with the other hand, and then performs a gentle clockwise or counterclockwise rotation.

1. Neck-rotating manipulation

(1) Neck-rotating manipulation in sitting position: The patient should take a sitting position with the neck relaxed. The practitioner stands behind the patient, holds the back of the top of the head with one hand, and supports the chin with the other hand, and exerts force in the opposite direction with both hands to slowly turn the patient's head to the left or right.

(2) Neck-rotating manipulation in supine position: The patient should take a supine position with the head relaxed. The practitioner should stand on the side, support the patient's head with the back of the upper forearm and hold the opposite shoulder at the same time. Moreover, the practitioner should support the top of the patient's head with the other hand, and then rotate the forearm to drive the patient's head to perform clockwise circular movements. Then alternate the hands, hold the patient's head with the other forearm, and perform a circular motion of the head in a counterclockwise direction, repeat the manipulation 3 to 5 times on each side.

2. Shoulder-rotating manipulation

(1) Supporting the elbow to rotate the shoulder: The patient should take a sitting position with shoulders relaxed, and naturally flex the affected limb. The practitioner stands on the affected side with the upper body leans slightly forward. Then, the practitioner supports the upper part of the patient's shoulder joint with one hand, holds the patient's elbow with the other hand (so that the forearm of the affected limb rests on the practitioner's forearm), and then performs clockwise or counterclockwise rotations

做肩关节的环转运动。

（3）握手摇肩法：患者取坐位，患肢自然放松、下垂，术者立于患者侧方，一手扶住其患肩的上部，另一手握住患肢的手腕部，而后做顺时针或逆时针方向的环转运动。

3. 肘关节摇法

患者取坐位或卧位，术者一手扶住患者肘部，另一手握住患肢腕部，而后做肘关节的顺时针或逆时针环转运动。

4. 腕关节摇法

术者一手握住患肢腕关节的上端，另一手握住其手掌部，先做腕关节的拔伸，而后将腕关节做顺时针或逆时针方向的环转摇动。

5. 腰部摇法

患者取坐位，腰部放松，术者坐或站于其后，用一手按住其腰部，另一手扶住患者对侧肩部，前臂按于颈项部，两手协同用力，将其腰部做缓慢的环转摇动。

6. 髋关节摇法

患者取仰卧位，患肢屈髋屈膝，术者站于患侧，一手扶住其膝部，另一手握住其踝部，两手协同动作，使其髋关节屈曲约90°，然后做顺时针方向或逆时针方向的环转运动。

slowly.

(2) Holding the elbow to rotate the shoulder: The patient should take a sitting position, relax the shoulder joint and naturally flex the affected limb. The practitioner should stand behind the patient, hold the upper part of the patient's shoulder with one hand, and the patient's elbow with the other hand, and then perform a circular motion of the shoulder joint.

(3) Holding the hand to rotate the shoulder: The patient should take a sitting position, relax and sag the affected limb naturally. The practitioner should stand on the side of the patient, support the upper part of the affected shoulder with one hand, and hold the wrist of the affected limb with the other hand, and then perform a clockwise or counterclockwise circular motion.

3. Elbow-rotating manipulation

The patient should take a sitting or lying position. The practitioner should hold the patient's elbow with one hand and the wrist of the affected limb with the other hand, and then perform a clockwise or counterclockwise circular motion of the elbow joint.

4. Wrist-rotating manipulation

The practitioner should hold the upper end of the wrist joint of the affected limb with one hand and the palm with the other hand, first pull and stretch the wrist joint, and then rotate the wrist joint clockwise or counterclockwise.

5. Waist-rotating manipulation

The patient should take a sitting position and relax the waist. The practitioner should sit or stand behind the patient, press the waist with one hand, support the opposite shoulder of the patient with the other hand, put the forearm on the neck, and uses both hands to make the waist conduct slow circular motions.

6. Hip-rotating manipulation

The patient should take a supine position and flex the hip and knee of the affected limb. The practitioner should stand on the side of the patient, hold the knee with one hand, and hold the ankle with the other hand. Both hands should work together to flex the hip to an angle about 90°, and then perform clockwise or counterclockwise circular movements.

7. 踝关节摇法

踝关节摇法，又称距小腿关节摇法。患者取仰卧位，或取坐位，下肢伸直，术者站于其足后，一手托住患者足跟，另一手握住足趾部，稍用力做牵引拔伸踝关节，并在此基础上做踝关节的环转运动。

7. Ankle-rotating manipulation

Ankle-rotating manipulation is also called talocrural-rotating manipulation. The patient should take a supine position or a sitting position with the lower limbs straightened. The practitioner should stand behind the patient's feet, support the heel with one hand, hold the toes with the other hand, pull and stretch the ankle joint with a little force, and then perform the circular motion of the ankle joint.

【要领】

（1）摇转的幅度由小到大。

（2）根据病情恰如其分地掌握摇转幅度的大小，做到因势利导，适可而止。

（3）摇转的幅度必须限制在正常关节生理许可范围之内，或在患者能忍受范围内进行。

（4）操作时，动作要缓和，用力要平稳，摇动速度宜缓慢。

肩部摇法：托肘摇肩法，术者须站于患者侧方，术者、患者皆屈肘90°，动作缓和平稳。

扶肘摇肩法，术者须站于侧后方，一手扶住其肘后部，贴身体做环转运动。

握手摇肩法，嘱患者患肢伸直放松，操作时环转幅度不应过大。

【Essentials】

(1) The amplitude of rotating should be from small to large.

(2) The amplitude of the rotation movements should be adjusted according to the severity of the disease, so as to achieve the best efficacy of the manipulation.

(3) Rotating manipulation should be carried out within the range permitted by the physiology or within the range that the patient can tolerate.

(4) When practicing the manipulation, the movements should be moderate, the force should be steady, and the rotating speed should be slow.

When practicing the shoulder-rotating manipulation, the practitioner should stand on the side of the patient, and both the practitioner and the patient need to bend their elbows to the angle of 90°. The movement should be gentle and stable.

When practicing the elbow-rotating manipulation, the practitioner should stand on the rear side of the patient, hold the back of the patient's elbow, and perform a circular motion.

When practicing the wrist-rotating manipulation, the

patient should relax and straighten the affected limb, and the movement should be in an appropriate range.

【应用】

摇法具有舒筋活血、滑利关节、松解粘连和增强关节活动功能等作用，多应用于颈项部、腰部以及四肢关节。

（1）坐位颈部摇法主要应用于防治落枕、颈椎病、颈项部软组织劳损等引起的颈项部酸痛、活动不利等症。

（2）卧位颈部摇法应用于颈项部酸痛、僵硬、活动不利等症。

（3）摇肩法常用于肩关节周围炎、肩关节粘连、骨折后遗症、中风后遗症所引起的肩关节酸痛、运动不利、功能障碍等症的防治。其中，扶肘摇肩法幅度最大，托肘摇肩法中等，握手摇肩法最小，临床应根据患者肩关节具体情况或疾病病程来选用适当的方法。

（4）肘关节摇法临床用于肘关节酸痛、运动不利、功能障碍等症的防治。

（5）腕关节摇法临床应用于腕关节伤筋、局部疼痛、活动不利等症的防治。

（6）腰部摇法临床常用于治疗腰背部酸痛，活动不利等症。

（7）髋关节摇法临床主要用于腰腿痛、髋关节伤筋或中风后遗症所引起的下肢运动不利以及髋关节慢性骨关节炎等病症治疗。

（8）踝关节摇法临床主要用于踝关节扭伤、伤筋引起的疼痛、活动不利等症的治疗。

【Applications】

Rotating manipulation has the effects of relaxing sinews and activating the blood, lubricating joint, removing accretion and enhancing joint movements. It is commonly used to treat diseases in the neck, waist and joint of limbs.

(1) Neck-rotating manipulation in sitting position is commonly used for the prevention and treatment of neck pain and unfavorable activities caused by stiff neck, cervical spondylosis, and neck soft tissue strain.

(2) Neck-rotating manipulation in supine position is commonly used for neck pain, stiffness, and unfavorable activities.

(3) Shoulder-rotating manipulation is often used for the prevention and treatment of shoulder joint aching pain, unfavorable movement and dysfunction caused by scapulohumeral periarthritis, shoulder joint adhesion, sequelae of fractures, and sequelae of stroke. Among these shoulder-rotating manipulations, the one with the hold of the elbow is in the largest amplitude, with the support of the elbow is in the medium, and with the hold of the hand is in the smallest. The appropriate manipulations should be selected according to the specific conditions of the patient's shoulder joint or the course of the disease.

(4) Elbow-rotating manipulation is often used for the prevention and treatment of elbow joint aching pain, unfavorable movement and dysfunctions.

(5) Wrist-rotating manipulation is often clinically used for the prevention and treatment of sinew injury of wrist joint, local pain and unfavorable movement.

(6) Waist-rotating manipulation is commonly used for aching pain in lower back and unfavorable activities.

(7) Hip-rotating manipulation is clinically used for the treatment of pain in the back and legs, sinew injury of

hip joints, unfavorable lower extremity movement caused by sequelae of stroke, and chronic osteoarthritis of the hip joints.

(8) Ankle-rotating manipulation is often clinically used for the treatment of pian caused by sinew injury or sprain of ankle joint, and unfavorable movement.

第三节 常规操作

Section Three Routine Manipulations

内功推拿治疗内、妇科疾病有一套完整的操作规律和手法程序，这套手法习惯上被称为“常规手法”。

一般顺序为头面部→颈项部→胸腹部→肩背腰部→肋胁部→上肢部→下肢部→头面部，最后以击法结束。

这套手法在辨证论治和辨病论治的基础上，临床应用时根据不同疾病适当加减变化。手法轻重因人而异，体弱者手法轻柔，体壮者手法可略重，或配合其他手法治疗。

There is a complete set of operating rules and manipulation procedures for the treatment of internal and gynecological diseases in Shaolin Internal Exercise and Tuina.

These manipulations are often performed in an order of head and face to neck to chest and abdomen to shoulder and back and waist to ribs to upper limbs to lower limbs to head and face and ended up with knocking manipulation.

Based on the pattern identification and treatment and disease identification and treatment, appropriate addition and subtraction should be made in clinical application. The severity of the manipulations varies from person to person. For patients with weak constitution, the manipulations should be gentle, and for patients with strong constitution, the manipulations should be slightly heavier, or combined with other manipulations.

一、操作步骤

Manipulation Procedures

（一）头面部

1. 五指抓头顶

患者正坐，两眼平视。术者站于患者左侧方，左手稳住前额，右手五

Head and Face

1. Grabbing the top of the head with five fingers

The patient takes a sitting position with eyes looking straight ahead. The practitioner stands on the left side

指分别放于头部五经（中指督脉，示指、环指放于膀胱经，拇指、小指放于胆经），而后同时屈曲各指骨间关节，由前向后脑移动至颈结节，分两侧三指拿向下至颈部。

2. 拿颈部

接上势，术者用三指拿法轻快地分别捏拿斜方肌的上部和左右胸锁乳突肌。

3. 推桥弓

继上势，术者拇指与其余四指分开呈“八”字形，四指置于颈部后侧起稳定作用，拇指由翳风穴向下沿胸锁乳突肌后缘做单方向抹至缺盆穴，呈一直线。左右交替进行。

4. 扫散法

术者一手扶头侧部，另一手拇指与其余四指分开呈“八”字形，并自然屈曲成90°，用拇指偏锋放于率谷穴处，四指放于后脑的脑空与风池穴处，然后做耳上由前向后下的单方向直线推动，以酸胀为度。

5. 分抹法

术者用两侧拇指与其余四指分开，四指放于头部两侧以稳定头部，两拇指由正中线向两侧分别抹前额、眉弓、上眼眶、眼球、下眼眶，以及迎香、人中、承浆等穴。

6. 合抹法

术者用两掌根由前向后抹于后脑两侧，然后内旋前臂，用小鱼际→掌根→大鱼际紧贴后脑向下转动，抹至两侧颈部。

of the patient, holds the forehead with the left hand, and respectively places the five fingers of the right hand on the five meridians of the head (the middle finger on the Du meridian, the index finger and the ring finger on the bladder meridian, and the thumb and little finger on the gallbladder meridian). Then, the practitioner flexes fingers and moves fingers from the front head to the back brain.

2. Grasping the neck

The practitioner uses three fingers to grasp the upper part of the trapezius muscle and the left and right sternocleidomastoid muscles respectively.

3. Pushing the bridge arch

The practitioner should separate the thumb from the other four fingers to form a splay shape. Place the four fingers on the back of the neck for stability, and use the thumb to smear downward from Yifeng (TE 17) along the posterior edge of the sternocleidomastoid muscle to Quepen (ST 12) in a straight line, and perform the manipulation between two sides.

4. Sweeping manipulation

The practitioner should hold the side of the patient's head with one hand, and place the thumb and the other four fingers of the other hand on Shuaigu (GB 8) and Naokong (GB 19) and Fengchi (GB 20) respectively, with the thumb separated from the remaining four fingers in a splay shape and naturally flexed to the angle of 90°. Then push in a straight line from front to back until soreness and distension is sensed by the patient.

5. Dividing-wiping manipulation

The practitioner separates the thumbs from the other four fingers, places the four fingers on the sides of the head for stability, and moves the two thumbs from the midline to the sides to wipe the forehead, eyebrows, upper eye sockets, eyeballs, lower eye sockets, Yingxiang (LI 20), Renzhong (GV 26), Chengjiang (CV 24) and other points respectively.

6. Combining-wiping manipulation

The practitioner wipes both sides of the back of the head from front to back with the roots of both palms, then rotate the forearm inward, and wipes downward with the hypothenar, palm root, thenar to the neck.

（二）躯干部

1. 擦前胸

术者站于患者左侧，用左手掌擦其胸前上部，由上而下至腹部（男女有别）。

2. 右手擦背部

继上势，术者转用右手擦其背部，由上而下至腰部（重点大椎、命门、腰阳关，以及八髎穴等）。

3. 左手擦背部

术者转到患者右侧，用左手擦其背部和腰部（与第二势方向相反）。

4. 擦胸前部

用右手横擦于胸前部，由上而下至腹部（与第一势方向相反）。

5. 擦两肺尖

术者站于患者后方，用四指擦其两侧肺尖，同时点揉膻中、中府、云门等穴，以酸胀为度。

6. 擦胃脘部

继上势，术者取坐位，手指并拢微屈，用手掌横擦患者胃脘部，以温热为度。

7. 擦胁肋部

术者站于其后，用双手擦患者两侧胁肋部，以温热为度。

The Trunk

1. Rubbing the front chest

The practitioner should stand on the left side of the patient and rub the upper part of the chest with the left palm, from top to bottom to the abdomen (males and females should be treated differently).

2. Rubbing the back with the right hand

The practitioner should rub the back with the right hand, from top to bottom to the waist [the key areas include Dazhui (GV 14), Mingmen (GV 4), Yaoyangguan (GV 3), and Eight Bone-Holes (BL 31–34)].

3. Rubbing the back with the left hand

The practitioner should turn to the right side of the patient and rub the back and waist with the left hand (the direction should be opposite to that of the second manipulation).

4. Rubbing the chest

The practitioner should rub the front chest with the right hand, from top to bottom to the abdomen (the direction should be opposite to that of the first manipulation).

5. Rubbing the apex region of both lungs

The practitioner should stand behind the patient, rub the apex region of both lungs with four fingers, and press and knead Danzhong (CV 17), Zhongfu (LU 1), and Yunmen (LU 2), at the same time, until the patient feels soreness.

6. Rubbing the abdomen

The practitioner should take a seated position, with the fingers close together and slightly bent, and rub the the gastral cavity region of the patient until feels warmth.

7. Rubbing the rib region

The practitioner should stand behind the patient and

rub the ribs on both sides of the patient with both hands until feels warmth.

（三）上肢部

1. 拿上肢

接上势，用三指拿施于三角肌（内、外、后三束）、上臂（肱二、三头肌）、前臂（伸肌群、屈肌群）。

2. 点揉

点揉极泉、小海、曲池、手三里、郄门、内关、合谷等穴。

3. 擦三阴三阳

掌擦法施患者手臂内侧（三阴）、手臂外侧（三阳），以热为度。

4. 理手背

术者以拇指螺纹面理拨患者手背。

5. 勒手指

术者站于受术者左侧前方，用拇指与示指第2节或者屈示、中指分开成钳状，依次夹住患者五指，从指根部至指端，做急速的滑拉动作。

6. 劈指缝

术者站于受术者左侧前方，一手握住患者腕部，让其屈肘，五指指端向上，并叉开五指，术者用另一手小指尺侧逐个劈击指缝。

7. 振拳面

患者上肢伸直，握拳。术者一手握其腕部，另一手用掌心击打患者近节指骨背侧3遍。操作时，击打方向必须沿着患者上肢纵轴方向。

8. 捻手指

术者站于患者左侧前方，拇指与示指指腹相对用力，依次捻搓其五指侧面或掌背面。

Upper Limbs

1. Taking the upper limbs

Following the above manipulations, the practitioner applies three fingers to the deltoid muscle (internal, external, and posterior muscles), upper arm (biceps and triceps), and forearm (extensor muscle group, flexor muscle group).

2. Point-kneading manipulation

Point-knead the Jiquan (HT 1), Xiaohai (SI 8), Quchi (LI 11), Shousanli (LI 10), Ximen (PC 4), Neiguan (PC 6), and Hegu (LI 4).

3. Rubbing along the three yin and three yang meridians

Palm-rubbing manipulation should be applied to the interior side of the patient's arm (three yin) and the lateral side of the arm (three yang) until the patient feels warmth.

4. Regulating the back of hands

The practitioner should regulate the back of the hand with the ribbed surface of the thumb.

5. Tightening fingers

The practitioner should stand the left front of the patient, and make rapid sliding and pulling movements on the patient's five fingers in turn from the base of the finger to the end of the finger.

6. Chopping between fingers

The practitioner should stand in the left front of the patient, hold the patient's wrist with one hand, ask the patient to bend the elbow with the fingertips face upwards, and chop between the five fingers with the ulnar side of the little finger of the other hand.

7. Vibrating the fist face

The patient should straighten his/her upper extremities and hold fists. The practitioner holds the patient's wrist

9. 运肩关节

术者成丁字步，站于患者左侧，两手掌相对，夹住患者的腕部，而后慢慢地将其左上肢向上、向前托起，同时位于下方的手逐渐翻掌，当其左上肢前上举至约160°时，虎口向下，并握住其腕部，另一手则由腕部沿上肢内侧下滑移至肩关节上部，此时可略停顿一下，两手协调用力，使患者肩关节向后做大幅度的环转运动。然后术者两手掌上下位置交换，以同样方法做肩关节向前的大幅度环转运动。

10. 搓抖肩与上肢

左右上肢交替进行，继而重复头面部操作。

搓肩关节以及上肢：术者两手掌相对用力夹住患者肩部，并略向上提起，然后由上而下，由肩部→上臂→前臂的顺序做快速搓揉或搓转动作，上下往返操作。

抖上肢：术者用双手或单手握住患者腕部或掌部，并将其上肢向前外方抬至60°左右，然后稍用力做连续的、小幅度的、频率较高的上下抖动。

11. 振囟门

术者手指自然松开，微屈，腕关节伸直，运用前臂力量，以掌根为着力点，击打头顶囟门穴。

12. 振大椎

医者腕关节伸直，屈伸肘关节用拳背平击大椎穴。

13. 振命门、腰阳关、八髎穴

用拳背横向击打命门、腰阳关和八髎等穴。

with one hand and hits the back of the patient's fists three times with the palm of the other hand. During manipulations, the practitioner should hit vertically.

8. Twisting fingers

The practitioner should stand in the left front of the patient, twist the sides of the patient's five fingers or the back of the palm in turn forcefully with the thumb and the index finger.

9. Rotating shoulder joints

The practitioner holds the upper arm of the patient with both hands and lifts it up from front to back. Taking the treatment of the left arm as an example, the practitioner holds the wrist of the patient's limb with one hand, and puts the back of the palm of the other hand under the wrist, and moves the wrist of the affected limb slowly forward and upward, from front to back. Then, take a reverse movement as soon as the upper arm is raised to about 160°. With that, the wrist support is turned into a wrist grip, and the other hand (the original wrist-holding hand) slides down along the forearm to the shoulder and presses it. At this time, the remaining wrist-holding hand pulls up, and the shoulder-pressing hand presses down, so that the affected limb is fully stretched.

10. Palm-twisting and shaking the shoulders and the upper limbs

The manipulation should be applied on the left and the right upper limbs alternately, and then repeat manipulations on head and face.

Palm-twisting shoulders and upper limbs: The practitioner should clamp the patient's shoulder with both palms facing each other, and lift shoulders slightly upwards, and then perform rapid kneading or twisting movements from top to bottom in the sequence of shoulder to upper arm to forearm. Perform the manipulations to and fro.

Shaking upper limbs: The practitioner should hold the patient's wrist or palm with both hands or single hand,

14. 拿肩井

用双手拇指指端同时拿两侧肩井以及肩部两侧，手法操作注意轻重缓急交替，宜有节律性，并要用指腹操作，忌用指端内抠。

15. 搓背部

术者双掌夹扶住患者腰背部肌肉，然后双手同时用力做快速的搓摩运动，同时做上下来回往返移动。

and lift the upper limb of the patient to the angle about 60 degrees forward and outward, and then make continuous, small-amplitude, high-frequency up-and-down shaking movements with slight force.

11. Vibrating the top of the head

The practitioner should loosen fingers naturally, bend fingers slightly, straighten the wrist joint, apply the strength of the forearm to hit the top of the head with the root of the palm as the focal point.

12. Vibrating Dazhui acupoint

The practitioner should straighten the wrist joint, and strike the Dazhui (GV 14) with the back of the fist by flexing and extending the elbow joint.

13. Vibrating Mingmen, Yaoyangguan, and Eight Bone-Holes acupoints

The practitioner hits the Mingmen (GV 4), Yaoyangguan (GV 3) and Eight Bone-Holes (BL 31–34) horizontally with the back of the fist.

14. Grasping Jianjing acupoint

When performing the manipulation, the practitioner holds the Jianjing (GB 21) and both sides of the shoulders at the same time with the fingertips of thumbs. It should be practiced rhythmically by alternating the force. Besides, the finger pulp should be used for manipulation to avoid forcefully grab inwards.

15. Palm-twisting the back

The practitioner should hold the patient's lower back muscles with both palms, and then perform a rapid twisting movement up and down.

（四）下肢部

1. 拿下肢

提拿大腿肌肉：内（内收肌）、前（股四头肌）、后内（半腱肌、半膜肌）、后外（股二头肌），以及小腿肌肉（小腿三头肌）。

Lower Limbs

1. Grasping the lower limbs

The practitioner lifts and grapes the muscles of the thigh, include adductors, quadriceps, semitendinosus, semimembranosus, biceps, and triceps of the calf.

2. 点揉穴位

点揉髀关、梁丘、风市、血海、足三里、阴陵泉、阳陵泉、委中、承山、三阴交诸穴。

3. 擦下肢

擦大腿（前、内、外侧）、小腿（外、内侧）。

4. 摇髋、膝关节

患肢屈膝屈髋，术者一手扶其膝部，另一手托或握其踝部，以髋关节为轴心做水平方向的环转运动；然后一手扶患者膝部，另一手托或握其踝部，以膝关节为轴心做垂直方向的环转运动。

5. 叩击下肢

用掌根、手掌、虎口、拳心等处，由上而下叩击两下肢，以酸胀为度。

6. 搓下肢

用两手掌夹住患肢，相对用力，自上而下搓揉下肢，并反复数次。

7. 抖下肢

术者两手握住患者踝部，做频率较快、小幅度、连续的抖动。

2. Kneading points

The acupoints include Biguan (ST 30), Liangqiu (ST 34), Fengshi (GB 31), Xuehai (SP 10), Zusanli (ST 36), Yinlingquan (SP 9), Yanglingquan (GB 34), Weizhong (BL 40), Chengshan (BL 57), Sanyinjiao (SP 6).

3. Rubbing the lower limbs

Rub thighs (front, inner, outer side), calves (outer and inner sides).

4. Rotating hip and knees

The patient bends the hip and knees. The practitioner should support the knee of the patient with one hand, and support or hold the patient's ankle with the other hand, and then perform a horizontal circular motion with the hip joint as the axis. Then hold the patient's knee with one hand, support or hold the ankle with the other hand to perform a vertical circular motion with the knee joint as the axis.

5. Tapping the lower limbs

Tap the lower limbs from top to bottom with palms, regions between the thumb and the index finger, or fists until the patient feels soreness.

6. Palm-twisting the lower limbs

Hold the affected limb with palms, rub the lower limbs from top to bottom, and repeat the movement several times.

7. Shaking the lower limbs

The practitioner should hold the patient's ankle with both hands, and perform rapid, small-amplitude, and continuous shaking movements.

二、注意事项

（1）擦法（或掌平推法）擦前胸时男女有别。

（2）手法操作，需根据疾病虚实，辨证施治。

Attentions

(1) Men and women should be treated differently when applying rubbing manipulation (or palm-pushing manipulation) on the front chest.

(2) Manipulations should be performed in terms of the

（3）操作时患者取正坐位，头顶平，两目前视。

（4）术者须呼吸自然，不可屏气。

（5）操作时用力柔和、均匀、持久，轻而不浮，重而不滞，防止冲击破皮。

（6）胃脘部擦法，术者稍偏后，手掌微曲呈抱着状。

（7）拿法操作时，需用螺纹面，不可用爪甲内扣，动作宜连贯灵活、轻快柔和。

（8）取穴准确，点揉准确，快速而灵活。

内功推拿常规操作是一个相对固定的套路，头面、躯干和上肢部操作需前后相连、一气呵成。病变与下肢部无关时可省略下肢操作。

内功推拿常规操作从头面到腰骶，涉及十二经和奇经八脉，有疏通经络、调和气血、荣灌脏腑之功效。治疗范围不仅适用于伤科和骨科方面的疾病，还广泛应用于内科的虚劳杂病、妇科经带诸症。

excess and deficiency of the disease, and give treatment after identifying patterns.

(3) During the manipulation, the patient should sit upright with the head raised and eyes looking straight forward.

(4) The practitioner should breathe naturally and not hold the breath.

(5) During the manipulations, it is advisable to manipulate gently and steadily, the force should be light but not floating, heavy but not stagnant, preventing the skin abrasion.

(6) When applying rubbing manipulation on the epigastric region, the practitioner should stand slightly backward, and the palm is slightly curved in a hugging position.

(7) When performing grasping manipulation, it's the ribbed surfaces of fingers that should be used to prevent hurts from nails. The movements should be consistent, flexible, light and soft.

(8) Be accurate to select acupoints and perform the point-kneading manipulation fast and flexibly.

Routine manipulations of Shaolin Internal Exercise and Tuina are fixed basically, so the manipulations on the head, trunk and upper limbs should be connected with each other and done in one go. Manipulations on the lower extremity can be omitted when there is no affected regions in there.

Manipulations of Shaolin internal exercise and Tuina involve the twelve meridians and the eight extraordinary meridians, from the head to the lumbar sacrum, and have the effects of dredging meridian and collateral, harmonizing qi and blood, and invigorating internal organs. The treatment is not only applicable to diseases in trauma and orthopedics, but also widely used in miscellaneous consumptive diseases and gynecological diseases in internal medicine.

第四节 常用穴位

Section Four Common Points

一、常用腧穴

Common Acupoints

1. 手太阴肺经

（1）中府

［定位］在胸部，横平第1肋间隙，锁骨下窝外侧，前正中线旁开6寸。

［防治］咳嗽，气喘，肩背痛。

（2）尺泽

［定位］在肘区，肘横纹上，肱二头肌腱桡侧缘凹陷中。

［防治］咳嗽，气喘，咽喉肿痛，肘臂挛痛等。

1. The lung meridian of hand-Taiyin (LU)

(1) Zhongfu (LU 1)

[Location] On the anterior thoracic region, at the same level as the first intercostal space, lateral to the infraclavicular fossa, 6 cun lateral to the anterior median line.

[Indications] Cough, panting, pain in the shoulder and the back.

(2) Chize (LU 5)

[Location] On the anterior aspect of the elbow, at the cubital crease, in the depression lateral to the biceps brachii tendon.

[Indications] Cough, panting, swelling and sore throat, elbow and arm cramps.

2. 手阳明大肠经

（1）合谷

［定位］在手背，第2掌骨桡侧的中点处。

［防治］头面五官病症，咽喉肿痛，面瘫，发热，各种疼痛。

（2）手三里

［定位］在前臂，肘横纹下2寸，阳溪与曲池连线上。

［防治］中风偏瘫，网球肘，前臂酸痛，面瘫。

（3）曲池

［定位］在肘区，尺泽与肱骨外上髁连线中点凹陷处。

2. The large intestine meridian of hand-Yangming (LI)

(1) Hegu (LI 4)

[Location] On the dorsum of the hand, radial to the midpoint of the second metacarpal bone.

[Indications] Diseases in five sense organs, swelling and pain in throat, facial paralysis, fever and various pains.

(2) Shousanli (LI 10)

[Location] On the posterolateral aspect of the forearm, on the line connecting LI5 with LI11, 2 cun inferior to the cubital crease.

[Indications] Hemiplegia caused by stroke, tennis elbow, forearm soreness, facial paralysis.

(3) Quchi (LI 11)

[Location] On the lateral aspect of the elbow, at

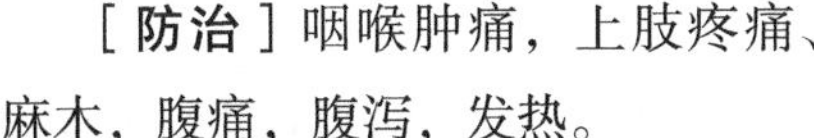

［防治］咽喉肿痛，上肢疼痛、麻木，腹痛，腹泻，发热。

（4）臂臑

［定位］在臂部，曲池上7寸，三角肌前缘处。

［防治］肩臂疼痛，颈项强痛，上肢不遂等。

（5）肩髃

［定位］在三角肌区，肩峰外侧缘前端与肱骨大结节两骨间凹陷中。

简便取穴法：曲臂外展，肩峰外侧缘呈现前后两个凹陷，前下方的凹陷即是本穴。

［防治］肩周炎，肩关节功能障碍，上肢疼痛，上肢萎软无力。

（6）迎香

［定位］在面部，鼻翼外缘中点旁，鼻唇沟中。

［防治］鼻塞不通，面瘫。

3. 足阳明胃经

（1）承泣

［定位］在面部，眼球与眶下缘之间，瞳孔直下。

［防治］目疾，口眼歪斜，面肌痉挛。

（2）四白

［定位］在面部，眶下孔处。

［防治］目疾，口眼歪斜，面肌痉挛，头痛，眩晕。

the midpoint of the line connecting LU5 with the lateral epicondyle of the humerus.

[Indications] Swelling and pain in throat, upper limb pain, numbness, abdominal pain, diarrhea, fever.

(4) Binao (LI 14)

[Location] On the lateral aspect of the arm, just anterior to the border of the deltoid muscle, 7 cun superior to Quchi (LI 11).

[Indications] Shoulder and arm pain, rigidity and pain of neck, upper limb paralysis, etc.

(5) Jianyu (LI 15)

[Location] On the shoulder girdle, in the depression between the anterior end of lateral border of the acromion and the greater tubercle of the humerus.

Simple methods for the location of acupoint:When the arm is abducted, two depressions appear, anterior and posterior to the acromion. LI 15 is located in the deeper depression anterior to the acromion.

[Indications] Scapulohumeral periarthritis, shoulder joints dysfunction, upper limbs pain, weakness and flaccidity of upper limbs.

(6) Yingxiang (LI 20)

[Location] On the face, in the nasolabial sulcus, at the same level as the midpoint of lateral border of the ala of the nose.

[Indications] Stuffy nose, facial paralysis.

3. The stomach meridian of foot-Yangming (ST)

(1) Chengqi (ST 1)

[Location] On the face, between the eyeball and the infraorbital margin, directly inferior to the pupil.

[Indications] Eye disorders, deviation of the mouth and eyes, facial spasm.

(2) Sibai (ST 2)

[Location] On the face, in the infraorbital foramen.

[Indications] Eye disorders, deviation of the mouth and eyes, facial spasm, headache and dizziness.

（3）地仓

［定位］在面部，口角旁开0.4寸。

［防治］口歪，流涎。

（4）颊车

［定位］在面颊部，下颌角前上方一横指（中指），闭口咬紧牙时咬肌隆起，放松时按之有凹陷处。

［防治］口歪，齿痛，颊肿。

（5）下关

［定位］在面部，颧弓下缘中央与下颌切迹之间凹陷中。

［防治］耳鸣，牙痛，口眼歪斜，牙关开合不利。

（6）天枢

［定位］在腹部，横平脐中，前正中线旁开2寸。

［防治］腹痛，腹胀，便秘，泄泻，月经不调，肥胖。

（7）梁丘

［定位］在股前区，髌底上2寸，股外侧与股直肌肌腱之间。

［防治］胃痛，膝肿痛，下肢不遂。

（8）足三里

［定位］在小腿前外侧，犊鼻下3寸，胫骨前嵴外1横指，犊鼻与解溪连线上。

［防治］胃肠病，虚劳消瘦，头晕，失眠，膝关节痛，小腿痛，偏瘫，癫狂。

（9）丰隆

［定位］在小腿外侧，外踝尖上8寸，胫骨前肌外缘；条口外侧一横指处。

［防治］头痛，眩晕，痰多咳嗽，下肢痿痹。

(3) Dicang (ST 4)

[Location] On the face, 0.4 cun lateral to the angle of the mouth.

[Indications] Deviation of the mouth, salivation.

(4) Jiache (ST 6)

[Location] On the face, one fingerbreadth (middle finger) anterosuperior to the angle of the mandible. When the mouth is closed and the teeth are clenched, this point is located at the prominence of the masseter and in the depression felt when the clenched teeth are released.

[Indications] Crooked mouth, toothache, swollen cheeks.

(5) Xiaguan (ST 7)

[Location] On the face, in the depression between the midpoint of the inferior border of the zygomatic arch and the mandibular notch.

[Indications] Tinnitus, toothache, deviation of the mouth and eyes, inability to open and close the teeth.

(6) Tianshu (ST 25)

[Location] On the upper abdomen, 2 cun lateral to the centre of the umbilicus.

[Indications] Abdominal pain, abdominal distension, constipation, diarrhea, irregular menstruation, obesity.

(7) Liangqiu (ST 34)

[Location] On the anterolateral aspect of the thigh, between the vastus lateralis muscle and the lateral border of the rectus femoris tendon, 2 cun superior to the base of the patella.

[Indications] Stomach pain, knee swelling and pain, lower extremity paralysis.

(8) Zusanli (ST 36)

[Location] On the anterior aspect of the leg, on the line connecting Dubi (ST 35) with Jiexi (ST 41), 3 cun inferior to Dubi (ST 35).

[Indications] Gastrointestinal disease, emaciation due to consumptive disease, dizziness, insomnia, knee pain, calf pain, hemiplegia, mania.

(9) Fenglong (ST 40)

[Location] On the anterolateral aspect of the leg, lateral border of the tibialis anterior muscle, 8 cun superior to the prominence of the lateral malleolus.

[Indications] Headache, dizziness, cough with excessive phlegm, paralysis of lower limbs.

4. 足太阴脾经

（1）三阴交

[**定位**] 在小腿内侧，内踝尖上3寸，胫骨内侧缘后际。

[**防治**] 腹痛，腹胀，腹泻，痛经，遗尿，小便不利，水肿，眩晕，失眠，月经不调，遗精，阳痿。

（2）阴陵泉

[**定位**] 在小腿内侧，胫骨内侧髁下缘与胫骨内侧缘之间的凹陷处。

[**防治**] 腹胀，泄泻，水肿，小便不利，膝痛。

（3）血海

[**定位**] 在股前区，髌底内侧端上2寸，股内侧肌隆起处。

[**防治**] 月经不调，湿疹。

4. The spleen meridian of foot-Taiyin (SP)

(1) Sanyinjiao (SP 6)

[Location] On the tibial aspect of the leg, posterior to the medial border of the tibia, 3 cun superior to the prominence of the medial malleolus.

[Indications] Abdominal pain, abdominal distension, diarrhea, dysmenorrhea, inhibited urination, dysuria, edema, dizziness, insomnia, irregular menstruation, nocturnal emission, impotence.

(2) Yinlingquan (SP 9)

[Location] On the tibial aspect of the leg, in the depression between the inferior border of the medial condyle of the tibia and the medial border of the tibia.

[Indications] Abdominal distension, diarrhea, edema, inhibited urination, knee pain.

(3) Xuehai (SP 10)

[Location] On the anteromedial aspect of the thigh, on the bulge of the vastus medialis muscle, 2 cun superior to the medial end of the base of the patella.

[Indications] Irregular menstruation, eczema.

5. 手少阴心经

（1）极泉

[**定位**] 在腋区，腋窝中央，腋动脉搏动处。

[**防治**] 胁肋痛，上肢疼痛、麻木。

（2）少海

[**定位**] 在肘前区，横平肘横纹，肱骨内上髁前缘。

[**防治**] 心痛，肘臂痛。

5. The heart meridian of hand-Shaoyin (HT)

(1) Jiquan (HT 1)

[Location] In the axilla, in the center of the axillary fossa, over the axillary artery.

[Indications] Pain in the subcostal region, pain in the upper limb, numbness.

(2) Shaohai (HT 3)

[Location] On the anteromedial aspect of the elbow, just anterior to the medial epicondyle of the humerus, at

（3）神门

［定位］在腕前区，腕掌侧远端横纹尺侧端，尺侧腕屈肌腱的桡侧缘。

［防治］心悸，失眠，高血压病。

6. 手太阳小肠经

（1）后溪

［定位］在手内侧，第5掌指关节尺侧近端赤白肉际凹陷中。

［防治］颈项强痛，手臂挛痛，目赤，咽喉肿痛。

（2）天宗

［定位］在肩胛区，肩胛冈中点与肩胛骨下角连线上1/3与下2/3交点凹陷中。

［防治］肩胛痛，上肢后侧痛，气喘。

（3）颧髎

［定位］在面部，颧骨下缘，目外眦直下凹陷中。

［防治］口眼歪斜，目疾，齿痛，颊肿，三叉神经痛。

（4）听宫

［定位］在面部，耳屏正中与下颌骨髁突之间的凹陷中。

［防治］耳疾，齿痛。

7. 足太阳膀胱经

（1）睛明

［定位］在面部，目内眦内上方

the same level as the cubital crease.

[Indications] Heartache, elbows and arms pain.

(3) Shenmen (HT 7)

[Location] On the anteromedial aspect of the wrist, radial to the flexor carpi ulnaris tendon, on the palmar wrist crease.

[Indications] Palpitations, insomnia, hypertension.

6. The small intestine meridian of hand-Taiyang (SI)

(1) Houxi (SI 3)

[Location] On the dorsum of the hand, in the depression proximal to the ulnar side of the fifth metacarpophalangeal joint, at the border between the red and white flesh.

[Indications] Rigidity and pain in the neck, arm cramp, red eyes, soreness in the throat.

(2) Tianzong (SI 11)

[Location] In the scapular region, in the depression between the upper one third and lower two thirds of the line connecting the midpoint of the spine of the scapula with the inferior angle of the scapula.

[Indications] Scapular pain, posterior upper limb pain, panting.

(3) Quanliao (SI 18)

[Location] On the face, inferior to the zygomatic bone, in the depression directly inferior to the outer canthus of the eye.

[Indications] Deviation of the mouth and eyes, eyes disease, toothache, cheek swelling, trigeminal neuralgia.

(4) Tinggong (SI 19)

[Location] On the face, in the depression between the anterior border of the center of the tragus and the posterior border of the condylar process of the mandible.

[Indications] Ear disease, toothache.

7. The bladder meridian of foot-Taiyang (BL)

(1) Jingming (BL 1)

[Location] On the face, in the depression between the

眶内侧壁凹陷中。

［防治］目疾，失眠。

（2）攒竹

［定位］在面部，眉头凹陷中，额切迹处。

［防治］头痛，目赤肿痛。

（3）天柱

［定位］在颈后部，横平第2颈椎棘突上际，斜方肌外缘凹陷中。

［防治］后头痛，颈项强痛，肩背腰痛，鼻塞。

（4）肺俞

［定位］在脊柱区，第3胸椎棘突下，后正中线旁开1.5寸。

［防治］咳嗽痰多，气喘胸痛，盗汗。

（5）心俞

［定位］在脊柱区，第5胸椎棘突下，后正中线旁开1.5寸。

［防治］胸闷，心慌，心律不齐，心烦，健忘，老年性痴呆，咳嗽。

（6）膈俞

［定位］在脊柱区，第7胸椎棘突下，后正中线旁开1.5寸。

［防治］呕吐，呃逆，咳嗽，盗汗，吐血，阴虚发热。

（7）肝俞

［定位］在脊柱区，第9胸椎棘突下，后正中线旁开1.5寸。

［防治］胁痛，脊背痛，目疾，癫痫。

（8）脾俞

［定位］在脊柱区，第11胸椎棘突下，后正中线旁开1.5寸。

［防治］中上腹不适、疼痛，腹胀，腹泻，四肢水肿，食欲减退，

superomedial parts of the inner canthus of the eye and the medial wall of the orbit.

[Indications] Eye disease, insomnia.

(2) Cuanzhu (BL 1)

[Location] On the head, in the depression at the medial end of the eyebrow.

[Indications] Headache, red and swelling and painful eyes.

(3) Tianzhu (BL 10)

[Location] In the posterior region of the neck, at the same level as the superior border of the spinous process of the second cervical vertebra (C2), in the depression lateral to the trapezius muscle.

[Indications] Headache, rigidity and pain in the neck, pain in the shoulder, back and waist, nasal congestion.

(4) Feishu (BL13)

[Location] In the upper back region, at the same level as the inferior border of the spinous process of the third thoracic vertebra (T3), 1.5 cun lateral to the posterior median line.

[Indications] Cough with copious sputum, panting, chest pain, night sweats.

(5) Xinshu (BL 15)

[Location] In the upper back region, at the same level as the inferior border of the spinous process of the third thoracic vertebra (T3), 1.5 cun lateral to the posterior median line.

[Indications] Oppression in the chest, palpitation, arrhythmia, upset, forgetfulness, senile dementia, cough.

(6) Geshu (BL 17)

[Location] In the upper back region, at the same level as the inferior border of the spinous process of the seventh thoracic vertebra (T7), 1.5 cun lateral to the posterior median line.

[Indications] Vomiting, hiccups, cough, night sweats, hematemesis, fever due to yin deficiency.

背痛，呕吐。

（9）胃俞

［定位］在脊柱区，第12胸椎棘突下，后正中线旁开1.5寸。

［防治］上腹痛，腹胀，肠鸣，呕吐。

（10）肾俞

［定位］在脊柱区，第2腰椎棘突下，后正中线旁开1.5寸。

［防治］遗精，阳痿，遗尿，月经不调，腰痛，耳鸣，水肿，气喘，全身乏力，腹泻。

（11）大肠俞

［定位］在脊柱区，第4腰椎棘突下，后正中线旁开1.5寸。

［防治］腰腿痛，腹胀，腹泻，便秘。

（12）八髎

［定位］在骶区，正对第1骶后孔中（上髎）。在骶区，正对第2骶后孔中（次髎）。在骶区，正对第3骶后孔中（中髎）。在骶区，正对第4骶后孔中（下髎）。

［防治］腰痛，腰骶痛，月经不调，痛经，遗精，阳痿，大小便不利，下肢萎软无力。

（13）委中

［定位］在膝后区，腘窝横纹中点。

［防治］下背痛，腰痛，股后肌肉痉挛，下肢萎软无力。

（14）承山

［定位］在小腿后区，腓肠肌两肌腹与肌腱交角处。

［防治］腰痛，小腿痉挛，痔疮，便秘，下肢肌肉疲劳酸痛。

(7) Ganshu (BL18)

[Location] In the upper back region, at the same level as the inferior border of the spinous process of the ninth thoracic vertebra (T 9), 1.5 cun lateral to the posterior median line.

[Indications] Pain in the subcostal region, pain in the back, eye disease, epilepsy.

(8) Pishu (BL 20)

[Location] In the upper back region, at the same level as the inferior border of the spinous process of the 11th thoracic vertebra (T 11), 1.5 cun lateral to the posterior median line.

[Indications] Middle and upper abdominal discomfort, pain, abdominal distention, diarrhea, limb edema, reduced appetite, back pain, vomiting.

(9) Weishu (BL 21)

[Location] In the upper back region, at the same level as the inferior border of the spinous process of the 12th thoracic vertebra (T 12), 1.5 cun lateral to the posterior median line.

[Indications] Upper abdominal pain, abdominal distention, bowel sounds, vomiting.

(10) Shenshu (BL 23)

[Location] In the lumbar region, at the same level as the inferior border of the spinous process of the second lumbar vertebra (BL 23), 1.5 cun lateral to the posterior median line.

[Indications] Nocturnal emissions, impotence, inhibited urination, irregular menstruation, lumbago, tinnitus, edema, panting, generalized weakness, diarrhea.

(11) Dachangshu (BL 25)

[Location] In the lumbar region, at the same level as the inferior border of the spinous process of the fourth lumbar vertebra (L 4), 1.5 cun lateral to the posterior median line.

[Indications] Lower back and leg pain, abdominal

（15）昆仑

［定位］在踝区，外踝尖与跟腱之间的凹陷中。

［防治］头痛，目赤肿痛，颈项强痛，肩背腰腿痛，脚跟痛，下肢肌肉疲劳酸痛。

distension, diarrhea, constipation.

(12) Baliao (BL 31–34)

[Location] In the sacral region, in the first posterior sacral foramen (Shangliao BL 31). In the sacral region, in the second posterior sacral foramen (Ciliao BL 32). In the sacral region, in the third posterior sacral foramen (Zhongliao BL 33). In the sacral region, in the fourth posterior sacral foramen (Xialiao BL 34).

[Indications] Lower back pain, lumbosacral pain, irregular menstruation, dysmenorrhea, nocturnal emissions, impotence, impaired urination and bowel movement, lower extremity weakness.

(13) Weizhong (BL 40)

[Location] On the posterior aspect of the knee, at the midpoint of the popliteal crease.

[Indications] Lower back pain, lumbago, muscle spasm in the posterior thigh, weakness of the lower limbs.

(14) Chengshan (BL 57)

[Location] On the posterior aspect of the leg, at the connecting point of the calcaneal tendon with the two muscle bellies of the gastrocnemius muscle.

[Indications] Lumbago, crus spasm, hemorrhoids, constipation, soreness in the lower limb muscles.

(15) Kunlun (BL 60)

[Location] On the posterolateral aspect of the ankle, in the depression between the prominence of the lateral malleolus and the calcaneal tendon.

[Indications] Headache, red, swelling and painful eyes, rigidity and pain in the neck, pain in the shoulder, back, waist and leg, heel pain, soreness in the lower limbs muscles.

8. 足少阴肾经

（1）涌泉

［定位］在足底部，屈足卷趾时足心最凹陷中；约当足底第2、第3趾蹼缘与足跟连线的前1/3与后2/3

8. The kidney meridian of foot-Shaoyin (KI)

(1) Yongquan (KI 1)

[Location] On the sole of the foot, in the deepest depression of the sole when the toes are flexed. When the toes are flexed, Yongquan (KI 1) is located approximately

交点凹陷中。

［防治］头痛，目赤肿痛，咽喉痛，失眠，便秘，小便不利，足心热。

（2）太溪

［定位］在足内踝区，内踝尖与跟腱之间凹陷中。

［防治］咽喉干痛，牙痛，耳鸣，月经不调，腰脊痛，失眠。

in the depression at the junction of the anterior one third and the posterior two thirds of the line connecting the heel with the web margin between the bases of the second and third toes.

[Indications] Headache, eye redness and pain, pain in throat, insomnia, constipation, inhibited urination, heat in the soles of the feet.

(2) Taixi (KI 3)

[Location] On the posteromedial aspect of the ankle, in the depression between the prominence of the medial malleolus and the calcaneal tendon.

[Indications] Sore dry throat, toothache, tinnitus, irregular menstruation, low back pain, insomnia.

9. 手厥阴心包经

（1）曲泽

［定位］在肘前区，肘横纹上，肱二头肌肌腱的尺侧缘凹陷中。

［防治］心悸，胃痛，呕吐，肘臂痛。

（2）内关

［定位］在前臂前区，腕掌侧远端横纹上2寸，掌长肌腱与桡侧腕屈肌腱之间。

［防治］胸闷心慌，胁痛，中上腹不适，呕吐，呃逆，失眠，上肢疼痛，手指麻木。

（3）劳宫

［定位］在掌区，横平第3掌指关节近端，第2、3掌骨之间偏于第3掌骨。

简便取穴法：握拳，中指尖下穴。

［防治］胸闷心慌，呕吐，口臭。

9. The pericardium meridian of hand-Jueyin (PC)

(1) Quze (PC 3)

[Location] On the anterior aspect of the elbow, at the cubital crease, in the depression medial to the biceps brachii tendon.

[Indications] Palpitation, stomach pain, vomiting, elbow and arm pain.

(2) Neiguan (PC 6)

[Location] On the anterior aspect of the forearm, between the tendons of the palmaris longus and the flexor carpi radialis, 2 cun proximal to the palmar wrist crease.

[Indications] Oppression in the chest, palpitation, pain in the subcostal region, middle and upper abdominal discomfort, vomiting, hiccups, insomnia, upper limb pain, numbness of fingers.

(3) Laogong (PC 8)

[Location] On the palm of the hand, in the depression between the second and third metacarpal bones, proximal to the metacarpophalangeal joints.

Simple methods for the location of acupoint: Make a fist, the point is under the tip of the middle finger.

[Indications] Oppression in the chest, palpitation, vomiting, ozostomia.

10. 手少阳三焦经

（1）外关

［**定位**］在前臂后区，腕背侧远端横纹上2寸，尺骨与桡骨间隙中点。

［**防治**］发热，头痛，耳鸣，胁肋痛，上肢疼痛。

（2）肩髎

［**定位**］在三角肌区，肩峰角与肱骨大结节两骨间凹陷处。

［**防治**］肩周炎，肩关节功能障碍，上肢疼痛，上肢萎软无力。

（3）翳风

［**定位**］在耳垂后方，当乳突与下颌角之间的凹陷中。

［**防治**］耳鸣，面瘫，落枕。

（4）耳门

［**定位**］在耳区，耳屏上切迹与下颌骨髁突之间的凹陷中。

［**防治**］耳鸣，牙痛，面瘫。

10. The Sanjiao meridian of hand-Shaoyang (TE)

(1) Waiguan (TE 5)

[Location] On the posterior aspect of the forearm, midpoint of the interosseous space between the radius and the ulna, 2 cun proximal to the dorsal wrist crease.

[Indications] Fever, headache, tinnitus, pain in the subcostal region, upper limb pain.

(2) Jianliao (TE 14)

[Location] On the shoulder girdle, in the depression between the acromial angle and the greater tubercle of the humerus.

[Indications] Scapulohumeral periarthritis, shoulder joints dysfunction, upper limbs pain, weak and flaccidity of upper limbs.

(3) Yifeng (TE 17)

[Location] In the anterior region of the neck, posterior to the ear lobe, in the depression anterior to the inferior end of the mastoid process.

[Indications] Tinnitus, facial paralysis, neck stiffness.

(4) Ermen (TE 21)

[Location] On the face, in the depression between the supratragic notch and the condylar process of the mandible.

[Indications] Tinnitus, toothache, facial paralysis.

11. 足少阳胆经

（1）瞳子髎

［**定位**］在面部，目外眦外侧0.5寸凹陷中。

［**防治**］目疾，头痛，口眼歪斜。

（2）听会

［**定位**］在面部，耳屏间切迹与下颌骨髁状突之间的凹陷中。

［**防治**］耳鸣，牙痛，面瘫。

（3）风池

［**定位**］在项后区，枕骨之下，胸锁乳突肌上端与斜方肌上端之间的凹陷中。

11. The gallbladder meridian of foot-Shaoyang (GB)

(1) Tongziliao (GB 1)

[Location] On the head, in the depression, 0.5 cun lateral to the outer canthus of the eye.

[Indications] Eyes disorder, headache, deviation of the mouth and eyes.

(2) Tinghui (GB 2)

[Location] On the face, in the depression between the intertragic notch and the condylar process of the mandible.

[Indications] Tinnitus, toothache, facial paralysis.

(3) Fengchi (GB 20)

[Location] In the anterior region of the neck, inferior to the occipital bone, in the depression between the origins

［防治］头痛，眩晕，颈项强痛，落枕，目疾，感冒，鼻塞。

（4）肩井

［定位］在肩胛区，第7颈椎棘突与肩峰最外侧点连线的中点。

［防治］颈项强痛，肩背痛，上肢无力。

（5）环跳

［定位］在臀部，股骨大转子最凸点与骶管裂孔连线的外1/3与内2/3交点处。

［防治］腰腿痛，下肢软弱无力，偏瘫。

（6）阳陵泉

［定位］在小腿外侧，腓骨头前下方凹陷中。

［防治］肌肉痉挛，偏瘫，膝关节肿痛，胁肋痛，口苦。

of sternocleidomastoid and the trapezius muscles.

[Indications] Headache, dizziness, rigidity and pain in the neck, neck stiffness, eyes disease, cold, nasal congestion.

(4) Jianjing (GB 21)

[Location] In the posterior region of the neck, at the midpoint of the line connecting the spinous process of the seventh cervical vertebra (C 7) with the lateral end of the acromion.

[Indications] Rigidity and pain in the neck, shoulder and back pain, upper limb weakness.

(5) Huantiao (GB 30)

[Location] In the buttock region, at the junction of the lateral one third and medial two thirds of the line connecting the prominence of the greater trochanter with the sacral hiatus.

[Indications] Pain in the waist and legs, weakness of lower limbs, hemiplegia.

(6) Yanglingquan (GB 34)

[Location] On the fibular aspect of the leg, in the depression anterior and distal to the head of the fibula.

[Indications] Muscle spasm, hemiplegia, knee joints swelling and pain, pain in the subcostal region, bitter taste in the mouth.

12. 足厥阴肝经

（1）太冲

［定位］在足背，第1、第2跖骨间，跖骨底结合部前方凹陷中，或触及动脉搏动。

［防治］头痛，眩晕，失眠，目赤肿痛，面瘫，胁痛，崩漏，小便不利，癫痫。

（2）期门

［定位］在胸部，第6肋间隙，前正中线旁开4寸。

［防治］胸胁胀痛，腹胀，呃

12. The liver meridian of foot-Jueyin (LR)

(1) Taichong (LR 3)

[Location] On the dorsum of the foot, between the first and second metatarsal bones, in the depression distal to the junction of the bases of the two bones, over the dorsalis pedis artery.

[Indications] Headache, dizziness, insomnia, red, swelling and painful eyes, facial paralysis, pain in the subcostal region, metrorrhagia and metrostaxis, inhibited urination, epilepsy.

(2) Qimen (LR 14)

[Location] In the anterior thoracic region, in the sixth

逆，乳痈。

intercostal space, 4 cun lateral to the anterior median line.

[Indications] Pain in the chest and the subcostal region, abdominal distension, hiccup, acute septic mastitis.

13. 督脉

（1）长强

[定位] 在会阴区，尾骨下方，尾骨端与肛门连线的中点处。

[防治] 痔疾，脱肛，泄泻，便秘，腰痛，尾骶骨痛。

（2）腰阳关

[定位] 在脊柱区，第4腰椎棘突下凹陷中，后正中线上。

[防治] 腰骶疼痛，下肢痿痹，月经不调，带下，遗精。

（3）命门

[定位] 在脊柱区，第2腰椎棘突下凹陷中，后正中线上。

[防治] 脊柱强痛，腰痛，阳痿，遗精，月经不调，腹泻，带下，全身乏力。

（4）大椎

[定位] 在脊柱区，第7颈椎棘突下凹陷中，后正中线上。

[防治] 头项强痛，背痛，热病，咳嗽，气喘，感冒，疟疾，癫痫，阴虚发热。

（5）百会

[定位] 在头部，前发际正中直上5寸。

[防治] 头痛，眩晕，失眠，脱肛，子宫脱垂。

（6）神庭

[定位] 在头部，前发际正中直上0.5寸。

[防治] 头痛，眩晕，失眠，鼻塞不通。

13. The governor vessel (GV)

(1) Changqiang (GV 1)

[Location] In the perineal region, inferior to the coccyx, midway between the tip of the coccyx and the anus.

[Indications] Hemorrhoids, prolapse of the rectum, diarrhea, constipation, low back pain, sacrocoxalgia.

(2) Yaoyangguan (GV 3)

[Location] In the lumbar region, in the depression inferior to the spinous process of the fourth lumbar vertebra (L 4), on the posterior median line.

[Indications] Lumbosacral pain, paralysis of lower limbs, irregular menstruation, abnormal vaginal discharges, nocturnal emission.

(3) Mingmen (GV 4)

[Location] In the lumbar region, in the depression inferior to the spinous process of the second lumbar vertebra (L 2), on the posterior median line.

[Indications] Pain and rigidity in the spine, lower back pain, impotence, nocturnal emission, irregular menstruation, diarrhea, abnormal vaginal discharges, fatigue.

(4) Dazhui (GV 14)

[Location] In the posterior region of the neck, in the depression inferior to the spinous process of the seventh cervical vertebra (C 7), on the posterior median line.

[Indications] Pain and rigidity in the head and the neck, back pain, fever, cough, panting, cold, malaria, epilepsy, fever due to yin deficiency.

(5) Baihui (GV 20)

[Location] On the head, 5 cun superior to the anterior hairline, on the anterior median line.

[Indications] Headache, dizziness, insomnia, prolapse of the rectum, prolapse of uterus.

（7）水沟（又名人中）

［定位］在面部，人中沟的上1/3与中1/3交点处。

［防治］昏厥，面瘫。

(6) Shenting (GV 24)

[Location] On the head, 0.5 cun superior to the anterior hairline, on the anterior median line.

[Indications] Headache, dizziness, insomnia, nasal congestion.

(7) Shuigou, also named Renzhong (GV 26)

[Location] On the face, at the junction of the upper one third and lower two thirds of the philtrum midline.

[Indications] Faint, facial paralysis.

14. 任脉

（1）关元

［定位］在下腹部，当脐中下3寸，前正中线上。

［防治］遗尿，小便不利，遗精，阳痿，月经不调，消化不良，腹泻，脱肛，体虚乏力。

（2）气海

［定位］在下腹部，脐中下1.5寸，前正中线上。

［防治］腹痛，遗尿，遗精，阳痿，腹泻，月经不调，体虚乏力。

（3）神阙

［定位］在脐区，脐中央。

［防治］腹痛，腹泻，虚脱。

（4）中脘

［定位］在上腹部，脐中上4寸，前正中线上。

［防治］中上腹不适、疼痛，腹胀，腹泻，消化不良，呕吐。

（5）膻中

［定位］在胸部，横平第4肋间隙，前正中线上。

［防治］胸闷，胸痛，心慌，气喘，乳汁少。

（6）天突

［定位］在颈前区，胸骨上窝中

14. The conception vessel (CV)

(1) Guanyuan (CV 4)

[Location] In the perineal region, at the midpoint of the line connecting the anus with the posterior border of the scrotum in males and the posterior commissure of labium majoris in females.

[Indications] Enuresis, inhibited urination, nocturnal emission, impotence, irregular menstruation, indigestion, diarrhea, prolapse of the rectum, lack of strength.

(2) Qihai (CV 6)

[Location] On the lower abdomen, 1.5 cun inferior to the centre of the umbilicus, on the anterior median line.

[Indications] Abdominal pain, enuresis, nocturnal emission, impotence, diarrhea, irregular menstruation, lack of strength.

(3) Shenque (CV 8)

[Location] On the upper abdomen, in the center of the umbilicus.

[Indications] Abdominal pain, diarrhea, fatigue.

(4) Zhongwan (CV 12)

[Location] On the upper abdomen, 4 cun superior to the center of the umbilicus, on the anterior median line.

[Indications] Upper abdominal discomfort, pain, abdominal distension, diarrhea, indigestion, vomiting.

(5) Danzhong (CV 17)

[Location] In the anterior thoracic region, at the same level as the fourth intercostal space, on the anterior median

央，前正中线上。

［防治］哮喘，咳嗽，咽喉肿痛，呃逆。

（7）承浆

［定位］在面部，颏唇沟的正中凹陷处。

［防治］面肿，流涎，面瘫。

line.

[Indications] Oppression in the chest, chest pain, palpitation, panting, scant breast milk.

(6) Tiantu (CV 22)

[Location] In the anterior region of the neck, in the center of the suprasternal fossa, on the anterior median line.

[Indications] Asthma, cough, swelling and sore throat, hiccup.

(7) Chengjiang (CV 24)

[Location] On the face, in the depression in the center of the mentolabial sulcus.

[Indications] Facial swelling, salivation, facial paralysis.

15. 经外奇穴

（1）印堂

［定位］在额部，当两眉头连线的中点。

［防治］头痛，失眠，鼻塞不通，鼻出血。

（2）太阳

［定位］在头部，当眉梢与目外眦之间，向后约一横指的凹陷中。

［防治］头痛，目疾，失眠。

（3）鱼腰

［定位］在头部，瞳孔直上，眉毛中。

［防治］失眠，眉棱骨痛，眼睑跳动，眼睑下垂，目赤肿痛。

（4）定喘

［定位］在脊柱区，横平第7颈椎棘突下，后正中线旁开0.5寸。

［防治］哮喘，咳嗽，落枕，肩背痛。

（5）夹脊

［定位］在脊柱区，当第1胸椎

15. Extra points

(1) Yintang (EX–HN 3)

[Location] On the forehead, the midpoint of the line connecting the two brows.

[Indications] Headache, insomnia, stuffy nose, nosebleed.

(2) Taiyang (EX–HN 5)

[Location] On the head, between the tip of the brow and the outer canthus of the eye, in a depression about a horizontal finger length backward.

[Indications] Headache, eye disease, insomnia.

(3) Yuyao (EX–HN 4)

[Location] On the head, directly above pupils, in the middle of eyebrows.

[Indications] Insomnia, pain in the supra-orbital bone, eyelid throbbing, eyelid drooping, red, swelling and painful eyes.

(4) Dingchuan (EX–B 1)

[Location] In the spinal area, horizontally below the spinous process of the seventh cervical vertebra (C 7), 0.5 cun lateral to the posterior midline.

[Indications] Asthma, cough, stiff neck, shoulder and

至第5腰椎棘突下两侧，后正中线旁开0.5寸。一侧17穴。

［防治］胸1～胸3：上肢不适；胸1～胸8：胸部不适；胸6～腰5：腹部不适；腰1～腰5：下肢不适。

（6）腰痛点

［定位］在手背，第2～第3及第4～第5掌骨之间，当腕横纹与掌指关节中点处，一手2穴，左右共4穴。

［防治］急性腰扭伤。

（7）四缝

［定位］在手指，第2～第5指掌面的近侧指间关节横纹的中央，一手4穴。

［防治］小儿疳积。

（8）膝眼

［定位］在髌韧带两侧凹陷处，内侧的称内膝眼，外侧的称外膝眼。

［防治］膝关节痛。

back pain.

(5) Jiaji (EX–B 2)

[Location] In the spinal area, beside the spinous process of the first thoracic vertebra (T 1) to the fifth lumbar vertebra (L 5), 0.5 cun lateral to the posterior midline. Seventeen points on one side.

[Indications] T 1 to T 3: upper extremity discomfort. T 1 to T 8: chest discomfort.T 6 to L 5: abdominal discomfort. L 1 to L 5: discomfort in the lower extremities.

(6) Yaotongdian (EX–UE 7)

[Location] On the back of the hand, between the second to third and fourth to fifth metacarpal bones, at the midpoint of the transverse crease of the wrist and the metacarpophalangeal joint, there are 2 acupoints in one hand, 4 acupoints in total.

[Indications] Acute lumbar muscle sprain.

(7) Sifeng (EX–UE 10)

[Location] On the fingers, in the middle of the transverse crease of the proximal interphalangeal joint on the palmar surface of the second to fifth fingers, 4 points in one hand.

[Indications] Infantile malnutrition with food stagnation.

(8) Xiyan (EX–LE 5)

[Location] In the depression on both sides of the patellar ligament, the inner side is called the inner Xiyan, and the outer side is called the outer Xiyan.

[Indications] Knee joints pain.

二、穴位选取原则

Principles for Point Selection

1. 根据穴位的局部作用取穴

一般称之为“局部取穴”，这是最常用、最简单的按摩取穴法。大多数的穴位都有主治局部病症的作用。

1. Based on its local functions

This is the most commonly used and simplest method of acupoint selection. Most acupoints have the role of treating local diseases.

2. 根据穴位的特殊作用取穴

根据前人的经验，有不少流传在民间的实用取穴方法，一般称为“经验取穴”。

3. 根据经络作用取穴

中医经络学说认为，穴位是通过所属的经络发挥作用的。经络所过，主治所及。根据病症的归经或经络循行部位的不同，先确定选用某一经络，然后在该经上选用作用较强的穴位。这种取穴方法往往不是在局部取穴，而是发挥穴位的远道作用，一般称之为“循经取穴”。

4. 根据神经节段作用取穴

脊神经的分布有节段性支配的特点。

5. 以痛为腧

以痛为腧，指根据手法触诊所探知的体表异常反应点来选取治疗点。这种异常反应点一般称为阿是穴，用手指按压该处常有酸、痛等主观反应，且可触及肌张力增高、结节、条索等软组织异常。内功推拿处理相关病症时，直接选用这些点，往往简单而有效。

6. 对称点取穴

对称点取穴是指在患侧疼痛部位（压痛点）的健侧对称点取穴。这种取穴方法有较好的止痛作用。

2. Based on its special functions

According to the experience of predecessors, there are many practical methods of selecting acupoints that have been spread among the folks. It is called “Selecting acupoints based on experiences”.

3. Based on functions of meridians

TCM meridian theory holds that acupoints work through the meridians they belong to. Treatments or manipulations should be performed on the areas related with meridians. Based on the differences among meridians that are related with diseases and symptoms, it is advisable to firstly determine a meridian, then select the acupoints with strong effect on this meridian. This method shows that points can not only treat local diseases, but also treat diseases in distant parts of the meridian. It is called selecting acupoints along with meridians.

4. Based on functions of nerve segments

Different nerve segments have different roles and innervate different body parts.

5. Based on the painful areas

It indicates that select points according to the sore and painful areas when applying palpation. These point with abnormal feelings are generally called the Ashi points. When pressing these points, patients can feel soreness and pain. Moreover, some soft tissue abnormalities can also be found by the practitioner during the application of palpation. It is effective and convenient for practitioners to take these points as the treated areas when applying internal exercise and tuina.

6. Based on the symmetric region

It refers to select symmetric acupoints at the unaffected side. Manipulate on the points selected by this method can relieve pain effectively.

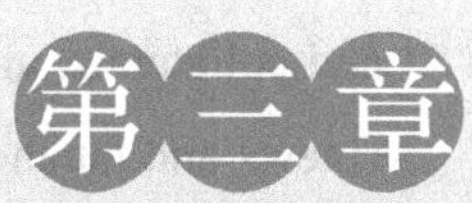

第三章 特色疗法

Chapter Three Special Treatments

第一节 Section one

棒击法 Stick-knocking Manipulation

棒击法是术者手握特制的桑枝棒的一端，用棒体平稳而有节奏地击打受术部位的一种操作方法。棒击法是内功推拿流派治疗疾病的一种重要方法，以中医经络与穴位理论为依据，通过刺激穴位、疏通筋络，达到治病和保健目的。棒击法讲究点、线、面的结合，点指人体穴位，线指人体经络，面指相应的经筋及皮部。一般在功法锻炼和手法治疗后配合棒击法，临床应用时需根据具体情况灵活掌握。马万龙、李锡九擅用此法治疗疾病，疗效甚佳。

棒击法是内功推拿流派的特色之一，既是一种治疗疾病的方法，又是一种强身保健功法。棒击法被武术家用于提高抗击打能力，而养生家则用于保健强身。击打法作为功法训练，源自明代出现的《易筋经》，主要工具有木杵、木槌、石袋击等。“木槌木杵用于肉处，骨缝之间悉宜石袋”。

棒击法属于中医外治法，《医宗金鉴・正骨心法要旨・器具总论》称其为振梃法，所用振梃是类似于擀面杖的木棒。治疗时用木棍微微振击软组织损伤四周，“使气血流通，得以四散，则疼痛渐减，肿硬渐消”。

For stick-knocking manipulation, practitioners need to steadily and rhythmically knock the specific parts of the body with a specially made mulberry stick. Among all tuina manipulations, this is an important one which based on meridian-collateral and acupoint methods of TCM and treats diseases as well as maintains people's health by stimulating acupoints and unblocking the meridian. Stick-knocking manipulation pays attention to the combination of points, lines, and planes. Points refer to acupoints of human body, lines represent meridians and collaterals, and planes mean corresponding meridian sinews and cutaneous regions. Generally, stick-knocking manipulation is applied as a complementary therapy after the treatments of TCM exercises and manipulations. Clinically, the application of this therapy depends on real circumstances. Ma Wanlong and Li Xijiu are two skillful practitioners of this therapy and have great achievements in this field.

As a distinctive therapy in Neigong Tuina (Shaolin Internal Exercise and Tuina), stick-knocking manipulation is applied for diseases treatment and life nurturing. Martial artists used it to improve people's resistance to hitting, and experts of life cultivation used it to maintain health and strengthen the body. As a TCM manipulation, knocking manipulation originates from the *Classic of Sinew Transformation* in the Ming Dynasty, "As for knocking tools, wooden pestle and wooden mallet are used in muscles and bags filled with stones are in joints". Therefore, at first, wooden pestle, wooden mallet, and bags filled with stones are main tools for knocking manipulation.

民国时期记载有揉打工具和具体程序，如《内功十三段图说》提出“揉打各法程序说”，初功开始用揉法揉遍全身，其后用散竹棒、木棒、铁丝棒等分层次对人体击打，“久则膜皮肤包裹肌肉皆腾起，浮至于皮，与筋齐坚，全无软陷，始为全功”。其作用是“因气坚而增重”，就是通过揉法使人体浅层“气坚”后，需进一步加力而深入，方用散竹棒击打。最后要“用散铁丝棒打之，打外虽属浅，而震入于内则属深矣，内外皆坚，方为全功”。这些描述的揉法和棒击可使身体内外皆“气坚”，实则“坚”皮、筋、骨三层。

内功推拿流派则将竹棒、木棒等拍打工具改进为桑枝棒，并创立了一套四肢和全身击打的常规套路。桑枝棒刚柔适中，有一定的韧性和弹性，击打声响也不像散竹棒那么大。在临床治疗中，不仅被用于疼痛麻木等肢体筋骨病症，还用于治疗肺结核等虚劳病症。桑枝棒击法已成为内功推拿的标志性手法之一。

Stick-knocking manipulation is an external therapy. In *Golden Mirror of Medicine: Essentials for Bone Orthopedics*, this therapy is called Zhentin Therapy, and Zhentin refers to a wooden bar shaped like a rolling pin. During treatment, practitioners use a wooden bar to slightly knock and vibrate around the soft tissue injury for “unblocking and circulating the qi and blood to relieve the pain and disperse swelling”.

There are records about specific procedures and tools for knocking and kneading in the time of the Republic of China. Introduction to *Different Stages of TCM Internal Exercise* documents the procedures of therapy, firstly kneading around the whole body, then using bamboo sticks, wooden sticks or wire rods to knock at the body, “After the practitioner knocking at the body for a while, membrane wrapped around the muscle will swell to the skin and be as hard as the sinews, with no soft area all over the body, indicating the ending of the manipulation.” After the qi is strengthened in the surface by kneading around the body, the practitioner applies bamboo stick to add strength and transmit the strength into deeper positions. Lastly, the practitioner needs to “Use wire rods to knock at the body. Although the knocking area is on the surface of the body, the strength will be transmitted inside deeply, making the body both firm inside and outside.” These descriptions show that kneading manipulation and stick-knocking manipulation can harden the skin, tendons and bones.

The Neigong Tuina school has improved those former tools into mulberry stick and created a routine of striking on the limbs and the whole body. With certain tenacity and elasticity, mulberry stick is in appropriate shape, and its sound of striking is not as loud as that of bamboo stick. In clinical treatment, it is not only employed in diseases like pain and numbness of limbs or tendons, but also used in deficiency overwork like tuberculosis. Now, the mulberry stick-knocking manipulation has been one of the signature therapies of Neigong Tuina.

一、桑枝棒制作方法

取长为 36 ～ 40 cm，粗 0.5 cm 的桑枝12 根，去皮阴干。把每根桑枝用棉线从一端紧密缠扎至另一端，然后用桑皮纸（每层一至两张）包绕，两端裹住，用棉线按顺序密密绕扎，12 根卷好的桑枝合在一起，然后再用桑皮纸和棉线卷紧扎好，手握之合适为度（虎口用力环握，拇指和中指相抵）。

做一内胆和外套，用质密且摩擦力较小的布料包裹，两头缝合即成内胆，外面缝上厚实而有弹性耐脏的布套，顶端用棒体横截面圆形，底端做一个可收口的细绳，即为外套，外套方便拆下换洗，即为桑枝棒。

Making of Mulberry Bar

Take 12 mulberry sticks with a length of 36 to 40 cm and a thickness of 0.5 cm, peel them off and dry them in the shade. Twine every twig tightly with cotton threads from one end to the other. Wrap each stick around mulberry paper (1–2 sheets per layer) and wind each stick with cotton threads again. Then put 12 sticks together and wrap and twine them with mulberry papers and cotton threads. Holding the mulberry stick bar in hand, if the thumb and middle finger can touch each other, it is the appropriate width.

Then make a pair of liner and cover. Wrap the bar with smooth and low-friction cloth, and sew the two ends to form a liner. Lastly, sew a thick, elastic and stain-resistant cloth cover on the outside, the top is rounded and the bottom is an opening that can be closed with string. The outer cover is easy to remove and wash.

二、桑枝棒使用方法

实施者，手握桑枝棒尾端，用棒体平稳而有节奏地击打受术部位。棒击力量要由轻到重，并适可而止。一般在一个部位连续击打3 ～ 5下即可。击打时，棒体接触面积要大，使棒体大部分平稳地击打受术部位，用力快速短暂，垂直击打体表。

棒击法：用手持棒击打，便于术者操作，减轻劳动强度，而且着力面积较大，具有一定穿透性。此

Application of Mulberry Bar

Practitioners need to steadily and rhythmically knock the specific parts of the body with a mulberry bar. The force should be from gentle to strong, and always in a moderate way. In addition, the force is quick and brief, knocking the body surface vertically. Generally, practitioners need to consistently knock 3 to 5 times at one position of the body. In the process, the knocking manipulation should be steady, and the contact area needs to be large enough.

Holding the stick by a hand is convenient and

外，击打时，声音爽朗而有节奏，患者精力集中，意气灌注有助于提高疗效。桑枝棒击打适用于肩、背、腰、四肢等肌肉丰厚部位，用于治疗软组织疼痛、肌肉紧张痉挛、风湿痹痛、头痛、头晕等病症。

labor-saving for practitioners to operate stick-knocking manipulation, making the contact area large enough to transmit the strength into the deep inside. In addition, during the process, the manipulation should be smooth and rhythmic, and the patient's qi and energy are concentrated, so as to improve the therapeutic efficacy. The mulberry stick-knocking manipulation is applicable to body parts with strong muscles like shoulder, back, waist, and limbs. It is an effective therapy for pain in soft tissues, muscle spasm, rheumatic arthritis, headache, dizziness.

三、棒击法操作常规

1. 头顶棒击法

患者取坐位，挺胸，上肢自然下垂。术者站在患者前方，左手扶助患者后颈部，嘱患者咬牙闭口，下颌微收，脊柱挺拔。术者右手持棒，用棒面击打头顶（百会、四神聪）3～5次。

头顶棒击法具有平肝潜阳，熄风宁脑，明目安神功效，侧重于治疗失眠、头晕等。

2. 大椎棒击法

患者取坐位，颈前屈。术者站在患者左侧，右手持棒，横棒与垂直线呈15°击打大椎穴3～5次。

大椎棒击法具有调节阴阳，温经通络，祛风散寒，振奋精神功效，侧重于治疗胸闷、神萎、上肢麻木、畏寒等。

3. 腰骶部棒击法

患者取坐位，术者略下蹲于患者左侧，右手持棒，横击腰骶部3～5次。

Routine Manipulations of Stick-knocking Therapy

1. Knocking on the head

The patient is in a sitting position with the chest up and the upper limbs hanging naturally. In addition, the patient needs to grit teeth and close mouth, tuck in his chin and sit upright. The practitioner stands in front of or behind the patient, holds patient's back of the neck with left hand, and knocks the patient's head [Baihui (GV20), Sishencong (EX–HN 1)] for 3 to 5 times.

This therapy has functions of pacifying the liver to subdue yang, subduing wind and quieting the brain, and improving vision and tranquilizing. It focuses on treating insomnia and dizziness.

2. Knocking on Dazhui (GV 14)

The patient is in a sitting position with the neck flexed forward. The practitioner stands on the patient's left side with a bar on the right hand. The bar is at a 15° angle to the back and used to knocks Dazhui (GV 14) 3 to 5 times.

This therapy has functions of regulating yin-yang, warming the meridian and freeing the collateral vessels, and uplifting spirits. It focuses on treating oppression in the chest, listlessness, numbness in the upper extremities, and

腰骶部棒击法具有疏通经络，调节二便，强身补肾功效。侧重于治疗便秘、慢性腹泻、阳痿、痛经、腰骶部疼痛、下肢麻木等。

4. 背部棒击法

患者取坐位，背略前屈。术者以“马档”或蹲位姿势于患者背后，右手持棒，击打患者两侧膀胱经外侧线T4至T10段。左右各3～5次。

背部棒击法具有调节脾胃，宽胸理气，疏通经络功效，侧重于治疗体虚纳差，胸闷，胃脘痛，背部疼痛、板滞等。

5. 胸部棒击法

患者取“弓箭步”或坐位姿势，挺胸。术者以“马档”或蹲位姿势面对患者，右手持棒，击打患者胸部膻中穴或左右中府、云门穴3～5次。

胸部棒击法具有宽胸降气，健肺肃肺，强身功效，侧重于治疗胸闷、咳嗽、喘息、体质虚弱等。

6. 下肢棒击法

髋关节棒击法：患者取侧卧位。以左侧髋关节为例，患侧在上紧屈左髋关节。术者站在患者腹侧，右手持棒，击打大转子或大转子周围3～5下。

大腿棒击法：患者取仰卧位或弓箭步，术者站在要击打患侧的正前方，右手持棒，沿大腿肌肉走行击打3～5次。

小腿棒击法：患者取“弓箭步”，以右侧小腿为例。术者站在患者右侧，右手持棒，击打小腿3～5次。

fear of cold.

3. Knocking on the waist

The patient is in a sitting position. The practitioner slightly squats on the patient’s left side with a bar on the right hand, and knocks the patient’s left side with a bar on the right hand. The bar is at a 15° angle to the back and used to knocks Dazhui (GV 14) 3 to 5 times.

This therapy has functions of soothing and unblocking the meridian and collateral vessels, regulating urination and defecation, tonifying the kidney and strengthening the body. It focuses on treating constipation, chronic diarrhea, impotence, dysmenorrhea, pain in the waist, and numbness in the lower extremities.

4. Knocking on the back

The patient is in a sitting position with the back slightly bent forward. The practitioner slightly squats on the patient’s back with a bar on the right hand, and knocks the lateral line of the bilateral bladder meridian from T 4 to T 10, 3 to 5 times in each side.

This therapy has functions of regulating the spleen, the stomach and the qi, soothing the chest and meridian and collateral vessels. It focuses on treating weak constitution, poor appetite, oppression in the chest, epigastric pain, back pain and dull expression.

5. Knocking on the chest

The patient is in a sitting position or bow and arrow step with the chest up. The practitioner slightly squats in front of the patient with a bar on the right hand, and knocks Danzhong (RN 17), or Zhongfu (LU 1) and Yunmen (LU 2) for 3 to 5 times.

This therapy has functions of soothing the chest, reducing qi, fortifying the lung and strengthening the body. It focuses on treating oppression in the chest, cough, panting and weak constitution.

6. Knocking on the lower extremities

Knocking on the hip joint: Take the left hip joint

下肢棒击法具有疏经通络，活血祛风，滑利关节的功效，侧重于治疗关节风湿疼痛，畏寒，关节活动不利、腓肠肌痉挛，小腿胀痛、麻木等。

for example. The patient lies down with the left hip joint flexed. The practitioner stands beside the patient with a bar on the right hand, and knocks the trochanter or the area around it for 3 to 5 times.

Knocking on the thigh: The patient is in a supine position or bow and arrow step. The practitioner stands in front of the patient with a bar on the right hand, and knocks the thigh 3 to 5 times.

Knocking on the calf: Take the right calf for example. The patient is in a bow and arrow step. The practitioner stands on the right side of the patient with a bar on the right hand, and knock the calf 3 to 5 times.

This therapy has functions of regulating meridians and collaterals, activating blood, dispelling wind, and lubricating the joints. It focuses on treating rheumatic pain of joints, aversion to cold, inconvenience of joints' movement, gastrocnemius muscle spasm, and distention, pain or numbness in calf.

四、辨证施棒

棒击法不同于推拿手法中的擦、推、被动等手法，其主要依靠棒击力对人体产生作用，因棒击的轻重而体现出补泻，所以棒击力量的大小对疗效起着重要作用。

运用棒击法，要严格遵循中医辨证施治的原则，从整体出发，视疾病的轻重、正气的盛衰，选择各种不同的部位，施以轻重不等的棒击力，这样才能收到较好的疗效。例如肺结核患者，气血均衰，以轻棒力可以增强脾胃功能，扶助正气，待气血渐盛，患者的体质已能承受重棒力时，方可适当加重棒击力量，

Application Differentiation

Stick-knocking manipulation differs from other tuina manipulations like liner-rubbing manipulation and pushing manipulation. It acts on the body by relying on the force of stick knocking. The force plays an important role because it will influence the tonifying and purging effect of the stick-knocking manipulation.

Pattern differentiation principle should be strictly abode by in the treatment. To improve the effectiveness, the practitioner should follow a holistic view and apply different forces at different positions after learning about the severity of diseases and the storage of healthy qi. Take tuberculosis patients with deficiency in both qi and blood for example. Slight knocking manipulation can strengthen patients' spleen and stomach, and reinforce the healthy qi.

加速体质恢复。如果开始就施之以重棒力，患者不仅难以承受如此力量，反而加重病情。

正确选择棒击部位是治病的关键。如支气管扩张可取大椎、背部、胸部等；胃脘痛可取背部；痛经可取腰骶部、足三里等；失眠可取囟门、大椎等；对于腰、髋关节等深部组织病变，推拿手法的力难以达到病变部位时可直接击打局部。

Only when the patients' qi and blood are abundant enough to withstand stronger force, can the operator increase the strength. Otherwise, the patient's condition will get worse owing to such strong force.

The position for stick-knocking manipulation is the key in treatment. For instance, Dazhui (GV 14), back and chest can be knocked for bronchiectasis, back for epigastric pain, waist and Zusanli (ST 36) for dysmenorrhea, and Dazhui (GV 14) for insomnia. In addition, when it comes to some tissues' lesion which the position of them is so deep that the force of manipulation is hard to be transmitted, the practitioner is allowed to directly hit the specific areas.

五、注意事项

棒击法是一种有效的治疗方法，运用得当，可大大加快疾病的恢复。但是，如果使用不当反而会加重病情。所以，使用此法治病，除了严格遵守相关禁忌证外，还要注意以下几点。

（1）治疗前嘱患者排解大小便。

（2）击打时，要先有“信棒”（即指打击时要先轻轻击两下，以引起患者注意，使其意气汇集击打部位），不击冷棒。

（3）除在大椎、八髎等处用横棒外，其余部位都要用顺棒，就是说棒身和肢体要平行。

（4）棒击时医生手腕要灵活，患者呼吸要调匀，击头顶时要让患者闭口咬牙，以免上下牙齿闭合伤及舌头。

（5）棒击频率不宜过频，隔天

Cautions

Stick-knocking manipulation is effective and can promote recovery if applied properly. Therefore, in addition to strictly obeying the relevant contradictions, attentions should also be paid to the following points.

(1) A reminder to the patient to urinate and defecate before treatment.

(2) Lightly tap on body surface to signal the start before implementing the knocking manipulation, which aims to get the patient's attention so that he can focus the energy and qi on the knocking position.

(3) The mulberry stick is horizontally applied when knocking Dazhui (GV 14) and Baliao (BL 31–34), but is vertically used when knocking other positions.

(4) The patient should breathe steadily, and the practitioner needs to be flexible in the wrists and ask the patient to keep the teeth gritted and the mouth closed to prevent hurting the tongue.

(5) Frequent manipulations are not allowed, once for every two days is appropriate.

治疗1次。

（6）小儿一般不用。后脑和肾区等部位严禁使用棒击法。

(6) This manipulation is not recommended for children and is prohibited in positions like back of the head and kidney area.

六、理论基础与作用机制

Theoretical Basis and Functional Mechanism

经络是人体结构的重要组成部分，具有联络人体脏腑器官，沟通内外上下、运行气血、调节阴阳及机体活动的作用。人体通过经络系统把五脏六腑、五官九窍、四肢百骸、筋脉皮肉等连接成为一个具有生命功能的整体。五脏六腑、经络之气输注于体表，经络是气血运行的枢纽。若是经络不通，气血则不畅，不通则痛，就会引发病患。通过辨证施治，对相应经络、穴位进行拍击敲打，使经络畅通，气血旺盛，以达“诸脉皆通，通则疾除”的效果。

“经脉者，人之所以生，病之所以成，人之所以治，病之所以起”“血气不和，百病乃变化而生”，认为经脉不通是万病的起因，而要治愈疾病则必须从疏通经脉开始。《医宗金鉴》曰：“气血郁滞，为肿为痛，宜用拍按之法，按其经络以通郁闭之气……其忠可愈。”

研究表明，人体肌肉每平方毫米的横切面上约有4 000条毛细血管，在平常安静的状态下仅有30～270条是开放状态，而在运动时毛细血管大量开放，此时开放数量可达安静时的20～50倍之多，因此，此时肌肉可获得比平时多得多的氧气

Meridian and collateral are important components of human body, with the fuctions of connecting our organs, regulating the lower part and the upper part of body, moving the qi and blood, and regulating yin-yang and body activities. Through this system, Five Zang-Organs and Six Fu-Organs, five sense organs and nine orifices, limbs and skeleton, and sinews and flesh are connected as a living whole. Meridian and collateral are the route for qi and blood transmission, if blocked, the moving of qi and blood cannot be smooth, people will feel pain and the illnesses will occur. TCM uses knocking manipulation on specific meridians, collaterals and acupoints of the human body after syndrome differentiation, with the purpose of making meridians and collaterals smooth and qi and blood abundant. By doing so, the meridians and collaterals are unblocked, the qi and blood are exuberant, and the diseases are cured eventually.

“It is through the twelve conduit vessels that a person comes to life, that the diseases become manifest, that a person is cured, and where the diseases emerge.” “When blood and qi are not in harmony, then a hundred diseases manifest.” Since ancient times, the block of meridians and collaterals are considered as the origin of diseases. Therefore, people believed that treatment must start from them. “When qi and blood are obstructed and cause pain, the patting and pressing manipulations should be applied along the meridians and collaterals to unblock them.” written in *Golden Mirror of Medicine*.

Research shows that there are 4 000 capillaries in

和养料。而全身毛细血管的大量开放会减轻心脏负担，降低血压，促进心脏功能改善，较好地防治心脑血管疾病及其他急慢性病症。

拍打疗法可疏通经络、行气活血、协调阴阳。气血畅通可令周身的组织器官得到充足的营养，使瘀阻之毒及代谢废物及时排出体外，从而祛病健身。拍打疗法可强健肌肉，灵活骨骼，增强活力，具体作用如下。

（1）舒筋通络：棒击法是消除疼痛和肌肉紧张痉挛的有效方法，主要机制为击打能加强局部血液循环，使局部温度升高；棒击直接刺激提高了局部组织的痛阈。

（2）活血化瘀：棒击法能促使击打部位的血液循环，增加组织的血流量。

（3）消炎止痛：击打后身体表面会出现类似刮痧自体溶血现象，可以刺激机体提高免疫功能，有消炎止痛的作用。

棒击法可疏通经络、行气活血、解痉止痛、消除疲劳、保健身体、防治疾病，还具有操作简单、安全可靠、无副作用、适用广泛、效果显著等众多优点，是一种值得临床推广和应用的自然疗法。

muscle's cross section per square millimeter, and only 30 to 270 of them are open in a quiet state, while in exercising, the number achieves 20 to 50 times than that in the quiet state. Therefore, muscles at that time get more oxygen and nutrients. Besides, the opening of large number of capillaries releases the heart burden, reduces blood pressure, promotes heart function, and better prevents and treats cardiovascular diseases and other chronic diseases.

The unblocking of qi and blood allows related organs to get abundant nutrients, and transmits stasis toxin and metabolic waste out of body. Knocking manipulation frees meridians and collaterals, moves qi and activates blood, and coordinates yin and yang. In addition, this therapy strengthens muscles, relaxes bones and enhances energy. These effects are illustrated in the followings.

(1) Relax sinews and activate collaterals: Knocking manipulation effectively relieves the pain and spasm of muscles. Its main mechanism is strengthening local blood circulation and increasing local body temperature through knocking. This therapy makes some local tissues be more tolerable to pain.

(2) Activate blood and resolve stasis: Knocking manipulation promotes blood circulation of the knocking position, increasing the blood flow of body tissues.

(3) Anti-inflammatory and relieve pain: Blood spots occur in body surface after knocking. It has functions of stimulating our body to improve immune function and relieve inflammation and pain.

As a natural therapy, in addition to unblocking meridians and collaterals, moving qi and activating blood, releasing spasm to stop pain, relieving fatigue, strengthening body, and preventing and treating diseases, knocking manipulation is also easy to apply, safe, reliable, effective with wide range of application and without side effects.

第二节 Section Two

膏摩

Gao Mo (Tuina Combined with Herbal Ointment)

膏摩又称“药摩法”“药物推拿”，是用药物配制成的介质，涂抹于施术部位，再施以推拿按摩手法，从而防治疾病的一种方法。膏摩是将推拿与药物配合运用的一种形式。之所以称为“膏摩”，一是因为“摩”是操作时常用方法，故作为推拿的简称；二是因为手法操作时，介质通常选用膏剂。除膏剂外，也可用水性、油性等介质。

膏摩在我国的发展源远流长，在许多史书中都有记载。长沙马王堆3号墓出土的帛书《五十二病方》中记载了我国推拿史上最早的药膏与膏摩。帛书中有以“车故脂”作为介质摩于患处治疗瘙痒的记载。虽然当时的制备方法还相当原始，但却为后世膏摩的发展奠定了基础。

《黄帝内经》记载了“马膏”治疗阳明经面瘫急性发作。汉代张仲景在《金匮要略》一书中首次提出了“膏摩”一词。并将其与针灸、导引等法并列，用于预防保健。认为“若人能养慎，不令邪风干忤经络。适中经络，未流传脏腑，即医治之。四肢才觉重滞，即导引、吐纳、针灸、膏摩，勿令九窍闭塞”。三国时期，华佗经常使用按摩手段治疗疾病，尤其是膏摩。据《三

Gao Mo, also called “Herbal Rubbing”, is a therapeutic method to apply herbal ointment on the surface of the body area to be treated, and always followed by tuina manipulations. This therapy combines tuina with herbal ointment. Its name originates from two reasons. One is that rubbing (Mo) is the brief expression of tuina, the other is that paste preparation (Gao) is always applied in the process. In addition, preparations of fluidity and ointment are also accepted.

With a long development history, Gao Mo is recorded in many ancient classics. The silk manuscript of *Formulas for Fifty-two Diseases* unearthed from number three of Mawangdui Han Tomb recorded the earliest application of herbal ointment and Gao Mo. It was recorded that Cheguzhi (seeds of an oil-rich plant) has been used for relieving itching. Although the processing way is quite primitive, it did lay a solid foundation for the development of Gao Mo in later generations.

Yellow Emperor's Canon of Medicine recorded “horse paste” treatment of Yangming channel facial paralysis acute attack. In the Han Dynasty, Zhang Zhongjing firstly introduced the word of Gao Mo in his *Essentials from the Golden Cabinet*, and listed it together with acupuncture and moxibustion and daoyin (guiding and stretching), marking it as a preventative therapy. The original text is “If people can cultivate right qi and take precautions against contraction of wind evil, they can prevent wind evil from disturbing the channels and network vessels. But if by chances wind evil strikes the channels and network vessels,

国志·魏书·华佗传》和《后汉书·华佗传》记载，他曾用倒悬、铍刀决脉、膏摩等法治顽固性头眩病。另据《诸病源候论》《外台秘要》《千金要方》等记载。华佗还将膏摩与火灸同用以治疗“伤寒始得一日在皮肤”。此外，《肘后备急方》中载有“疗百病”的“华佗虎骨膏”等，对后世医家的影响极其深远。《神农本草经》一书中提到了用“雷丸”做摩膏除小儿百病。这是膏摩用于小儿疾病的最早记载，从中可见膏摩至少在汉代已被古医家应用于儿科。

晋代的葛洪十分重视膏摩疗法，是第一位系统论述膏摩的证、法、方、药的医家。尤其对于膏摩施术的记载更加详细、完备。另外，葛洪还在《肘后备急方》中介绍了以蜜作为介质摩身，治疗时行疮疡。东晋末年的《刘涓子鬼遗方》书中记载了近十首膏摩方，用于治疗外科病症，并体现了对痈疽病的辨证论治思想。隋末唐初的孙思邈所著的《备急千金要方》中记载了许多预防和治疗小儿疾患的膏摩方。如《备急千金要方·少小婴孺方》中的五物甘草生摩膏方、丹参赤膏、摩生膏、豉、衣中白鱼、米粉盐等。

王焘所著的《外台秘要》一书中记载了大量的膏摩方名，并且大都注明了膏摩方的出处，为后世研究膏摩的发展史提供了很重要的参考价值。北宋初期的《太平圣惠方》一书囊括了有史以来最多的膏摩方，并体现了专方专用的特点。书中共

a physician must treat it immediately, before it flows into the bowels and viscera. As soon as the limbs feel heavy and stagnant, treat the patient with conduction, inhalation and exhalation, acupuncture and moxibustion, or paste rubbing to prevent the nine orifices from becoming blocked". In the Three Kingdoms Period, Hua Tuo usually applied rubbing manipulation, especially the Gao Mo. It was said in *Records of the Three Kingdoms* and *Book of the Later Han* that Hua Tuo had used therapies like Gao Mo for intractable dizziness treatment. Besides, other TCM classics as *Treatise on the Origins and Manifestations of Various Diseases* and *Arcane Essentials from the Imperial Library* also recorded that Hua Tuo had combined Gao Mo with fire moxibustion to treat cold damage. In addition, *Emergency Formulas to Keep Up One's Sleeve* stated the Hua Tuo Tiger Bone Paste, a widely-applicated paste which profoundly influences the later physicians. Lei Wan (Thunder Pill) mentioned in *Shen Nong's Classic of the Materia Medica* is the earliest record of the application of Gao Mo for curing children's diseases. From these, we learned that at least in the Han Dynasty, Gao Mo had been applied in pediatrics.

In the Jin Dynasty, Ge Hong stressed the Gao Mo therapy and was the first physician who systematically analyzed its pattern, treatment, formula and materia medica. He also described its application process in detail. Moreover, Ge Hong introduced its application in treating sore and ulcer. In the end of the East Jin Dynasty, Liu Juanzi's *Ghost-Bequeathed Formulas* mentioned ten formulas of Gao Mo for external treatment, and demonstrated the pattern differentiation on abscess. In the end of the Sui Dynasty and the beginning of the Tang Dynasty, Important Formulas Worth a *Thousand Gold Pieces for Emergency* wrote by Sun Simiao recorded many formulas of Gao Mo for preventing and treating pediatric diseases, such as Five Ingredients Massaging Ointment, Danshen Chigao (a rubbing paste made by Danshen).

有膏摩方、药摩方近百首。北宋末年的《圣济总录》不仅记载了许多临床有效的骨伤膏摩方，而且还进一步将膏摩纳入骨伤治疗的三大程序之一，理论上进行了总结，扩大了膏摩在骨伤科的应用。

明代《普济方》载有膏摩方数十种，如五物甘草生摩膏、太傅白膏、延年蒴翟膏等。大多可见于此书前的各篇历史文献中，可以说是对疗效好的经典膏摩的又一次整理总结。明代王肯堂编写的《证治准绳》中也记载了膏摩方数则，如摩腰膏、摩风膏、防己膏等。清代吴尚先编著的外治法专著《理瀹骈文》一书详细介绍了将药物熬膏，或敷或擦，或摩或浸或熏的方法。这就使古代的膏摩、药膏得到了空前的发展。

民国陆锦笙著的《溪外治方选》，载有推拿外治方数十则，有众多用药物推拿之法，突破了前人用药膏摩患处的“膏摩”框框，无论在用药方面，还是在用手法方面均更加灵活多变，适应证范围也更为广泛。

内功推拿流派在临床中广泛运用膏摩治疗疾病，应用膏摩介质不但可以加强手法作用，提高治疗效果，而且还可起到润滑和保护皮肤的作用。

Arcane Essentials from the Imperial Library wrote by Wang Tao also stated many formulas' name of Gao Mo with their origins, providing references for later generations. In the Northern Song Dynasty, with almost a hundred formulas of Gao Mo and herbal rubbing, *Formulas from Benevolent Sages Compiled during the Taiping Era* included the largest number of Gao Mo formulas, and introduced their purposes specifically. In the end of the Northern Song Dynasty, *Comprehensive Recording of Divine Assistance* contained many effective Gao Mo formulas on bone injury, included Gao Mo as one of the three treatment procedures of bone injury and summarized its theories, enlarging its application in the field of orthopedics and traumatology.

In the Ming Dynasty, dozens of Gao Mo were recorded in *Formulas for Universal Relief* such as Five Ingredients Massaging Ointment, Longevity Shuozhai Ointment. *Standards for Diagnosis and Treatment* of Wang Kentang also mentioned several Gao Mo formulas. In the Qing Dynasty, *Rhymed Discourse on External Remedies* compiled by Wu Shangxian introduced the methods of how to boil the medicine into the paste and how to apply, rub, soak into, and use herbal paste. These classics all facilitate the development of Gao Mo.

In the Republic of China, *Selected Formulas Used for External Treatment* recorded dozens Tuina formulas, among which some formulas are more flexible and widely-used.

The school of Neigong Tuina widely used Gao Mo in clinical treatments. In addition to enhancing the effect of manipulations, it also smooths and protects our skin.

一、常用介质

Common Medium

膏摩使用方剂有单方和复方之分。常应用的介质有葱姜水、滑石

Formulas of Gao Mo are different in the number of their ingredients. One named single formula and the other

粉、麻油、冬青膏及各种药物制成的药膏。其他如松节油、舒筋活络药水、红花油均可应用。一般无毒性的植物油均可因地制宜选用。推拿临床中常用的介质如下。

冬青膏：将冬绿油（水杨酸甲脂）与凡士林混合称冬青膏。用擦法或按揉法时常用此膏，可加强透热效果。

葱姜水：用葱白和生姜捣碎取汁涂少许按摩（或将葱姜用酒精浸泡），能加强温热发散作用，常用来治疗小儿虚寒证（在夏季治疗小儿发热时用清水）。

滑石粉：一般在夏季应用。夏季易出汗，在出汗部位运用手法时，容易使皮肤破损，局部敷以滑石粉，可保护患者和医者的皮肤。

麻油：运用擦法时涂上少许麻油，可加强手法的透热效果。

called compound formula. Common mediums include scallion-ginger juice, talcum powder, sesame oil, and various herbal pastes. Besides, turpentine oil, sinews-relaxing and collaterals-activating potion and red flower oil also can be applied. Generally, people can choose different plant oils without toxin based on their local conditions. And some mediums which commonly applied in clinic are introduced as follows.

Holly ointment: a paste compounding methyl salicylate with Vaseline. This paste is commonly used to enhance the effect when performing linear-rubbing manipulation and pressing-kneading manipulation.

Scallion-ginger juice: mashing scallion white and fresh ginger together, or immersing scallion white and ginger in alcohol. This juice strengthens the warming and dispersing effect of tuina, and is appropriate for treating deficiency cold pattern of children (clean water should be used for treating children's fever in summertime).

Talcum powder: usually used in summer. People tend to sweat in summer, and our skin is easier to be broken if the manipulation area is sweaty. Therefore, talcum powder is recommended for the skin protection for both patients and practitioners.

Sesame oil: the warming effect can be strengthened when sesame oil is applied in linear-rubbing manipulation.

二、使用方法

临床操作时，先按处方配制成软膏，然后将膏少许涂抹于体表施术部位上，再进行推拿按摩治疗。一般多用擦法、摩法、平推法和按揉法。在应用膏摩的方法时，有时还需要借助一些器具，如《圣济总录》曰："以铁熨斗，摩顶一二千

Manipulations

In clinical Manipulations, practitioners firstly make paste according to the prescriptions, then apply the paste to the skin, and start to manipulate. Linear-rubbing, circular-rubbing, flat-pushing and pressing-kneading are the most common manipulations. In application, some tools are needed. *Comprehensive Recording of Divine Assistance* stated that "use iron to rub the top of the head for one or

下。”“以铁匙挑一钱许，涂顶上，细细用铁匙研之。”

two thousand times” and “apply one qian ointment to the top of the head and use an iron spoon to rub it”.

【临床应用举例】

颈部膏摩操作方法：第1步，患者坐位或俯卧位（胸部垫以软枕），使颈项部皮肤充分暴露。第2步，将药膏涂于颈项部正中，用柔和的一指禅推法或拇指按揉法操作于风府穴至大椎穴部位。由上而下，紧推慢移，力量适中，在风府穴及大椎穴稍作停留。第3步，将药膏涂在颈部双侧斜方肌处，以一指禅推法或拇指按揉法操作于风池穴、阿是穴及颈夹脊等部位。

沿风池穴至肩井穴由上而下拇指直推10次。小鱼际擦于颈肩部，以透热为度。第4步，将药膏涂于上背部，用一指禅推法、拇指按揉法、掌揉法或掌根揉法施于肩胛提肌、斜方肌、冈下肌等处。沿斜方肌肌纤维方向施以小鱼际擦法，以透热为度。第5步，拿风池、颈部斜方肌、肩井，以局部产生酸胀感为度。

【Clinical Examples】

Manipulation of Gao Mo on the neck. Firstly, the patient needs to sit or in a prone position (with a soft pillow under the chest), and completely exposes the neck area. Secondly, the practitioner applies the ointment to the middle of the patient’s neck. Yi Zhi Chan-pushing manipulation or the pressing-kneading manipulation with thumbs from Fengfu (GV 16) to Dazhui (GV 14) with appropriate force and makes a short stay on these two points. Thirdly, the practitioner applies the ointment to the bilateral trapezius muscle of the patient’s neck and employs the Yi Zhi Chan-pushing or the pressing-kneading manipulation with thumbs on Fengchi (GB 20), Ashi point and Jingjiaji (EX–B 2).

Employ straight-pushing manipulation from the Fengchi (GB 20) to Jianjing (GB 21) with thumbs for 10 times. Employ the hypothenar-rubbing manipulation on the shoulder and neck position to warm the skin. Fourthly, apply the ointment to the upper area of the patient’s back and employ the Yi Zhi Chan-pushing or the pressing-kneading manipulation with thumbs or palms on areas of levator scapulae, trapezius muscle and infraspinatus. Fifthly, grasp Fengchi (GB 20), bilateral trapezius muscle of the neck and Jianjing (GB 21) until the patient feels soreness and swelling.

三、临床应用

Clinical Application

本疗法适用范围很广，广泛用于内、外、妇、儿、伤及五官等科，治疗风湿痹痛、中风偏瘫、口眼歪斜、痛风、骨损肿痛、伤筋、闭经、

This therapy is widely used in the fields of internal medicine, surgery, obstetrics and gynecology, pediatrics, traumatology, ophthalmology and otorhinolaryngology, and so on. It is applied for treating wind-damp impediment

便秘、夜啼、惊风、目暗赤痛、喉中息肉等症。

pain, wind stroke hemiplegia, deviated eye and mouth, pain wind, pain and swelling of the bone, sinews injury, amenorrhea, constipation, night crying, infantile convulsion, dim vision, redness and pain of the eyes, laryngeal polyp, and so on.

四、注意事项

Cautions

（1）膏摩方多含有毒物成分，故不可入口。

（2）施用膏摩时，应注意防止损伤皮肤。

（3）介质无论选用何种剂型，均宜选取适量。过多（太湿）或过少（太燥），均不便于手法操作。

（4）急性传染性疾病、各种感染性疾病、各种出血、严重的内科疾病、休克、外伤出血及骨折早期、截瘫初期等不宜使用膏摩疗法。精神病或其他不配合者，也禁用本法。

(1) There are ingredients with toxicity in most Gao Mo formulas, please do not put it in your mouth.

(2) When applying Gao Mo, take care to prevent your skin from breaking.

(3) No matter what medium you choose, please make sure that the amount is appropriate, for too much (wet) or too little (dry) will both hinder the Manipulations.

(4) Gao Mo is not recommended for the treatment of acute infectious diseases, bleeding, critical medical diseases, shock, early stage of bone fracture and paraplegia, and so on. People with mental disorders or not cooperating with practitioners are prohibited from doing this therapy.

五、常用膏摩方

Common Formulas

【单方】

（1）葱白：辛，温。入肺、胃经。发表、解毒。用于推、摩、揉、擦。捣烂取汁，或将葱白浸泡在酒或95%乙醇内，取其浸出液。

（2）生姜：辛，温。入肺、胃经。通血脉、祛寒气、行药力。用以推、摩、揉、擦。亦可用生姜、葱白同捣取汁，或同时浸入酒或95%乙醇之中，取浸出液使用。

（3）麻油：甘，凉。入大肠经。

【Single formula】

(1) Scallion white (葱白, *Alli Fistulosi Bulbus*): It is pungent in flavour and warm in nature, and affects lung and stomach meridians. It can effuse the exterior and detoxify. It is mostly applied for pushing, circular-rubbing, kneading and linear-rubbing manipulations. Mash the scallion white to collect its juice, or immerse it in wine or 95% alcohol to get its lixivium.

(2) Fresh ginger (生姜, *Rhizoma Zingiberis Recens*): It is pungent in flavour and warm in nature, and affects lung and stomach meridians. It can unblock blood vessels,

润燥，生肌、通便、解毒。用以推、摩、揉、擦。

（4）酒：甘、苦、辛，有毒。入心、肝、肺、胃经。通血脉、祛寒气、行药力，以推、摩、揉、擦。

（5）滑石：甘、淡，寒。入胃、膀胱经。清热、利窍、润燥、渗湿。研粉用以推、摩、揉、擦。

（6）薄荷油：辛，凉，无毒。疏风清热。用以涂抹、推、摩。

（7）蓖麻油：甘、辛，平，有小毒。开窍通关，行经络，止诸痛，消肿，去脓，拔毒。用以推、摩、揉、擦。

（8）蛋清：甘，微寒，无毒。除热，止烦咳，解热毒。用以推、摩、擦、抹。

（9）新汲水：甘，冷，无毒。祛邪，调中、下热气，解闭，祛毒。用以推、摩、擦、抹。

dispel cold, and help the functioning of medicinal. It is mostly applied for pushing, circular rubbing, kneading and rubbing manipulations. Mash the fresh ginger and scallion white together to collect the juice, or immerse them in wine or 95% alcohol to get the lixivium.

(3) Sesame oil: It is sweet in flavour and cool in nature, and enters the large intestine meridian. It can moisten dryness, regenerate new tissues, promote bowel movements, and remove toxins. It is mostly applied for pushing, circular rubbing, kneading and rubbing manipulations.

(4) Liquor: It is sweet, bitter and pungent in flavour, has poison, and affects heart, liver, lung and stomach meridians. It can unblock blood vessels, dispel cold and help the functioning of medicinal. It is mostly applied for pushing, circular rubbing, kneading and linear rubbing manipulations.

(5) Huashi (滑石, *Talcum*): It is sweet and tasteless in flavour and cold in nature, and affects stomach and bladder meridians. It can clear heat, facilitate passage through the orifices, moisten dryness, and drain dampness. Grind Huashi into power and apply it for pushing, circular rubbing, kneading and linear rubbing manipulations.

(6) Mint oil: It is pungent in flavour, cool in nature, and without poison. It can disperse wind and clear heat. It is mostly applied for wiping, pushing and circular rubbing manipulations.

(7) Caster oil: It is sweet and pungent in flavour, neutral in nature, and has slight poison. It can open the orifices, unblock meridians and collaterals, alleviate edema, expel pus, and draw out toxin. It is mostly applied for pushing, circular rubbing, kneading and linear rubbing manipulations.

(8) Egg white: It is sweet in flavour, slight cold in nature, and without poison. It can relieve fever and cough, and remove heat toxin. It is mostly applied for pushing, circular rubbing, kneading and rubbing manipulations.

(9) Fresh well water: It is sweet in flavour, cold in nature, and without poison. It can eliminate the pathogenic

（10）食盐：咸，寒。入胃、肾、大小肠经。涌吐，凉血，清火，解毒。研末，用以推、擦。

（11）麝香：辛，温。入心、脾、肝经。开窍，辟秽，通络，散瘀。研末，用以推、摩、擦、抹。

（12）珍珠：甘、咸，寒。镇心安神，养阴熄风，清热坠痰，退翳明目，解毒生肌。研粉，用以摩、擦。

（13）醋：酸、苦，温。入肝、胃经。散瘀，止血，解毒，杀虫。用以推、抹、摩、擦。

（14）胡荽：辛，温。微毒。消谷，调补五脏，通心窍，辟秽毒。取胡荽汁或煎汤，用以推、揉、摩、抹。

（15）木香：辛，温，无毒。入肝经。消毒，健脾消食，调气，引药。研末，用以推、摩。

factors, regulate the middle, remove the heat qi and blocks, and detoxify. It is mostly applied for pushing, circular rubbing, linear rubbing and wiping manipulations.

(10) Salt: It is salty in flavour, cold in nature, and affects stomach, kidney, small and large intestine. It can induce vomit, cool the blood, clear the heat, and detoxify. Grind salt into power and apply it for pushing and wiping manipulations.

(11) Shexiang (麝香, *Moschus*): It is pungent in flavour, warm in nature, and affects heart, spleen and liver meridians. It can open the orifices, dispel filth, unblock collaterals, and dissipate stasis. Grind Shexiang into power and apply it for pushing, circular rubbing, linear rubbing and wiping manipulations.

(12) Pearl (珍珠, *Margarita*): It is sweet and salty in flavour, and cold in nature. It can settle the heart and tranquilize, nourish yin and extinguish wind, clear the heat and resolve phlegm, remove nebula and improve vision, and detoxify and promote tissue regeneration. Grind Zhenzhu into power and apply it for circular rubbing and linear rubbing manipulations.

(13) Vinegar: It is sour and bitter in flavour, warm in nature, and affects liver and stomach meridians. It can dissipate stasis, stop bleeding, detoxify, and kill bugs. It is mostly applied for pushing, wiping, circular rubbing and linear rubbing manipulations.

(14) Husui (胡荽, *Herba Coriandri Sativi cum Radice*): It is pungent in flavour, warm in nature, and with slight poisons. It can regulate and replenish Five Zang-Organ, unblock the heart orifices, and dispel filth and toxin. Collect its juice or make it in decoction, and apply these juice for pushing, kneading, circular rubbing and wiping manipulations.

(15) Muxiang (木香, *Radix Aucklandiae*): It is pungent in flavour, warm in nature, without poison, and affects liver meridian. It can detoxify, fortify the spleen and

（16）花椒：辛，温，有毒。祛风邪，除寒痹，温中明目。取花椒末、汁，或煎取淑油，用以推、摩、擦、抹、揉、搓。

（17）蒜：辛，温，有小毒。入脾、肾经。消谷，理胃，温中，祛邪除痹。用汁推、摩、擦、抹、揉、搓。

（18）肉桂：辛、甘，热。入肾、脾、膀胱经。补元阳，暖脾胃，除积冷，通血脉。浸麻油中，用于推、摩。

（19）桃仁：苦、甘，平。入心、肝、大肠经。破血行瘀，润燥滑肠。桃仁侵去皮尖，研细加泥，和蜜，用时温水化开，可摩治皮肤皲裂。

（20）蜂蜜：甘，平。入肺、胃、大肠经。止痛解毒。用以推、摩、揉、擦。

promote digestion, regulate qi, and guide medicinal. Grind Muxiang into powder and apply it for pushing and circular rubbing manipulations.

(16) Huajiao (花椒, *Pericarpium Zanthoxyli*): It is pungent in flavour, warm in nature, and has poisons. It can dispel wind, resolve cold impediment, and warm the middle and improve vision. Collect its powder and juice or fry it for oil, and apply these for circular rubbing, linear rubbing, wiping, kneading and palm-twisting manipulations.

(17) Garlic: It is pungent in flavour, warm in nature, with slight poisons, and affects spleen and kidney meridians. It can swift digestion, regulate the stomach, warm the middle, and eliminate the pathogenic factors and impediment. The garlic juice is mostly applied for pushing, circular rubbing, linear rubbing, wiping, kneading and palm-twisting manipulations.

(18) Rougui (肉桂, *Cortex Cinnamomi*): It is pungent and sweet in flavour, warm in nature, and affects kidney, spleen and bladder meridians. It can tonify the original yang, warm the spleen and stomach, eliminate accumulation and cold, and unblock blood vessels. Immerse it in sesame oil and then apply it for pushing and circular rubbing manipulations.

(19) Taoren (桃仁, *Semen Persicae*): It is bitter and sweet in flavour, neutral in nature, and affects heart, liver and large intestine meridians. It can break and expel blood stasis, and moisten dryness and smooth the intestines. Remove coat and radicle of peach seeds, grind seeds into powder and mix them with soil and honey. When applying, melt this paste with warm water and supplemented with circular rubbing manipulation to treat chapped skin.

(20) Fengmi (蜂蜜, *Honey*): It is sweet in flavour, neutral in nature, and affects lung stomach and large intestine meridians. It can relieve pain and detoxify. It is mostly applied for pushing, circular-rubbing kneading and linear-rubbing manipulations.

【复方】

（1）苍悟道士陈元膏疗百病方：当归、天雄、乌头各三两，芎䓖、朱砂各二两，干姜、附子、雄黄各二两半，桂心、白芷各一两，松脂八两，地黄二斤（捣，绞去汁）。

十三物别捣，雄黄、朱砂为末，以酽苦酒三升合地黄渍药一宿，取猪脂八斤，微火煎十五沸，白芷黄为度，绞去滓，内雄黄、朱砂末，搅令调和，密器贮之。

腹内病，皆对火摩病上，日二三度，从十日乃至二十日，取病出差止。(《肘后备急方・卷八》)

【Compound formula】

(1) Taoist Chenyuan Pain-alleviating Ointment: Danggui (当归, *Radix Angelicae Sinensis*) 3 liang, Tianxiong (天雄, *Radix Aconiti carmichaeli*) 3 liang, Wutou (乌头, *Aconitum carmichaeli debx*) 3 liang, Chuanxiong (川芎, *Rhizoma Ligustici Chuanxiong*) 2 liang, Zhusha (朱砂, *Cinnabaris*) 2 liang, Ganjiang (干姜, *Rhizoma Zingiberis*) 2.5 liang, Fuzi (附子, *Radix Aconiti Lateralis Preparata*) 2.5 liang, Xionghuang (雄黄, *Realgar*) 2.5 liang, Guixin (桂心, *Cassia Bark*) 1 liang, Baizhi (白芷, *Radix Angelicae Dahuricae*) 1 liang, Songzhi (松脂, *Gum Rosin*) 8 liang, Shengdihuang (生地黄, *Radix Rehmanniae Recens*) 2 jin (churned and pounded to remove juice).

Pound the above Chinese herbal medicines respectively and blend these drugs together except for Xionghuang and Zhusha. Soak the medicinal mixture with Dihuang and 3 shen vinegar for a night. Decoct the medicinal mixture with 8 jin lard in low heat. After boiling for 15 times, the Baizhi in the decoction turns to yellow. Remove the residues, mix the decoction with Xionghuang and Zhusha, and store this mixture in a sealed container.

For abdominal pain, patient can massage the painful area with this ointment for 2 to 3 times a day, lasting 10 to 20 days until the pain is relived. (From volume 8 of the *Emergency Formulas to Keep Up One's Sleeve*)

（2）神明白膏：当归、细辛各三两，吴茱萸、芎䓖、蜀椒、白术、前胡、白芷各一两，附子三十枚。

中风恶气、头面诸病、青盲风、烂眦鼻、耳聋、寒齿痛，痈肿疽痔、金疮、癣疥悉主之。

九物切、煎，猪脂十斤，炭火煎一沸即下，三上三下，白芷黄，膏成，去滓，密贮。

病在外，皆摩傅之。中风恶气、

(2) Spirit-clearing White Ointment: Danggui (当归, *Radix Angelicae Sinensis*) 3 liang, Xixin (细辛, *Herba Asari*) 3 liang, Wuzhuyu (吴茱萸, *Fructus Evodiae*) 1 liang, Chuanxiong (川芎, *Rhizoma Ligustici Chuanxiong*) 1 liang, Shujiao (蜀椒, *Pricklyash Peel*) 1 liang, Baizhu (白术, *Rhizoma Atractylodis Macrocephalae*) 1 liang, Qianhu (前胡, *Radix Peucedani*) 1 liang, Baizhi (白芷, *Radix Angelicae Dahuricae*) 1 liang, Fuzi (附子, *Radix Aconiti Lateralis Preparata*) 30 pieces.

It is applicable for many illnesses, such as wind

头面诸病、青盲风、烂眦鼻、耳聋、寒齿痛，痈肿疽痔、金疮、癣疥悉主之。(《肘后备急方·卷八》)

stroke and pathogenic qi, head and facial illnesses, vision declining, nose ulcer, deafness, toothache, abscess, furuncle, deep-rooted ulcer, haemorrhoid, incised wound, and mange.

Cut the above Chinese herbal medicines and decoct them with 10 jin lard. Once boiling, remove the container from the coals and repeat this process for 3 times. Ultimately, the Baizhi in the decoction should be in yellow. Remove the residues, and store this decoction in a sealed container.

For external illnesses, patient can massage the painful area with this ointment. (From volume 8 of the *Emergency Formulas to Keep Up One's Sleeve*)

（3）卫候青膏：当归、瓜蒌根、干地黄、甘草、蜀椒各六两，半夏七合，桂心、芎䓖、细辛、附子各四两，黄芩、桔梗、天雄、藜芦、皂荚各一两半，厚朴、乌头、莽草、干姜、人参、黄连、寄生、续断、戎盐各三两，黄野葛二分，生竹茹六升，巴豆二十枚，石楠、杏仁各一两。

治百病，久风头眩，鼻塞，清涕，泪出，霍乱吐逆，伤寒咽痛，脊背头项强、偏枯拘挛，或缓或急，或心腹久寒，积聚疼痛，咳逆上气，往来寒热，鼠漏瘰疬，历节疼肿，关节尽痛，男子七伤，胪胀，腹满，羸瘦不能饮食，妇人生产遗疾诸病，疥恶疮痈肿，阴蚀，黄疸，发背，马鞍牛领疮肿方。

猪脂三斗，苦酒一斗六升。上三十一味，诸药以苦酒渍一宿，以猪脂微火上煎之，三上三下，膏成。病在内，以酒服，如半枣。在外，摩，日三。(《备急千金要方·卷

(3) Weihou Green Ointment: Danggui (当归, *Radix Angelicae Sinensis*) 6 liang, Gualougen (瓜蒌根, *Mongolian Snakegourd Root*) 6 liang, Shengdihuang (生地黄, *Radix Rehmanniae Recens*) 6 liang, Gancao (甘草, *Radix Glycyrrhizae*) 6 liang, Shujiao (蜀椒, *Pricklyash Peel*) 6 liang, Banxia (半夏, *Rhizoma Pinelliae*) 7 he, Guixin (桂心, *Cassia Bark*) 4 liang, Chuanxiong (川芎, *Rhizoma Ligustici Chuanxiong*) 4 liang, Xixin (细辛, *Herba Asari*) 4 liang, Fuzi (附子, *Radix Aconiti Lateralis Preparata*) 4 liang, Huangqin (黄芩, *Radix Scutellariae*) 1.5 liang, Jiegeng (桔梗, *Radix Platycodonis*) 1.5 liang, Tianxiong (天雄, *Radix Aconiti carmichaeli*) 1.5 liang, Lilu (藜芦, *Veratrum nigrum Linn*) 1.5 liang, Zaojia (皂荚, *Gleditsia sinensis Lam*) 1.5 liang, Houpo (厚朴, *Cortex Magnoliae Officinalis*) 3 liang, Chuanwu (川乌, *Radix Aconiti*) 3 liang, Mangcao (莽草, *Illicium henryi Diels*) 3 liang, Ganjiang (干姜, *Rhizoma Zingiberis*) 3 liang, Renshen (人参, *Radix Ginseng*) 3 liang, Huanglian (黄连, *Rhizoma Coptidis*) 3 liang, Sangjisheng (桑寄生, *Herba Taxilli*) 3 liang, Xuduan (续断, *Radix Dipsaci*) 3 liang, Rong salt 3 liang, Gegen (葛根, *Radix Puerariae*) 2 fen, Zhuru (竹茹, *Caulis Bambusae in Taenia*) 6 shen, Badou (巴豆, *Fructus Crotonis*) 20 pieces, Shinan (石

七·风毒脚气》）

楠, *Photiniae Folia*) 1 liang, Xingren (杏仁, *Semen Armeniacae Amarum*) 1 liang.

It is said that Weihou green ointment is applicable for hundreds of diseases, including dizziness, stuffy and running nose, tears for no reasons, vomiting resulted by cholera, cold damage, sore throat, headache with neck rigidity, spastic paralysis caused by stroke, other chronic and acute diseases, pain in heart and abdomen caused by coldness, cough, alternating fever and chills, scrofula, severe and migratory joint pain and swelling, seven damages, abdominal distension, emaciation with diet prohibition, various diseases caused by women's childbirth, scabies, abscess, vulvar ulceration, and yellow deep-rooted ulcer.

Soak the above Chinese medicines with 1 dou 6 shen vinegar for one night. Then, decoct them with 3 dou lard. Once boiling, remove the container from the coals and repeat this process 3 times. For diseases inside the body, patients should take the paste with liquor; for diseases outside, patients should use the ointment to massage the site 3 times a day. (From volume 7 of the *Important Formulas Worth a Thousand Gold Pieces for Emergency*)

（4）摩膏方：蓖麻子（去皮，研）一两半，草乌头（生，为末）半两，乳香（研）一钱。

治打仆内损疼痛。

上三味，一切和匀，量多少，入炼成猪脂研为膏。每取少许，涂伤处，炙手摩之，令热取效，如痛甚不可摩。(《圣济总录·卷第一百四十五·打仆损伤》)

(4) Massage Ointment: Bimazi (蓖麻子, *Semen Ricini*) 1.5 liang (peeled and ground), Caowutou (草乌头, *Radix Aconiti Agrestis*) 0.5 liang (raw and powdered), Ruxiang (乳香, *Olibanum*) 1 qian (ground).

It is applicable for sprain on tendons and bones.

Mix the above three kinds of medicine, and decoct them with lard.

During application, take a small amount of the ointment and apply it to the wound, rub hands hot and then massage the wound to help promote absorption. But massage is prohibited if the wound is too painful. (From volume 145 of *Comprehensive Recording of Divine Assistance*)

（5）生肌膏方：大黄、芎䓖、芍药、黄芪、独活、当归、白芷以

(5) Tissue-regenerating Ointment: Dahuang (大黄, *Radix et Rhizoma Rhei*) 1 liang, Chuanxiong (川

上各一两，慈白二两（另方一两），生地黄一两（另方二两）。

治痈疽金疮。

上九味合，以猪脂三升煎，三上三下，白芷色黄膏成，绞去滓，磨之，多少随其意。(《刘涓子鬼遗方·卷二》)

芎, *Rhizoma Ligustici Chuanxiong*) 1 liang, Baishao (白芍, *Radix Paeoniae Alba*) 1 liang, Huangqi (黄芪, *Radix Astragali seu Hedysari*) 1 liang, Duhuo (独活, *Radix Angelicae Pubescentis*) 1 liang, Danggui (当归, *Radix Angelicae Sinensis*) 1 liang, Baizhi (白芷, *Radix Angelicae Dahuricae*) 1 liang, Xiebai (薤白, *Bulbus Allii Macrostemonis*) 2 liang / 1 liang, Shengdihuang (生地黄, *Radix Rehmanniae Recens*) 1 liang/ 2 liang.

It is applicable for abscess, deep-rooted ulcer, and incised wound.

For this prescription, 2 liang Xiebai matches 1 liang Shengdihuang, or 1 liang Xiebai matches 2 liang Shengdihuang. Decoct the above Chinese medicines with 3 shen lard. Once boiling, remove the container from the coals and repeat this process 3 times. Ultimately, the Baizhi in the decoction should be in yellow. Remove the residues, and grind it into ointment. When applying, the amount of ointment depends on the case. (From volume 2 of *Liu Juan-zi's Ghost-Bequeathed Formulas*)

（6）青膏方：当归、芎䓖、蜀椒、白芷、吴茱萸、附子、乌头、莽草各三两。

治伤寒头痛项强，四肢烦疼。

上八味，以醇苦酒渍之再宿，以猪脂四斤煎，令药色黄，绞去滓，以温酒服枣核大三枚，日三服，取汗，不知稍增。可服可摩。如初得伤寒一日，苦头痛背强，宜摩之佳。(《备急千金要方上·卷九·伤寒上》)

(6) Green Ointment: Danggui (当归, *Radix Angelicae Sinensis*) 3 liang, Chuanxiong (川芎, *Rhizoma Ligustici Chuanxiong*) 3 liang, Shujiao (蜀椒, *Pricklyash Peel*) 3 liang, Baizhi (白芷, *Radix Angelicae Dahuricae*) 3 liang, Wuzhuyu (吴茱萸, *Fructus Evodiae*) 3 liang, Fuzi (附子, *Radix Aconiti Lateralis Preparata*) 3 liang, Chuanwu (川乌, *Radix Aconiti*) 3 liang, Mangcao (莽草, *Illicium henryi Diels*) 3 liang.

It is applicable for cold damage, headache with neck rigidity, and intense pain in limbs.

Soak the above Chinese medicines with vinegar for two nights. Decoct them with 4 jin lard until the color of the decoction turns to yellow, then remove the residues. This ointment can be used orally or topically. When taken orally, take 3 pieces a time with warm liquor for 3 times a day, and each piece is as big as a date kernel. The effect of the medicine is characterized by sweating, and the dosage can be increased if the effect is not obvious. When applied topically, it is suitable to be used in the first day of cold damage, and if the patient has the symptoms of headache and back rigidity, massage these regions with this ointment is the best. (From volume 9 of *Important Formulas Worth a Thousand Gold Pieces for Emergency*)

（7）摩腰方：巴戟一两，附子一两（生，去皮、脐），阳起石一两（细研），硫黄一两（细研），雄雀粪一两，川椒一两（去目），干姜一两，木香一两，菟丝子一两（酒浸三日，曝干，别捣为末），韭子一两（微炒）。

治久冷腰痛。

捣箩为末，以真野驼脂熬成油，滤去膜，待冷，入诸药末，和丸如弹子大。洗浴了，取一丸分作四丸，于腰眼上，热炙，手摩之。（《太平圣惠方·卷四十四·治久腰痛诸方》）

(7) Waist-massaging Ointment: Bajitian (巴戟天, *Radix Morindae Officinalis*) 1 liang, Fuzi (附子, *Radix Aconiti Lateralis Preparata*) 1 liang (raw and peeled), Yangqishi (阳起石, *Actinolite*) 1 liang (ground), Liuhuang (硫黄, *Sulfur*) 1 liang (ground), Xiongquefen (雄雀粪, *feces of Passer montanus saturatus Stejieger or Passer rutilans rutilans* (*Temminck*)) 1 liang, Chuanjiao (川椒, *Zanthoxyli Pericarpium*) 1 liang (without seeds), Ganjiang (干姜, *Rhizoma Zingiberis*) 1 liang, Muxiang (木香, *Radix Aucklandiae*) 1 liang, Tusizi (菟丝子, *Semen Cuscutae*) 1 liang (first soaked in liquor for 3 days, then expose to dry, and ground into powder), Jiucaizi (韭菜子, *Semen Allii Tuberosi*) 1 liang (fried).

It is applicable for waist pain caused by long time coldness.

Grind the above medicines, and sift the mixture through a fine sieve. Boil camel fat into oil, and filter the membrane above the oil. Cool the oil and mix it into the medicinal mixture, and make the paste into some small round balls. After showering, take a ball and divide it into 4 smaller balls, put them on the waist and massage with warming. (From volume 44 of *Formulas from Benevolent Sages Compiled during the Taiping Era*)

（8）木防己膏：木防己半升，茵芋五两。

治产后中风。

上二味，以苦酒九升，渍一宿，猪膏四升，煎三上三下，膏成，炙手摩千遍。（《备急千金要方·卷三·妇人方上》）

(8) Orbicular Snailseed Root Ointment: Mufangji (木防己, *Radix Cocculi Orbiculati*) 0.5 shen, Yinyu (茵芋, *Skimmiae Reevesianae Caulis et Folium*) 5 liang.

It is applicable for wind attack after childbirth.

Soak the above Chinese medicines with 9 shen vinegar for a night, then decoct them with 4 shen lard. Once boiling, remove the container from the coals and repeat this process 3 times. When applying this ointment, warm the hands first, and massage the treated area for thousands of times. (From volume 3 of *Important Formulas Worth a Thousand Gold Pieces for Emergency*)

（9）五物甘草生摩膏方：甘草、防风各一两，白术二十铢，雷丸二两半，桔梗二十铢。

治少小新生肌肤幼弱，喜为风邪所中，身体壮热，或中大风，手足惊掣。

以不中水猪肪一斤煎为膏。以煎药，微火上煎之，稍息视稠浊，膏成去滓。取如弹丸大一枚，炙手以摩儿百过。寒者更热，热者更寒，小儿虽无病，早起常以膏摩囟上及手足心，甚辟寒风。（《备急千金要方·卷五上·少小婴孺方上》）

(9) Five Ingredients Massaging Ointment: Gancao (甘草, *Radix Glycyrrhizae*) 1 liang, Fangfeng (防风, *Radix Saposhnikoviae*) 1 liang, Baizhu (白术, *Rhizoma Atractylodis Macrocephalae*) 20 zhu, Leiwan (雷丸, *Omphalia*) 2.5 liang, Jiegeng (桔梗, *Radix Platycodonis*) 20 zhu.

It is applicable for wind attack, high fever, and jerking of the hands and feet in small children.

Decoct these medicines with 1 jin lard until the mixture turns into thick paste, then remove the residues. Take the ointment as big as a pellet, warm the hands, and massage the body of the children for over a hundred times. This manipulation treats cold with heat and treats heat with clod. For children without illness, apply the ointment to massage on their top of the head and center areas of the hands and feet can dispel the cold wind. (From volume 5 of *Important Formulas Worth a Thousand Gold Pieces for Emergency*)

（10）治少小鼻塞不通及涕出方：杏仁半两，蜀椒、附子、细辛各六铢。

上四味以醋五合，渍药一宿，明旦以猪脂五合，煎令附子色黄，膏成去滓，待冷以涂絮道鼻孔中，日再兼摩顶上。（《备急千金要方·卷五下·少小婴孺方下》）

(10) Ointment for Stuffy and Runny Nose in Children: Kuxingren (苦杏仁, *Semen Armeniacae Amarum*) 0.5 liang, Shujiao (蜀椒, *Pricklyash Peel*) 6 zhu, Fuzi (附子, *Radix Aconiti Lateralis Preparata*) 6 zhu, Xixin (细辛, *Herba Asari*) 6 zhu.

Soak these Chinese medicines with 5 he vinegars for a night, and decoct them with 5 he lards in the next day until the color of Fuzi turns into yellow. Remove residues and set aside for cooling. This ointment can be applied to the nostrils and the top of the head with massaging. (From volume 5 of *Important Formulas Worth a Thousand Gold Pieces for Emergency*)

第三节 热敷

Section Three Hot compress

热敷法是采用药物和适当的辅料经过加热或辅助以形态的束缚，敷于患部或腧穴。它借助温热之力，将药物渗透皮毛腠理，循经运行，内达脏腑，从而产生防治疾病的作用。热敷法是中医独特有效的外治法之一，由于操作简单，取材方便，费用低廉，安全性高，临床应用广泛。

药物外敷疗法的产生与人类用植物、泥浆之类涂敷伤口的自发行为有关，随着局部按压和敷药重复操作，发现具有止血、止痛、消肿，甚至加速创伤的愈合的作用，此类经验不断总结和发展逐步形成一种外治疗法。

古代的热敷方法很多，诸如药熨、汤熨、酒熨、葱熨、铁熨、盐熨、土熨等。《五十二病方》和《黄帝内经》中记载的“熨”法就是热敷法。《灵枢·经筋》曰：“足阳明之筋……颊筋有寒，则急引颊移口；有热则筋弛纵缓不胜收，故僻。治之以马膏，膏其急者，以白酒和桂，以涂其缓者，以桑钩钩之，即以生桑灰置之坎中，高下以坐等，以膏熨急颊。”

根据热敷用具湿度的特点，热敷可分干热敷和湿热敷。干热敷就是用黄豆、盐、沙、土、药等炒热

Hot compress is a common external therapy in Chinese medicine to treat diseases through heat stimulation on specific positions or acupuncture points. Through heat stimulation, medicine penetrate into the skin and interstices, and ultimately achieve the internal organs through meridians and collaterals, so as to prevent and treat diseases. It is one of the unique and effective TCM external therapies. And it is widely applied, for it is easy to operate, accessible, affordable, and safe.

The origin of hot compress is related to people's spontaneous behavior of coating wound with plants, mud and so on. After several times of pressing and applying medicine to the wound, people found that these methods are able to stop bleeding, relieve pain, disperse swelling and even speed up the recovery of the wound. Therefore, after continuous summing up of experience and development, this external therapy was formed.

There are many categories of hot compress in ancient times, such as hot compress with medicine, with hot water, with liquor, with scallion white (stalk), with iron powder, with salt, with mud, and so on. The "Yun (熨)" method in *Formulas for Fifty-two Diseases* and the *Yellow Emperor's Canon of Medicine* all refers to hot compress. It was recorded in the chapter 13 of *Ling Shu* that "If there is cold in the cheek tendon, it will contract the cheek and mouth; if there is heat in the cheek, the tendon will become flaccid and the mouth will become wry. This disease can be treated by horse fat which is applied to the contracted regions. The mixture of white liquor with cinnamon is applied to the flaccid regions to adjust distortion. Then a

放于袋中敷于患处。湿热敷是将热敷毛巾等用具浸泡在熬煮好的药液内，绞干取出，趁热敷在患处。内功推拿流派临床治疗以湿热敷为常用。根据不同的热敷方法，热敷用具可以灵活变通。民间也往往就地取材选用泥坯、砖加热后浇醋裹上毛巾做热敷。此外，热敷也可以用一个布袋做敷料收纳容器，将熬煮中药的渣滓收纳于布袋以做热敷，布袋有收纳药物作用，还可以提供形状塑造，以之做热敷可以调整脊柱生理弧度，也有支撑作用。

piece of mulberry stick is used as a hook which is attached to the angle of the mouth. And then mulberry charcoal is burnt in a basin which is put at the level of a place that the patient is able to warm his or her cheek with it. At the same time, horse fat is applied to the affected regions over the cheeks."

Hot compress can be categorized into dry hot compress and wet hot compress. Soybean, salt, sand, mud and medicine are stir-fried and put into bags for dry hot compress. While wet hot compress is to soak towels in hot decoctions, then wring out the wet towel and put it on the area to be treated. For the school of Neigong Tuina, wet hot compress is more common in clinical treatment. Various tools are employed in different categories of hot compress. In grassroots level, people usually choose to heat clay or a brick, pour vinegar on them and wrap towel around them to perform hot compress. Besides, cloth bags are also recommended to be containers for hot compress. Dregs of decoctions are storied in the cloth bag for hot compress. Cloth bags can contain medicine and the shape of cloth bag can be changed to adjust the curvature of the spine.

一、操作方法

热敷法分为干热敷和湿热敷，可以单独操作，也可以在推拿之后操作。

1. 干热敷法

干热敷一般用布袋收纳，布袋制作可以用两层A4纸大小的布，三边缝合，一端用绳子做收口，方便使用。

热敷辅具材料可选黄豆、粗盐、沙、中药、小鹅卵石等。加热方法多种（微波炉加热、蒸汽熏蒸、锅内炒热均可），放入布袋，收口固

Manipulations

Hot compress can be categorized into dry hot compress and wet hot compress. It can be operated alone or after tuina.

1. Dry hot compress

Cloth bags are usually employed in dry hot compress. Sew two pieces of A4-sized cloth together, and choose one side as the opening where can be easily opened and closed by using ropes.

Choose soybean, crude salt, sand, materia medica, or small pebbles as the materials stuffed in the bag. Heat those materials in a container (microwave, steamer, or

定，趁热敷于特定部位。也可以将60～70℃的热水灌满热水袋后装入暖水袋，用布套或用布包裹于敷于患处。

2. 湿热敷法

将选好的药物用布袋装好收口扎紧，放入砂锅内或铝锅内，加适量清水，煮沸5～10分钟，趁热将毛巾浸透绞干，折成方形或长条，贴敷患病部位，待毛巾不太热时，换另一块毛巾操作。可用三个毛巾轮换。每次热敷时间不宜超过30分钟，每日2次。本法常用于擦法之后，使得局部毛孔开放，随机热毛巾敷上，并施以轻拍法，以增加热量渗透，待患者感到热量稍减，可以施加按压法，以使中心热药汁带热量渗透而出，以延长单次热敷时间。亦可将熬煮的药渣布袋趁热取出，裹以毛巾，少许挤干药汁，趁热垫于腰背之下，已达热敷效果。

另外，亦可采用药饼（糊）热敷法。将药物直接捣烂调拌面粉做成饼并放入笼上蒸熟，或将药物研成细末，调拌辅料做成饼或糊状，加热后敷于治疗部位；也可捣烂新鲜药物或调拌油料类药物直接捏饼；也可以将糊剂或饼剂着于患处，用艾绒搓柱放其上，点燃后加热操作，类似临床隔物灸的操作。

pot). Put them in the bag, close the bag, and put the bag in a specific position of the body. You can also fill a hot water bag with hot water at 60 to 70 degrees, and put it on the affected area with a cloth wrapped around.

2. Wet hot compress

Put the materia medica in a cloth bag, place the bag in a pot with some water and boil it for 5 to 10 minutes. Soak towels into hot decoctions, then wring out the wet towel and put it on the affected area. Change the towel when it is not hot enough. The treatment time shouldn't longer than 30 minutes once, and it is appropriate to apply the hot compress two times a day. This method is usually employed after the linear rubbing manipulation. First stimulate the opening of pores and then apply the hot towel with patting manipulation. When patients feel the reduction of the heat, practitioners can apply pressing manipulation to squeeze the hot decoction. Or the practitioner can take the bag out and wrap it with a towel, squeeze it and put it under the waist of the patient.

Moreover, other four methods can be applied for hot compress. Pound those Chinese medicines, mix medicines with flour to make cakes and put them on a steamer. Grind Chinese medicines into powder, mix them with other supplements to shape cakes or pastes, and put pastes on the area to be treated after heating. Pound fresh herbs or blend oily herbs to shape cakes. Medicinal cakes and pastes can be directly put on the affected area with lighted moxa sticks on them. This manipulation is similar to that of indirect moxibustion.

二、施术部位和体位

Affected Areas and Body Positions

热敷部位多为病变局部，颈项、肩背、腰部、腹部、四指关节部位

Hot compress can be applied in neck, shoulder and back, waist, abdomen, and knuckles. Based on TCM

均可操作。根据中医理论选择腧穴部位进行热敷，如阳痿可选肾俞、命门等。

热敷体位可根据患者情况灵活选用，可采用仰卧位、俯卧位、侧卧位、坐位或俯伏坐位，以稳固、持久、舒适为度。

theories, this therapy can be used in specific acupoint. For diseases like impotence, hot compress should be used in Shenshu (BL 23) or Mingmen (GV 4).

During the manipulation of hot compress, patients can be in supine position, prone position, side position, or sit position. Patients should make sure that the position is stable, long-lasting and comfortable.

三、适应证

热敷可以治疗软组织损伤所引起的病痛，如常见的肩周炎、网球肘、腰椎间盘突出症等各种闭合性损伤及关节炎所引起的疼痛。热敷还应根据中医脏腑理论、经络学说辨证选用，对慢性内科、妇科、男科疾病，如某些慢性胃肠道疾病、急性乳腺炎早期、阳痿、不育、痛经、卵巢多发性囊肿、宫寒不孕、早期尚未排脓的疖肿、淋巴结炎、麦粒肿、牙痛、尿潴留、术后腹胀等病症有治疗作用。

Indications

Hot compress can treat pains caused by soft tissue injuries, such as frozen shoulder, tennis elbow, and lumbar disc herniation. In addition, it is also effective for treatment of diseases of chronic internal medicine, gynecology and male medicine, such as chronic gastrointestinal diseases, acute mastitis in early stages, impotence, sterility, dysmenorrhea, ovarian multiple cysts, infertility, swollen boil in early stages, lymphadenitis, stye, toothache, urinary retention, postoperative abdominal distention.

四、注意事项

（1）注意保暖，预防受凉。本法一般在室内进行施药，但在冷天或严寒季节施药时，室内宜空调加温，或覆盖衣被保温。尤其体虚患者、老年人及小儿更为重要。

（2）热敷局部乙醇消毒，防止烫伤溃破后感染。

（3）毛巾必须折叠平整，使热量均匀透入，且不易烫伤皮肤。

Cautions

(1) Keep warm and be careful not to catch cold. This therapy is usually operated indoors. Therefore, please open the air conditioners to keep warm in cold seasons, or cover with thick coat and blanket, especially for children, the old, and weak patients.

(2) Please disinfect the local position with alcohol before applying hot compress, so as to prevent bacterial infections.

(3) Towels need to be folded neatly, so as to allow the

（4）湿热敷时可隔着毛巾做拍法，待热稍减可用轻按法，切忌用揉法。被敷部位一般不再施加其他手法，否则容易破皮，所以热敷手法均在手法操作结束之后。

（5）热敷毛巾的干湿与药液温度高低密切相关。药液温度较高时，应迅速取出用力绞拧毛巾，使得毛巾越干越好；药液温度不烫手后，药汁可以略多些，以不滴水为度。

（6）热敷的温度应以患者耐受为限，要防止发生烫伤和晕厥。对于年长、糖尿病末梢感觉异常者尤需注意。

（7）关节扭伤初期（36 小时以内）禁用热敷，因热敷可能加重出血和肿胀。

heat penetrate into the skin evenly.

(4) Wet hot compress can be accompanied with patting manipulation. If the temperature of towel is appropriate, pressing manipulation is also allowed in the treatment process, but kneading manipulation is strictly prohibited. With the principle that do not abrade the skin, hot compress is always applied after tuina manipulations.

(5) The degree of wet towels for hot compress should depend on the temperature of the decoction. When the decoction temperature is high, the towel should be drier. If the towel is not that hot, it doesn't need to be so dry, just not dripping is enough.

(6) The temperature of hot compress should be differentiated from person to person, and burns and fainting should be prevented. Therefore, practitioners need to pay more attention to the old, patients with diabetes, and those who are sensitive to temperature.

(7) This therapy is prohibited in the early stage (within 36 hours) of joints sprain, for hot compress may strengthen the bleeding and swelling.

五、作用原理

Mechanism

热敷法具有温和通的功效，温以散寒、通以活血，在中医理论的指导下，通过辨证选用中草药，并借用温热之力，可使药性直达病所，从而更加充分地发挥中药所具有的补气血、祛风寒、活血通络、化瘀止痛等各种作用。寒得解，气血和，则痛止，脏腑功能得到调节。热敷疗法还具有经络调整作用，在体表给药，药物之性味由经络入脏腑，输布全身，直达病所，达到补虚泻实、调整阴阳、治疗疾病的目的。

Hot compress has functions of warming and unblocking. Under the guidance of TCM theories, TCM physicians select herbs and make their natures affect the position directly through warming and heating, showing the herb's roles of tonifying qi and blood, dispelling wind coldness, circulating blood and unblocking collaterals, and transforming stasis and alleviating pain. If the coldness is dispelled and the qi and blood are harmonious, the pain will be alleviated and the functions of internal organs will be regulated. Hot compress also has functions of regulating meridians and collaterals. After applying materia medica on the body surface, properties and flavors of herbs can

现代医学认为，热敷能使局部皮肤温度升高，血管扩张，毛细血管内皮细胞间隙加宽，通透性增加，药物被有效吸收，从而更好地发挥药物的作用；热敷通过促进毛细血管、淋巴管的扩张，能改善局部血液循环及淋巴循环，促进新陈代谢，改善局部组织营养和全身功能，加速水肿和炎性物质的吸收，促使损伤组织的修复；温热刺激还可以缓解肌紧张、肌痉挛，达到解痉止痛的目的；温热刺激还能够活跃网状内皮系统的吞噬能力，提高人体免疫力；温热能够使人体紧张情绪放松，调节自主神经功能。

热敷法也有采用特殊刺激作用的药物。药物本身刺激体表局部，加之温热物理作用，使局部血管扩张，加速血液循环而改善周围组织的营养，可起到消炎退肿的作用。某些刺激性较强的药物，强烈刺激外周感觉神经，可通过神经反射激发机体的调节作用，从而使机体的某些抗体形成，提高机体的免疫力。

affect internal organs through meridians and collaterals, spreading over the whole body to treat diseases. It helps achieving aims of tonifying the deficiency and discharging the excess, regulating yin-yang, and treating illnesses.

Experts of modern medicine state that hot compress increases the skin temperature, enlarges blood vessels, and widens capillary endothelial cell gap to make medicinal be absorbed more effectively. Moreover, through stimulating the enlargement of capillaries and lymphatic vessels, hot compress improves the local circulation of blood and lymph, facilitates the metabolism, enhances the local tissue's nutrition and the whole body's functions, speeds up the elimination of edema and inflammation, and strengthens the recovery of injured tissues. In addition, hot compress relieves convulsions and stops pain, activates phagocytic function of reticuloendothelial system and boosts human immunity, and relieves the pressure and regulates autonomic nervous functions.

Practitioners also can apply medicinal with stimulating effects in hot compress. Local position is stimulated by medicinal, and blood vessels in that area are dilated because of warming. In this way, blood circulation will speed up and bring more nutrients for surrounding tissues, thus alleviating inflammation and dispersing swelling. Some medicinal with strong stimulant can spur the peripheral sensory nerves and inspire the regulation function of our body. In this way, some antibodies are formed and people's immunity is boosted.

六、湿热敷方药

Formulas and Chinese Medicines of Wet Hot Compress

湿热敷法是内功推拿流派有代表特色的操作流程之一。一般选用具有祛风散寒、温经通络、活血止痛作用的中草药。临床根据不同疾

Medicines with the functions of dispelling wind and dissipating cold, warming meridians and unblocking collaterals, and circulating blood and stopping pain are

病的病因病机，在中医理论的指导下，按照辨证论治的原则选用。临床中可根据病情选用下述药物。

（1）活血化瘀类药物：当归、乳香、没药、川芎、鸡血藤、桃仁、红花、牛膝、降香、赤芍、苏木、血竭等。

（2）祛风除湿类药物：独活、威灵仙、防己、秦艽、木瓜、徐长卿、海桐皮、透骨草、海风藤、千年健、松节、伸筋草、忍冬藤等。

（3）散寒止痛类药物：桂枝、麻黄、生姜、防风、羌活、附子、干姜、肉桂、吴茱萸、花椒、丁香等。

always used in wet hot compress. In clinical practice, physicians usually choose medicines according to the etiological factors and pathogenesis of different diseases under the guidance of TCM theories and based on the pattern identification treatment principles. The followings are some Chinese medicines in practice.

(1) Activate blood and resolve stasis: Danggui (当归, *Radix Angelicae Sinensis*), Ruxiang (乳香, *Olibanum*), Moyao (没药, *Myrrha*), Chuanxiong (川芎, *Rhizoma Ligustici Chuanxiong*), Jixueteng (鸡血藤, *Caulis Spatholobi*), Taoren (桃仁, *Semen Persicae*), Honghua (红花, *Flos Carthami*), Niuxi (牛膝, *Radix Achyranthis Bidentatae*), Jiangxiang (降香, *Lignum Dalbergiae Odoriferae*), Chishao (赤芍, *Radix Paeoniae Rubra*), Sumu (苏木, *Lignum Sappan*), Xuejie (血竭, *Sanguis Draconis*).

(2) Dispel wind and eliminate dampness: Duhuo (独活, *Radix Angelicae Pubescentis*), Weilingxian (威灵仙, *Radix Clematidis*), Fangji (防己, *Radix Stephaniae Tetrandrae*), Qinjiao (秦艽, *Radix Gentianae Macrophyllae*), Mugua (木瓜, *Fructus Chaenomelis*), Xuchangqing (徐长卿, *Radix Cynanchi Paniculati*), Haitongpi (海桐皮, *Cortex Erythrinae*), Tougucao (透骨草, *Herb of Tuberculate Speranskia*), Haifengteng (海风藤, *Caulis Piperis Kadsurae*), Qiannianjian (千年健, *Rhizoma Homalomenae*), Songjie (松节, *Lignum Pini Nodi*), Shenjincao (伸筋草, *Herba Lycopodii*), Rendongteng (忍冬藤, *Caulis Lonicerae*).

(3) Dissipate cold and relieve pain: Guizhi (桂枝, *Ramulus Cinnamomi*), Mahuang (麻黄, *Herba Ephedrae*), Fresh ginger (生姜, *Rhizoma Zingiberis Recens*), Fangfeng (防风, *Radix Saposhnikoviae*), Qianghuo (羌活, *Rhizoma et Radix Notopterygii*), Fuzi (附子, *Radix Aconiti Lateralis Preparata*), Ganjiang (干姜, *Rhizoma Zingiberis*), Rougui (肉桂, *Cortex Cinnamomi*), Wuzhuyu (吴茱萸, *Fructus Evodiae*), Huajiao (花椒, *Pericarpium Zanthoxyli*), Dingxiang (丁香, *Flos Caryophylli*).

（4）行气通经类药物：木香、香附、沉香、檀香、橘皮、桑枝、路路通、冰片、地龙、丝瓜络等。

（5）强筋壮骨类药物：补骨脂、自然铜、续断、天麻、鳖甲、杜仲等。

热敷方组成时，可在以上各类药物中，每类选取2～4味，全方由12～14味药物组成，每味药用量10～30 g。

现介绍推拿伤科常用的2个热敷方，以供临床参考使用。

（1）传统推拿热敷方：红花10 g，桂枝15 g，乳香10 g，没药10 g，苏木50 g，香樟木50 g，宣木瓜10 g，老紫草15 g，伸筋草15 g，钻地风10 g，路路通15 g，千年健15 g。主治扭伤、挫伤、风湿疼痛、局部怕冷、关节酸痛等。

（2）简化推拿热敷方：香樟木50 g，豨莶草30 g，桑枝50 g，虎杖根50 g。主治因扭挫伤而引起的疼痛肿胀，并治肢体酸楚等。

(4) Move qi and unblock the meridian: Muxiang (木香, *Radix Aucklandiae*), Xiangfu (香附, *Rhizoma Cyperi*), Chenxiang (沉香, *Lignum Aquilariae Resinatum*), Tanxiang (檀香, *Lignum Santali Albi*), Jupi (橘皮, *Tangerine Peel*), Sangzhi (桑枝, *Ramulus Mori*), Lulutong (路路通, *Fructus Liquidambaris*), Bingpian (冰片, *Bomeolum Syntheticum*), Dilong (地龙, *Lumbricus*), Sigualuo (丝瓜络, *Retinervus Luffae Fructus*).

(5) Strengthen sinew and invigorate bone: Buguzhi (补骨脂, *Fructus Psoraleae*), Zirantong (自然铜, *Pyritum*), Xuduan (续断, *Radix Dipsaci*), Tianma (天麻, *Rhizoma Gastrodiae*), Biejia (鳖甲, *Carapax Trionycis*), Duzhong (杜仲, *Cortex Eucommiae*).

When forming formulas, 2 to 4 medicines can be selected in every types. Hence, there are 12 to 14 medicines in one formula, and 10 to 30 g of each medicinel.

There are two common formulas of hot compress for clinical practice.

(1) Traditional hot compress formula: Honghua (红花, *Flos Carthami*) 10 g, Guizhi (桂枝, *Ramulus Cinnamomi*) 15 g, Ruxiang (乳香, *Olibanum*) 10 g, Moyao (没药, *Myrrha*) 10 g, Sumu (苏木, *Lignum Sappan*) 50 g, Xiangzhangmu [香樟木, *Cinnamomum camphora* (L.) *Presl*] 50 g, Xuanmugua (宣木瓜, *Fruit of Common Flowering quince*) 10 g, Laozicao (老紫草, *Radix Sinkiang Arnebia*) 15 g, Shenjincao (伸筋草, *Herba Lycopodii*) 15 g, Zuandifeng (钻地风, *Root-bark of Chinese Hydrangeavine*) 10 g, Lulutong (路路通, *Fructus Liquidambaris*) 15 g, Qiannianjian (千年健, *Rhizoma Homalomenae*) 15 g. This formula is suitable for the treatment of sprain, contusion, wind-dampness pain, fear of cold in specific positions, aching pain of joints, and so on.

(2) Simplified hot compress formula: Xiangzhangmu [香樟木, *Cinnamomum camphora* (L.) *Presl*] 50 g, Xixiancao (豨莶草, *Herba Siegesbeckiae*) 30 g, Sangzhi (桑枝, *Ramulus Mori*) 50 g, Huzhanggen (虎杖根, *Rhizoma Polygoni Cuspidate*) 50 g. This formula is suitable for the treatment

of pain and swelling caused by sprain and contusion, and body soreness.

第四节 熏蒸

Section Four Fumigation

熏蒸是指用中药煮沸之后产生的蒸汽熏蒸患者全身或局部，利用药性、水和蒸汽等刺激作用来达到防病治病的一种方法。熏蒸疗法属于中医常用的外治方法之一，是以中医学基本理论为指导，通过局部体表的经皮吸收到达病所，根据不同的熏蒸药物方可起到滋养津液、滋润肌肤、健脾和胃、壮肾利水、舒筋活络、强筋壮骨等作用。

熏蒸疗法历史久远，马王堆汉墓出土的《五十二病方》已记载熏洗方8首，用熏蒸治疗痔瘘、烧伤、毒虫咬伤等多种病症。秦汉时期开始了对熏蒸理论的探索，《黄帝内经》有言“善治者治皮毛，其次治肌肤。”认为疾病乃邪气由外入侵所致，对疾病的治疗也应从外而解。

《黄帝内经》还记载了用椒、姜、桂和酒煮熏治疗痹证的关节肿胀、疼痛、伸展不利等症状。东汉时期，张仲景在《金匮要略》中记载使用熏蒸治疗大量疾患，充分发挥了其简、廉、效的特点，如雄黄熏蒸治疗狐惑蚀于肛，苦参汤熏洗狐惑，蚀于下部则咽干。唐宋金元时期，熏蒸疗法已广泛用于内、外、

Fumigation is a therapeutic method involves fuming the diseased area or the whole body with the vapor of a boiling decoction and by utilizing both the medicinal and heat effects to prevent and treat diseases. The medicinal vapor achieve the root of diseases through being absorbed by the open interstices, so as to nourish fluid and humor, moisten skin, fortify the spleen and harmonize the stomach, invigorate the kidney and induce diuresis, relax sinews and activate collaterals, and enhance sinews and bones.

Fumigation therapy has a long history. There are 8 fumigation formulas recorded in *Formulas for Fifty-two Diseases* unearthed from Mawangdui Han Tomb, stating that fumigation is effective for the treatment of hemorrhoid and fistula, burns, poisonous insect bite, and so on. The exploration of fumigation theories was started from the Qin and the Han Dynasties. *The Yellow Emperor's Canon of Medicine* mentions that "Excellent doctors treat diseases when pathogenic factors have just invaded the skin and hair; ordinary doctors treat diseases when pathogenic factors have deepen into the muscles." That is, diseases were caused by pathogenic qi, therefore, the treatment should begin from the external, too.

Moreover, *The Yellow Emperor's Canon of Medicine* also recorded that ginger can be boiled with wine in fumigation to treat swelling, pain, and extension disorder of joints caused by impediment. In the eastern Han Dynasty, Zhang Zhongjing's *Essentials from the Golden*

妇、儿、皮肤五官等疾病的防治中。《千金方》将熏蒸疗法分为烟熏法、气熏法、淋洗法等细门，并加以病例佐述。明清时期熏蒸疗法趋于成熟，王肯堂的《证治准绳》、陈实功的《外科正宗》、张介宾的《景岳全书》大量记载了中药熏蒸治疗各类疾病。

内功推拿流派将熏蒸疗法广泛应用于临床实践，不仅用于临床治疗，也用于养生保健。熏蒸疗法还有利于功法训练过程中的身体功能恢复。

Cabinet had the records of fumigation in clinical treatment, showing that this therapy was simple, cheap and effective. In the Tang, Song, Jin, and Yuan Dynasties, fumigation was commonly applied in the treatments and prevention of diseases of internal medicine, surgery, obstetrics and gynecology, pediatrics, and so on. In *Important Formulas Worth a Thousand Gold Pieces*, fumigation therapy was classified into smoke fumigation, qi fumigation, douche, and so on, with cases of diseases listed alongside. In the Ming and the Qing Dynasties, fumigation therapy has been more mature. Many classics in this time talked about fumigation, such as *Standards for Diagnosis and Treatment* of Wang Kentang, *Orthodox Lineage of External Medicine* of Chen Shigong, *The Complete Works of Zhang Jing-yue* of Zhang Jiebin, etc.

For the school of Neigong Tuina, fumigation can be employed in both clinical treatment and life cultivation. Moreover, fumigation can help the body recovery during TCM exercises.

一、操作方法

Manipulations

1. 传统熏蒸法

把药物放在器具里（不锈钢、瓷或瓷砂器具）。然后加水煮沸，找好合适的姿势，把要蒸熏的部位放在器具以上用蒸汽熏蒸，注意避免烫伤，熏蒸时间20～30分钟，最后关火。

2. 药浴机熏蒸法

把药物放在药浴机的中药煮蒸器中煎煮，设置相关参数。药浴机自动控温，自动进水，补水，排水，还配有方便治疗的清洁淋浴花洒和立体音响，熏蒸与音乐疗法相结合，

1. Traditional fumigation

Put Chinese medicines into containers made by stainless steel, porcelain or porcelain sand, then boil them with water. The patient needs to lie down in an appropriate posture, makes the vapor archive on the diseased areas while preventing burns. Twenty to 30 minutes was enough for the treatment, and don't forget to turn off the fire.

2. Fumigation with medicinal bath machine

Put medicines into the boiling container for decocting and set related parameters. This machine will automatically control the temperature and feed and drain water. Moreover, it is equipped with shower and stereo, combines music with treatment, making the effect more significant.

使临床效果更加显著。

二、适应证

熏蒸疗法在内功推拿中用于功法训练早期及训练过程的修复，在临床疾病中常用于：① 风湿类疾病：风湿关节炎、类风湿关节炎、肩周炎、强直性脊柱炎等；② 骨伤类疾病：腰椎间盘突出症、退行性骨关节病、各种急慢性软组织损伤；③ 皮肤类疾病：神经性皮炎、各种癣、疥疮、湿疹、皮肤瘙痒症、扁平疣等；④ 内科：感冒、咳嗽、糖尿病、失眠、神经官能症、血栓闭塞性脉管炎、慢性肠炎；⑤ 妇科：痛经、闭经等。

Indications

Fumigation is commonly applied for the recovery in training process and the early stage of TCM exercise. In clinical treatment, it is usually used for: ① Rheumatic diseases, such as rheumatoid arthritis, scapulohumeral periarthritis, ankylosing spondylitis. ② Orthopedic diseases, such as lumbar disc herniation, degenerative osteoarthropathy, various acute or chronic injuries of soft tissues. ③ Skin diseases, such as neurodermatitis, dermatomycosis, scabies, eczema, pruritus, flat wart. ④ Internal diseases, such as cold, cough, diabetes, insomnia, neurosis, thromboangitis obliterans, chronic enteritis. ⑤ Gynecological diseases, such as dysmenorrhea, amenorrhea.

三、注意事项

（1）使用熏蒸浴具，注意消毒。

（2）实施熏蒸疗法，应注意安全、防止烫伤。各种用具牢固稳妥，热源应当合理放置，药物不应接触患者皮肤。小儿及智力低下、年老体弱者熏蒸时间不宜过长，并需家属陪同。

（3）熏蒸后及时补充水分，适量饮用温开水 300 ～ 500 mL。冬季治疗结束后注意保暖。

（4）治疗期间对辛辣、油腻、甘甜等类食物摄入应适当。不宜使用各种化妆品、洗面奶等。过饥、过饱、过度疲劳，以及饭前饭后30

Cautions

(1) Please remember to disinfect tools used in fumigation.

(2) Please pay attention to the temperature and prevent burns when operating this therapy. All equipment needs to be solidly placed, especially the container of hot water. Please remember that patients' skin should not touch medicines and decoctions in treatment, and children and patients who are old, weak, or have intellectual problems should not be treated for too long at a time and need to be accompanied with their family members.

(3) Patients need to drink 300 to 500 mL water after fumigation, and pay attention to keep warm in winter.

(4) Patients should not eat too much spicy, pungent, greasy, or sweet food, and should not apply makeups and facial cleaners during the treatment. Patients who are over

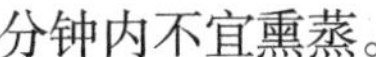

分钟内不宜熏蒸。

（5）注意熏蒸的禁忌证。经期及孕妇、温热感觉障碍者、有严重出血倾向者、皮肤过敏者禁止熏蒸；特殊疾病、皮肤破损处不宜熏蒸。

hungry, overfed and over exhausted are not advisable for fumigation. Do not fumigate within 30 minutes before or after meals.

(5) Fumigation is prohibited for people who are in period, have disorders in feeling temperature, and easy to bleeding and allergy; and is not recommended for people who have special diseases and skin injuries.

四、熏蒸方

Formulas for Fumigation

（1）强身健体熏蒸方：当归20 g，黄芪30 g，独活25 g，川羌活15 g，伸筋草10 g，透骨草15 g，秦艽15 g，桂枝10 g，苍术10 g，杜仲20 g，桑寄生10 g，威灵仙12 g，干姜20 g。

（2）活血祛瘀熏蒸方：全当归20 g，赤芍15 g，白芍15 g，炒桃仁20 g，牡丹皮20 g，生姜15 g，川军15 g，苏木10 g，红花10 g，紫草10 g，乳香15 g，没药15 g，乌药10 g，秦艽20 g，汉防己10 g，雷公藤20 g，狗脊10 g。

(1) Formulas for strengthening the body: Danggui (当归, *Radix Angelicae Sinensis*) 20 g, Huangqi (黄芪, *Radix Astragali seu Hedysari*) 30 g, Duhuo (独活, *Radix Angelicae Pubescentis*) 25 g, Qianghuo (羌活, *Rhizoma et Radix Notopterygii*) 15 g, Shenjincao (伸筋草, *Herba Lycopodii*) 10 g, Tougucao (透骨草, *Speranskiae seu Impaticntis Herba*) 15 g, Qinjiao (秦艽, *Radix Gentianae Macrophyllae*) 15 g, Guizhi (桂枝, *Ramulus Cinnamomi*) 10 g, Cangzhu (苍术, *Rhizoma Atractylodis*) 10 g, Duzhong (杜仲, *Cortex Eucommiae*) 20 g, Sangjisheng (桑寄生, *Herba Taxilli*) 10 g, Weilingxian (威灵仙, *Radix Clematidis*) 12 g, Ganjiang (干姜, *Rhizoma Zingiberis*) 20 g.

(2) Formulas for activating blood and dispelling stasis: Quandanggui (全当归, *Angelicae Sinensis*) 20 g, Chishao (赤芍, *Radix Paeoniae Rubra*) 15 g, Baishao (白芍, *Radix Paeoniae Alba*) 15 g, stir-fried Taoren (桃仁, *Semen Persicae*) 20 g, Mudanpi (牡丹皮, *Cortex Moutan Radicis*) 20 g, Fresh ginger (生姜, *Rhizoma Zingiberis Recens*) 15 g, Dahuang (大黄, *Radix et Rhizoma Rhei*) 15 g, Sumu (苏木, *Lignum Sappan*) 10 g, Honghua (红花, *Flos Carthami*) 10 g, Zicao (紫草 *Radix Arnebiae*) 10 g, Ruxiang (乳香, *Olibanum*) 15 g, Moyao (没药, *Myrrha*) 15 g, Wuyao (乌药, *Radix Linderae*) 10 g, Qinjiao (秦艽, *Radix Gentianae Macrophyllae*) 20 g, Fangji (防己, *Radix Stephaniae Tetrandrae*) 10 g, Leigongteng (雷公藤, *Radix*

（3）海桐皮汤熏蒸方：海桐皮15 g，透骨草15 g，乳香15 g，没药10 g，当归（酒洗）10 g，川椒15 g，川穹10 g，红花10 g，威灵仙10 g，白芷10 g，甘草5 g，防风10 g。

（4）祛风除湿熏蒸方：制川乌、制草乌、羌活、独活、伸筋草、秦艽、四叶参、丁香各30 g，桂枝、木瓜、黄芪、石斛、姜半夏、丹参、姜黄各15 g。

（5）关节疼痛（痰阻络脉证）熏蒸方：威灵仙15 g，清半夏12 g，白芥子10 g，嫩桑枝30 g，伸筋草15 g，透骨草15 g，细辛10 g，苏木15 g，红花15 g，川牛膝15 g，海风藤10 g，制乳香、没药各10 g。

Folium seu Flos Tripterygii Wilfordii) 20 g, Gouji (狗脊, *Rhizoma Cibotii*) 10 g.

(3) Formulas of Erythrina Decoction: Haitongpi (海桐皮, *Cortex Erythrinae*) 15 g, Tougucao (透骨草, *Speranskiae seu Impaticntis Herba*) 15 g, Ruxiang (乳香, *Olibanum*) 15 g, Moyao (没药, *Myrrha*) 10 g, Danggui (当归, *Radix Angelicae Sinensis*) (processing with wine) 10 g, Chuanjiao (川椒, *Zanthoxyli Pericarpium*) 15 g, Chuanxiong (川芎, *Rhizoma Ligustici Chuanxiong*) 10 g, Honghua (红花, *Flos Carthami*) 10 g, Weilingxian (威灵仙, *Radix Clematidis*) 10 g, Baizhi (白芷, *Radix Angelicae Dahuricae*) 10 g, Gancao (甘草, *Radix Glycyrrhizae*) 5 g, Fangfeng (防风, *Radix Saposhnikoviae*) 10 g.

(4) Formulas for dispelling wind and eliminating dampness: Processed Chuanwu (川乌, *Radix Aconiti*) 30 g, Processed Caowu (草乌, *Radix aconiti agrestis*) 30 g, Qianghuo (羌活, *Rhizoma et Radix Notopterygii*) 30 g, Duhuo (独活, *Radix Angelicae Pubescentis*) 30 g, Shenjincao (伸筋草, *Herba Lycopodii*) 30 g, Qinjiao (秦艽, *Radix Gentianae Macrophyllae*) 30 g, Siyeshen (四叶参, *Codonopsitis Lanceolatae Radix*) 30 g, Dingxiang (丁香, *Flos Caryophylli*) 30 g, Guizhi (桂枝, *Ramulus Cinnamomi*) 15 g, Mugua (木瓜, *Fructus Chaenomelis*) 15 g, Huangqi (黄芪, *Radix Astragali seu Hedysari*) 15 g, Shihu (石斛, *Herba Dendrobii*) 15 g, Processed Banxia (半夏, *Rhizoma Pinelliae*) 15 g, Danshen (丹参, *Radix Salviae Miltiorrhizae*) 15 g, Jianghuang (姜黄, *Rhizoma Curcumae Longae*) 15 g.

(5) Formulas for joints pain (pattern of phlegm obstructing collaterals): Weilingxian (威灵仙, *Radix Clematidis*) 15 g, Banxia (半夏, *Rhizoma Pinelliae*) (processing with alum) 12 g, Baijiezi (白芥子, *Semen Sinapis Albae*) 10 g, Tender Sangzhi (桑枝, *Ramulus Mori*) 30 g, Shenjincao (伸筋草, *Herba Lycopodii*) 15 g, Tougucao (*Herba* 透骨草, *Speranskiae seu Impaticntis*) 15 g, Xixin (细辛, *Herba Asari*) 10 g, Sumu (苏木, *Lignum Sappan*) 15 g, Honghua (红花, *Flos Carthami*) 15 g, Chuanniuxi (川牛膝, *Radix Cyathulae*)

（6）关节疼痛（寒湿内停证）熏蒸方：当归 20 g，黄芪 20 g，独活 25 g，羌活 15 g，伸筋草 10 g，透骨草 15 g，秦艽 15 g，桂枝 10 g，制附片 10 g，苍术 10 g，杜仲 20 g，桑寄生 10 g，露蜂房 10 g，威灵仙 12 g，干姜 20 g。

15 g, Haifengteng (海风藤, *Caulis Piperis Kadsurae*) 10 g, processed Ruxiang (乳香, *Olibanum*) and processed Moyao (没药, *Myrrha*) 10 g.

(6) Formulas for joints pain (pattern of internal obstruction of cold-damp): Danggui (当归, *Radix Angelicae Sinensis*) 20 g, Huangqi (黄芪, *Radix Astragali seu Hedysari*) 20 g, Duhuo (独活, *Radix Angelicae Pubescentis*) 25 g, Qianghuo (羌活, *Rhizoma et Radix Notopterygii*) 15 g, Shenjincao (伸筋草, *Herba Lycopodii*) 10 g, Tougucao (透骨草, *Herba Speranskiae seu Impaticntis*) 15 g, Qinjiao 秦艽, *Radix Gentianae Macrophyllae*) 15 g, Guizhi (桂枝, *Ramulus Cinnamomi*) 10 g, Cangzhu (苍术, *Rhizoma Atractylodis*) 10 g, Duzhong (杜仲, *Cortex Eucommiae*) 20 g, Sangjisheng (桑寄生, *Herba Taxilli*) 10 g, Lufengfang (露蜂房, *Vespae Nidus*) 10 g, Weilingxian (威灵仙, *Radix Clematidis*) 12 g, Ganjiang (干姜, *Rhizoma Zingiberis*) 20 g.

五、作用原理

Mechanism

中药熏蒸疗法将温热效应和药物作用相结合，使机体产生协同和增效作用，发挥显著、持久的生理、药理效应。熏蒸过程的热效应是由源源不断的热药蒸汽以对流和传导的方式直接作用于人体的，而药疗效应或是由熏蒸药物中逸出的中药粒子作用于体表直接产生杀虫、杀菌、消炎、止痒、止痛等作用；或是经透皮吸收入体通过激动组织细胞的受体或参与调节新陈代谢水平等生化过程发挥药疗作用。中药熏蒸过程中，丰富热能和对症药物持续作用于人体，便出现一系列生理、药理效应。

1. 促进血液循环

药理实验研究表明，熏蒸疗法

Fumigation therapy combines warming and medicine effect, making the physiological and pharmacological effects more visible and long-lasting. The warming effect directly acts on the body by convection and conduction of steam, and the medicine effect depends on those medicinal components to directly kill worms and bacteria, relieve inflammation, itch, and pain. Meanwhile, those medicinal components can be absorbed into the body through the skin and participate in biochemical process like metabolism.

1. Promote blood circulation

Pharmacological experiments shown that fumigation improves hemorheology of animal models, decreases blood viscosity, and improves the microcirculation. Thermal stimulation causes the body capillary to fully dilate and open. Rapid increase in peripheral blood volume leads to redistribution of stored blood, which in turn triggers

可改善模型动物血液流变学，降低血液黏滞度和改善微循环的作用。热是一种物理因子，可刺激引起周身体表毛细血管网充分扩张、开放，外周血容量迅速增多，导致体内储血重新分布，进而引发全身血液大循环。在疏通腠理、舒张血管、通达血脉、促进血液循环的同时能增进药物的吸收，而随着红花、丹参、川芎、当归等活血化瘀药物的吸收并发挥药效，又使因热效应产生的活血化瘀作用更加突出，更加持久。

2. 促进药物的吸收

皮肤是人体最大的器官，面积大、毛孔多，除具有防御外邪侵袭的保护作用外，还具有分泌、吸收、渗透、排泄、感觉等多种功能，是人体与外界进行交换的器官。中药熏蒸的药物治疗作用直接与皮肤相关，对皮肤体表的痈疽疮疡及各种皮肤病，熏蒸药物的有效成分可直接在接触的肌肤部位产生药效或在向体内转运的透皮吸收过程即发挥其抑菌消炎、杀虫止痒、活血化瘀、消肿止痛等作用。

3. 产生“发汗”效应

发汗为中医治病基本手法之一，具有解表祛邪、祛风除湿、利水消肿、排泄体内有害物质的功能。同时发汗可有效调节体内水液输布、运行和排泄。而中药熏蒸疗法所产生的热药蒸汽，促使汗腺活动增加，汗液分泌增多，并能恢复部分汗腺、皮脂腺的功能；汗液排泄还能带走部分积蓄在体内的毒素和沉积物，清除体内毒素对机体各脏器的损伤，

a general circulation of blood throughout the body. This process could unblock interstices, dilate and unblock blood vessels, improve blood circulation and enhance the medicine absorption. Meanwhile, with the absorption of blood-activating and stasis-resolving medicines like Honghua (红花, *Flos Carthami*), Danshen (丹参, *Radix Salviae Miltiorrhizae*), Chuanxiong (川芎, *Rhizoma Ligustici Chuanxiong*), and Danggui (当归, *Radix Angelicae Sinensis*), the effect of blood activating and stasis resolving will be more visible and long-lasting.

2. Promote the absorption of Chinese medicinal

Skin is the largest organ of human body with many pores. In addition to the prevention of external pathogen, skin also owns functions of secretion, absorption, penetration, excretion, and sensory, which shows that skin is an organ where the exchanges happen between the body and the outer environment. During the fumigation process, Chinese medicines are directly contacting with skin. Hence, for various skin diseases like sore and ulcer, active ingredients of the Chinese medicinal perform functions in the ways of directly applying to the skin or penetrating the skin into the body, with the purpose of repressing bacteria and decreasing inflammation, killing worms and relieving itch, unblocking blood and resolving stasis, and dispersing swelling and relieving pain.

3. Promote sweating

Sweating is one of the basic TCM treatments, with the functions of releasing the exterior and eliminating the pathogenic factors, dispelling wind and eliminating dampness, inducing diuresis to alleviating edema and excreting harmful substances inside the body. Sweating regulates the distribution, transportation, and excretion of water inside the body. Medicinal vapor which produced by fumigation promotes sweat gland activities and sweat secretion, and even restores some sweat and sebaceous glands. Moreover, sweating also takes away some toxin

可用于尿毒症、慢性肾功能不全等临床治疗。

4. 神经、经络调节作用

人体皮肤分布着丰富的神经感受器和腧穴，而人体信息的传递，正是由这些感受器和腧穴分别通过神经纤维和十二经络组成的信息网络，时刻保持着皮肤→内脏→大脑间频繁的信息传递与调节过程来完成。也即外周传入感觉神经在脊髓段与内脏传入神经发生了交织与联系，从而使传导的信号相互影响。因此，临床上常发现内脏病变时，某一区域皮肤痛觉变得敏感起来，还有可能发生牵涉痛或反射性肌痉挛。

5. 抗炎、免疫作用

现代药理研究表明，中药熏蒸疗法可通过调节致炎因子和肿瘤坏死因子，减轻炎性反应，缓解局部肿胀。在中药熏蒸温热作用下，增加体内脑啡肽的含量，小动脉及毛细血管周围出现白细胞总数增加，网状内皮系统功能加强，大小吞噬细胞的吞噬功能加强，淋巴细胞的转化加强，使机体的免疫功能提高，从而使化脓性炎症病灶早日局限化、成熟，促使坏死物质迅速脱落、代谢排出。并增进正常新陈代谢作用，使生理机能发挥极致意识趋于安定而达到身心平衡状态。

6. 止痛作用

熏蒸疗法通过热与药的共同作用，可以加速血液、淋巴循环，加强代谢物的排泄，促进炎性致病因子的吸收与排泄。能增强人体体液免疫和细胞免疫能力，较快缓解肌

inside the body, reducing harms they posed on organs. Therefore, it is applied for clinical treatments of uremia and chronic renal insufficiency.

4. Regulatory function of nerves and meridians

There are many sensory receptors and acupuncture points in the skin. It is these receptors and acupoints which connect with nerves and twelve meridians that accomplish the exchanges of information inside the body. Peripheral afferent sensory nerves connect with visceral afferent nerves in the spinal cord segment, so that the conducted signals interact with each other. Therefore, when visceral lesions are found in clinical treatments, certain regions of skin are becoming sensitive, or even painful and have spasms at the same time.

5. Anti-inflammatory and immunological functions

Modern pharmacological researches shown that by regulating inflammatory factors and tumor necrosis factors, fumigation reduces inflammatory response and relieves local swelling. Under the circumstances of warming, the amount of enkephalins inside the body and leukocytes around the small arteries and capillaries increased, functions of reticuloendothelial system, phagocytosis, and lymphocyte enhanced, and ultimately strengthened the body's immune system. Therefore, purulent inflammatory lesions will be mature in earlier times, prompting rapid shedding and metabolic discharge of necrotic material. Meanwhile, normal metabolism is enhanced, maximizing physiological functions and settling mind, so as to achieve the balanced state.

6. Relieve pain effect

With the combination of warming and Chinese medicines, fumigation speeds up the circulation of blood and lymph, enhances the excretion of metabolites, and promotes the absorption and excretion of inflammatory pathogenic factors. In addition, fumigation strengthens the humoral immunity and cellular immunity, relieves muscles

肉及周围软组织紧张，加速人体对中药的吸收，使局部致痛物质迅速消失，从而使疼痛缓解。当感觉神经受到刺激产生的信号作为一种与痛觉信号同时传入脊髓神经再传至大脑中枢时，熏蒸治疗可干扰神经通路传递的此痛觉信号，可降低其兴奋性，减弱其传至大脑中枢时的强度，使主观上的痛觉感受减轻。同时，熏蒸加剧了体内神经传递介质或其他相关分子、离子的运动，从而在分子或离子水平上阻碍或干扰了痛觉信号传导过程，也起了治痛作用。

and surrounding soft tissues, accelerates the absorption of Chinese medicinal by human body, and makes the local pain-causing substances disappear rapidly, thus relieving the pain. When being stimulated, sensory nerves will produce a kind of signal which can be transmitted to spinal nerve and then to the brain center as a pain signal. Fumigation is taken as a treatment to disrupt this pain signal, lower its excitability, weaken its intensity when transmitted to the brain center, thus subjectively relieving pain. Meanwhile, fumigation intensifies the movement of neurotransmitter mediators or other related molecules and ions in the body, obstructing the transmission process in the level of molecules and ions, which also shows its pain-reliving function.

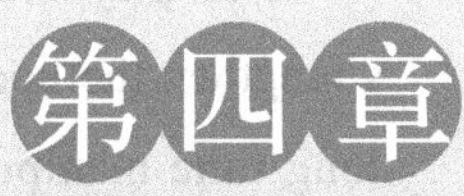

练功法

Chapter Four
Shaolin Internal Exercise

第一节 Section One

概述 Introduction

内功推拿就是在少林内功基础上发展起来的一种推拿疗法。少林内功是内功推拿主要的练功内容和方法，是内功推拿流派的重要组成部分。它强调患者通过锻炼少林内功与接受推拿治疗相结合，同时要求推拿医师和患者均要练习少林内功。

功法训练对推拿专业人员来说，有利于增强体质与保证手法长时间操作的力量与耐力，预防职业性疾病，并有助于掌握手法技巧。对患者而言，功法训练或功能锻炼，可巩固和延伸推拿手法疗效，并向康复领域延伸。通过功法手法的良性刺激可以激发经络系统的自身整体调整功能，帮助人体的生命活动恢复到正常状态。对于虚损明显的患者，更需要坚持用一点时间练功，待脏腑和气血功能增强后再增加手法治疗。因此，内功推拿有“先练后推”的要求。

少林内功其实是一种内外兼练的功法。不仅“内练一口气”，而要“外练筋骨皮”，着重锻炼下肢的“霸力”和上肢的“灵活性”。临床应用时，则是参照专业人员功法锻炼的方法，根据不同疾病制订功法处方，按照三因制宜的原则指导患者锻炼，虚证以患者耐受为度，实证以汗出为宜。

Shaolin internal exercise and tuina is a kind of tuina therapy based on Shaolin internal exercise. As the main content and method in Shaolin internal exercise and tuina, Shaolin internal exercise is an important component of the school of internal exercise and tuina. It stresses that patients should do Shaolin internal exercise and accept tuina manipulations at the same time and both physicians and patients need to exercise Shaolin internal exercise to build up their body.

For physicians, the exercise can help them to strengthen the body, maintain strengths and endurance of long-time manipulations, prevent occupational diseases and grasp manipulation skills. For patients, the exercise can help them to improve tuina efficacy and speed recovery. The appropriate stimulation of exercise and manipulations can activate the overall adjustment functions of the meridian and collateral systems and help restore the body's vital activities to a normal state. Patients with chronic consumptive conditions need to exercise more. After the function of their internal organs and qi and blood is enhanced, give them manipulation treatment. Therefore, “exercising first, accepting tuina manipulations second” is the prerequisite for Shaolin internal exercise and tuina.

In fact, Shaolin internal exercise requires both internal and external exercise. That means the “Shaolin internal exercise aims to cultivate internal qi inside and strengthen tendons, bones and skins outside, ” with the focus of strengthening the stability of lower limbs and flexibility of upper limbs. In clinical treatment, the exercise is referred to the professionals' exercise, and prescriptions are formulated according to different diseases, seasons, locations, and people. Patients with deficiency pattern should exercise according to their personal healthy conditions; and patients with excess pattern should exercise to sweat.

一、推拿练功的主要作用

1. 强身健体修神，充沛气血内劲

推拿练功通过调身、调息、调心，做到“内练一口气，外练筋骨皮”，达到内外兼修，强身健体修神、充沛气血内劲的效果。

推拿练功有形神双修功效，使推拿医师具备充足的体力、良好的精神状态。通过推拿练功，可使推拿医师气血旺盛、经筋脉络畅通，十分有益于推拿从业人员始终保持“阴平阳秘”的最佳工作状态。长期推拿练功，也可以使推拿医师增强内功，逐步产生内劲，进而有效发挥推拿手法效应。

2. 医练结合，增强疗效

古人云：“上工治未病，下工治已病。”推拿临床工作中，正是按照这一说法，不仅重视疾病的治疗，还注意预防疾病的发生和发展，尤其是传统练功中亦有着很好的体现。其中一些动作很适合患者练习，有利于消除疾病，是一种扶正祛邪和调动患者积极性的好方法。如前推八匹马、倒拉九头牛等动作，两手自胁肋两侧向前推出，使中气蓄行于中焦，故能健脾和胃，促进胃肠功能，使摄纳增加，化生有源，气

Main Functions of Shaolin Internal Exercise and Tuina

1. Strengthen the body to exercise the mind and flourish the qi and body

By regulating body, breath and mind, Shaolin internal exercise and tuina help patients cultivate internal qi inside and strengthen tendons, bones and skins outside, and make qi and blood abundant.

Shaolin internal exercise and tuina have the efficacy of cultivating the body and mind, making tuina practitioners full of energy. The practice of Shaolin internal exercise and tuina can make the practitioner's qi and blood abundant and the meridians and collaterals smooth, which is very beneficial for the practitioner to maintain the relative equilibrium of yin and yang. Long-term Shaolin internal exercise and tuina can also enable tuina practitioners to enhance their internal strength and gradually produce internal force, making tuina manipulations have greater efficacy.

2. Combination of exercise and tuina manipulations can improve therapeutic effect

Ancients says that "The superior practitioner initiates a cure where there is no disease yet, he does not cure where there is a disease already." It is according to this statement that people do not pay attention to the treatment but also the prevention of the occurrence and development of diseases. This view is particularly reflected in traditional exercise. Some of the exercises are very suitable for

血充沛。

3. 提高推拿专业技能，预防职业性疾病

推拿手法的功力、技巧是疗效差异的关键，良好的手法必须是“均匀、柔和、持久、有力”的，这就需要推拿医生有一定的指力、臂力、腰腿力等身体的整体力量和手法所规定的手形、步形，推拿是一种脑力和体力相结合的劳动，因此，推拿医生在具备良好心理素质的同时，还必须具备良好的身体素质，推拿练功为推拿医生具备上述条件打下了基础。推拿练功强调练习肢体姿势与动作，学习有序的呼吸方法和有益的情志控制力，从中培养推拿实践中规范的步法、身法、手法和眼法，达到四法合一的境界，进而充分协调发挥推拿医师身体各部功能，提高推拿操作功效，有效地预防推拿职业性疾病。少林内功的下肢裆势练习，使推拿师下盘稳固灵活、步法协调，关节筋肉柔顺韧性，能够胜任长时间的不同操作体姿；上肢动作练习使推拿师手部内气充实，运劲自如；长期均匀节律的呼吸法和意念控制的学习，可以让推拿师呼吸功能流畅，练习推拿操作中气、意、劲协同发挥的最佳操作模式。

patients to practice, which is conducive to reinforcing the healthy qi and eliminating the pathogenic factors and motivating patients' interests in exercise. For example, in the exercise of Qian Tui Ba Pi Ma (Pushing Eight Horses Forward) and Dao La Jiu Tou Niu (Pulling Nine Oxen Backward), people push two hands forward from the rib cage, so that the middle qi is stored in the middle energizer. Therefore, it can strengthen the spleen and harmonize the stomach, improve the function of the stomach and intestines, increase the intake of nutrients, and make the qi and blood abundant.

3. Improve the professional skills of tuina and prevent occupational diseases

The force and skills are critical to improve the manipulation efficacy. Good manipulations must be "even, soft, long-lasting and powerful", which means that tuina practitioners should have certain strength, such as finger strength, arm strength, waist and leg strength, and the hand forms and step form required by manipulations. As tuina requires both mental and physical strength, tuina practitioners should have good mental and physical quality. Shaolin internal exercise and tuina have helped them to lay the good foundation for giving tuina manipulations to patients. Shaolin internal exercise and tuina emphasize the practice of body stances and gestures, and how to breathe naturally and control the mind. In this way, the step form, body techniques, hand forms and eye techniques can be cultivated at the same time. Thus, it can fully coordinate the functions of all parts of the body of tuina practitioners, improve the efficacy of tuina manipulations, and effectively prevent occupational diseases. The exercise of lower limbs in Shaolin internal exercise enables tuina practitioners to have stable and flexible lower plate, coordinated step forms, and soft and flexible joints and tendons, so that he or she can maintain in different stances for a long time. The exercise of upper limbs makes tuina practitioners' hands full of strength. And the long-time learning of even and rhythmical breathing and intentional control allows the tuina practitioner to breathe smoothly and achieve the coordination of middle qi, intention and force.

二、少林内功的特点

少林内功与一般的静坐类、导引类的功法不同，它要求在练功时呼吸自如，四肢特别是手脚要用足力量，做到"练气不见气"，以力带气，气贯四肢。在练功时，强调下实上虚，着重锻炼两下肢的"霸力"和上肢的"内劲"。要求上身正直，下肢稳重，足跟踏实，五趾抓地，站如松树，稳而牢固。上肢在进行各种姿势锻炼时，要求凝劲于肩、肘、腕、指。呼吸自然，与上肢动作相协调，达到"外紧内松"。练功时要求力达四肢腰背，气随力行，注于经脉，使气血循行畅通，濡养四肢百骸和五脏六腑，增强内功。

少林内功的要领：蓄劲指端，以力贯气；下肢霸力，气贯四肢；出声发力，外紧内松；呼吸自然，意念集中。上肢动作练习时，可采用"嘿"字出声，配合指掌发力。出声发力要求声音短促，丹田运气，气声浑厚。

少林内功动作明确、锻炼全面、针对性很强。徒手练功中，首先强调步型、裆势，要求通过下肢各种屈曲、起伏动作，使下肢肌肉、韧带以及腹肌、腰肌、背肌等都得到

Features of Shaolin Internal Exercise

Different from quiet qigong and daoyin, Shaolin internal exercise requires free breathing and full strength in four limbs, especially in the hands and feet, so as to "practice with qi without seeing qi", and lead qi to the limbs with strength. In exercise, it stresses weight support of lower limbs and weight free of upper limbs, with the purpose of strengthening the stability of lower limbs and flexibility of upper limbs. Make the upper body upright, the lower limbs stable and the heels solid. In addition, stand firmly with toes grasping the ground and heels touching the ground tightly, like a stable and firm pine tree. It is asked to focus the strength on the shoulders, elbows, wrists and fingers when doing the exercise of upper limbs. Breathe naturally and coordinate with the upper limb movements. In exercise, make qi flow with strength to achieve four limbs, back, waist, meridians and collaterals, so as to promote the circulation of qi and blood, nourish the four limbs, the internal organs, and strengthen internal force.

The key points of Shaolin internal exercise: focus the strength on the fingertips and lead qi to the limbs with strength; focus on the stability of lower limbs and make qi circulate in four limbs; store up strength when speaking out loudly; breathe naturally and concentrate the mind. When doing the exercise of upper limbs, speak "Hi" loudly and store up strength in fingers and palms. Speak out shortly, rapidly and deeply, and circulate qi with Dantian.

一个全面的锻炼，长期练习，可使下肢肌肉亢实，力量大增；还有许多动作都是以手掌的动作为基础，掌从胁肋下擦推而出，徐徐有力，两手起落多有螺旋翻转，使前臂肌肉产生一个拧转裹抱的过程，形成拧劲、争劲，螺旋劲等，通过各部肌肉的伸展收缩，相互争衡，可使指掌、上肢肌肉力量得到更大的锻炼。

少林内功动静结合、意气相随。少林内功中动功与静功密切结合，在动态练习时要"动中求静"，即在进行练功动作的同时，要求呼吸自然、全神贯注，保持精神的宁静；在保持固定姿势时要求"静中有动"，即在体表安静的状态下，保持气息运动的。所以，少林内功不仅具有外练筋骨皮的作用，也有内练精气神的功效。

Shaolin internal exercise is targeted with clear and comprehensive actions. It emphasizes the step form and stances and requires a variety of flexibility and ups and downs of the lower limbs, so that the lower limb muscles, ligaments and abdominal muscles, waist muscles, back muscles, etc. can get a comprehensive exercise. And the long-term practice can make the lower limb muscles hyperactive and strong; there are many movements that are based on the action of the palm. Push the palm from the ribs, make two hands up and down, so that the fingers, palms and muscles of upper limbs can be exercised.

Shaolin internal exercise emphasizes the combined motion and stillness and moving with qi. In movement it requires a peaceful mind, that is when doing Shaolin internal exercise, people should breathe naturally and concentrate the mind. In stillness it requires stable breath movement, that is when keeping a fixed stance, people should keep their breath under control. Therefore, Shaolin internal exercise strengthens the muscles, bones, and skin and internal exercise at qi.

三、少林内功的主要锻炼内容

Main Content of Shaolin Internal Exercise

1. 基本裆势

站裆、马裆、弓箭裆、并裆、大裆、悬裆、低裆、坐裆、磨裆和亮裆十个裆势。

2. 上肢动作锻炼法

前推八匹马、倒拉九头牛、凤凰展翅、霸王举鼎、顺水推舟、怀中抱月、仙人指路、平手托塔、运掌合瓦、风摆荷叶、双手托天，单凤朝阳、海底捞月、顶天抱地、力劈华山、乌龙钻洞、饿虎扑食、三起三落和单掌拉金环等。

1. Basic stances

Standing Stance, Horse Stance, Bow Stance, Folding Stance, Splitting Stance, Squatting-Splitting Stance with Hands on the Waist, Lower Stance, Lower Stance, Sitting Stance, Mill Stance and Flash Stance.

2. Upper limbs exercise

Qian Tui Ba Pi Ma (Pushing Eight Horses Forward), Dao La Jiu Tou Niu (Pulling Nine Oxen Backward), Feng Huang Zhan Chi (Chinese Phoenix Spreading its Wings), Ba Wang Ju Ding (Hegemonic King Supporting Tripot), Shun Shui Tui Zhou (Pushing Boat along Water-Flowing), Huai Zhong Bao Yue (Embracing the Moon), Xian Ren Zhi

3. 双人锻炼法

推把上桥、双龙搅水、双虎夺食、箭腿压法和八走势等。

Lu (Immortal Guiding Way), Ping Shou Tuo Ta (Holding Tower with Flat Hand), Yun Zhang He Wa (Turning Palm to Fold Tile), Feng Bai He Ye (Wind Blowing Lotus Leaf), Shuang Shou Tuo Tian (Supporting the Sky with Two Hands), Dan Feng Chao Yang (Single Phoenix Facing the Sun), Hai Di Lao Yue (Scooping the Moon from Sea Bottom), Ding Tian Bao Di (Supporting the Sky and Embracing the Earth), Li Pi Hua Shan (Splitting Hua Mountain with Vigorous Efforts), Wu Long Zuan Dong (Black Dragon Crawling into Cave), E Hu Pu Shi (Hunger Tiger Pouncing on its Prey), San Qi San Luo (Three Ups and Three Downs) and Dan Zhang La Jin Huan (Drawing Golden Ring with One Palm).

3. Exercise in pairs

Tui Ba Shang Qiao, Shuang Long Jiao Shui (Two Chinese Dragons Stirring the Water), Shuang Hu Duo Shi (Two Tigers Fighting over Food), Jian Tui Ya Fa and Ba Zou Shi.

四、少林内功的练习方法

少林内功练习强度的安排一般应由小到大，在保持练功质量的基础上，完成一定的数量。在临床治疗过程中，一般以锻炼者微汗为宜。为防止肌肉、韧带等损伤发生，在练功前必须进行适当的准备活动，准备活动与正式练功之间要有2～3分钟的间隔休息。练功后做整理活动（包含一些呼吸运动和较缓和的全身运动），量不可太大，并且逐步由大到小，练功期间注意饮食营养（质量和摄入量）及睡眠休息，以保证身体的需要和练功的预期效果。

Practice Method of Shaolin Internal Exercise

The intensity of Shaolin internal exercise should be added gradually, and the quality of exercise should be ensured. During clinical treatment, it is generally appropriate for exercisers to sweat slightly. To prevent injuries of muscles and ligament, appropriate warm-up activities before Shaolin internal exercise are required. And there should be a rest interval of 2 to 3 minutes between warm-up activities and formal practice. Do warm-down activities after practice (including some respiratory exercises and gentle whole-body exercises) and the amount should not be excessive. And attention should also be paid to diet, nutrition (quality and intake) and sleep rest in practice to meet the needs of the body and achieve the expected efficacy.

少林内功各裆势和上肢动作可灵活组合练习，可以一个裆势单独练习，也可结合一个上肢动作练习，也可以一个裆势结合多个上肢动作练习，或形成套路连续练习（表4-1）。体质差者或初练者可先单练，练至体力增强或动作熟练后再成套锻炼。单练时每个动作应重复3～7次，成套锻炼时，每个动作应重复3～5次。各人可根据具体情况，适量锻炼。

在套路练习后，再配合双人练、棒击法和内功推拿常规操作，加深理解少林内功的功法内涵。

All stances in Shaolin internal exercise can be combined with the upper limb movements flexibly. We can practice a stance alone, or we can practice a stance with an upper limb movement or with multiple upper limb movements. Or we can form a set of continuous practice (Table 4–1). People with poor physical conditions or beginners can do a single practice first, and then complete sets of exercises when they have increased strength or become familiar with the actions. In single exercise, each action should be repeated 3 to 7 times, and each action should be repeated 3 to 5 times when exercising in sets. Different people should exercise according to their specific healthy conditions.

After exercise in sets, people can combine with double workouts, stick-knocking manipulation and routine manipulations to have a better understanding of Shaolin internal exercise.

五、少林内功的临床应用

Clinical Application of Shaolin Internal Exercise

临床应用少林内功强调辨证施用。在治疗虚劳等病证时，要求功法与手法密切结合，患者必须加强练功，选择站裆势结合前推八匹马、倒拉九头牛等动作姿势，以后逐渐加强马裆势、弓箭裆势、大裆势锻炼，并选择两手托天、霸王举鼎等动作。在治疗肺结核、哮喘、肺气肿等病证时，一般在手法治疗1个疗程后，指导患者先练习站裆势，适当选练前推八匹马、倒拉九头牛。第2疗程后，可以练习马裆势、弓箭裆势，并选练风摆荷叶、两手托天等动作。高血压、失眠、胃脘痛等病症可以根据患者实际情况，指导

Clinical application of Shaolin internal exercise emphasizes the treatment based on syndrome differentiation. In the treatment of deficiency and other diseases, it requires close integration of exercise and manipulations. And patients must strengthen their practice, choosing standing stance combined with Qian Tui Ba Pi Ma (Pushing Eight Horses Forward) and Dao La Jiu Tou Niu (Pulling Nine Oxen Backward). And later they should gradually strengthen the exercise of horse stance, bow stance and splitting stance with hands backward and choose the movement of Shuang Shou Tuo Tian (Supporting the Sky with Two Hands) and Ba Wang Ju Ding (Hegemonic King Supporting Tripot). In the treatment of tuberculosis, asthma, and emphysema, patients are instructed to practice standing stance and then choose the exercise of Qian Tui Ba Pi Ma

表4-1 少林内功下肢裆势与上肢动作组合练习方法
Table 4-1 The exercise methods of upper limbs and lower limbs in Shaolin internal exercise

上肢动作 Upper limbs exercise	下肢裆势 Lower limbs stances					
	站裆势 Standing Stance	马裆势 Horse Stance	弓箭裆势 Bow Stance	并裆势 Folding Stance	大裆势 Splitting Stance	低裆势 Lower Stance
前推八匹马 Qian Tui Ba Pi Ma (Pushing Eight Horses Forward)	√	√	√	√	√	√
倒拉九头牛 Dao La Jiu Tou Niu (Pulling Nine Oxen Backward)	√	√	√	√	√	√
凤凰展翅 Feng Huang Zhan Chi (Chinese Phoenix Spreading its Wings)	√	√	√	√	√	√
霸王举鼎 Ba Wang Ju Ding (Hegemonic King Supporting Tripot)	√	√	√	√	√	√
顺水推舟 Shun Shui Tui Zhou (Pushing Boat along Water-Flowing)	√	√	√	√	√	√
仙人指路 Xian Ren Zhi Lu (Immortal Guiding Way)	√	√	√	√	√	√
顶天抱地 Ding Tian Bao Di (Supporting the Sky and Embracing the Earth)	√	√				
海底捞月 Hai Di Lao Yue (Scooping the Moon from Sea Bottom)	√	√				
三起三落 San Qi San Luo (Three Ups and Three Downs)	√					
平手托塔 Ping Shou Tuo Ta (Holding Tower with Flat Hand)	√	√	√	√	√	√
饿虎扑食 E Hu Pu Shi (Hunger Tiger Pouncing on its Prey)	√					
风摆荷叶 Feng Bai He Ye (Wind Blowing Lotus Leaf)	√	√	√	√	√	√

注：√代表该下肢裆势可与该上肢动作组合练习。
Note: √ Represents that Lower limbs stances can be combined with the upper limbs exercise for practice.

少林内功锻炼。一般在练功结束后，休息片刻再接受常规推拿手法治疗。

在内功推拿临床工作中，不仅重视治病，而且更注重防病，少林内功中的一些练功方法可以强壮身体，预防疾病的发生和发展。少林内功对于人体的影响是整体的，无论是医生还是患者都可以通过推拿功法的练习培育人体正气，达到“正气存内，邪不可干”的目的。

推拿练功已成为推拿学的一个重要的组成部分，它不仅是推拿医生增强上肢、下肢、腰腿部等身体各部力量、提高手法技巧动作的主要方法之一，也是患者达到扶助正气、强壮身体、治疗疾病的方法之一。

(Pushing Eight Horses Forward) and Dao La Jiu Tou Niu (Pulling Nine Oxen Backward) after receiving one course of manipulation treatment. After the second course of manipulation treatment, patients can practice horse stance and bow stance with Feng Bai He Ye (Wind Blowing Lotus Leaf) and Shuang Shou Tuo Tian (Supporting the Sky with Two Hands). Patients with hypertension, insomnia, stomach and epigastric pain can do Shaolin internal exercise according to their physical conditions. Generally, after the end of the exercise, patients should have a rest for a few moments before receiving routine tuina manipulations.

In the clinical treatment, Shaolin internal exercise and tuina do not only pay attention to the treatment of diseases, but also pay more attention to the prevention of diseases. Some practices in Shaolin internal exercise can strengthen the body and prevent the occurrence and development of diseases. Shaolin internal exercise has a holistic effect on the human body. Both physicians and patients can cultivate the healthy qi through exercise. In this way, there is sufficient qi inside the body that pathogenic factors cannot invade the body.

Internal exercise has become an important component of the school of tuina. It is not only one of the main methods for tuina physicians to enhance the strength of various body parts such as upper limbs, lower limbs, waist and legs, and to improve their manipulation skills, but also one of the methods for patients to reinforce the healthy qi, strengthen the body and treat diseases.

六、少林内功锻炼的注意事项

Attention for Training Shaolin Internal Skills

（1）练功要端正态度，树立信心，明确锻炼的目的，要有不怕困难，勤学苦练，持之以恒的精神。

（2）练功宜在饭后1个多小时进

(1) We should have a good attitude and male clear the purpose of exercise. And we also need to be confident and diligent.

(2) It is advisable to practice Shaolin internal exercise

行，饥饿时和饱食后不宜练功。环境宜在室内进行，避免汗出当风。衣着宜宽松，须穿软底鞋（以布底鞋最为适宜）。

（3）练功前应认真做好准备活动，以防止肌肉、韧带、关节在运动中出现损伤。

（4）练功时要求动作准确，姿势舒适自然，呼吸均匀、平稳、缓慢、意守丹田，不可屏气。练功时应专心一致，排除杂念，养成全神贯注的习惯，以防产生不良后果。

（5）练功结束时，应做全身或局部的整理放松运动，以消除疲劳、促进体力恢复。

（6）女子经期也应酌情练功。

more than one hour after meals, and it is not advisable to practice when we feel hungry or after we have a full meal. Besides, we need to exercise indoors to avoid getting cold. Dress should be loose and soft-soled shoes should be worn (cloth-soled shoes are most suitable).

(3) Warm-up activities should be done carefully to prevent injuries of muscles, ligaments and joints before exercise.

(4) When practicing Shaolin internal exercise, it is required that the movement is accurate, gestures are comfortable and natural, the breathing is even, smooth and slow. Sink qi to Dantian and do not hold your breath. Fully concentrate the mind, exclude distracting thoughts, and develop a habit of full concentration to prevent adverse consequences.

(5) At the end of practice, we should do whole or local warm-down activities to dissipate fatigue and restore physical strength.

(6) Women should reduce the exercise during menstruation periods.

七、练功的运动量

练功运动量是指人体在练功过程中所能完成的生理负荷量。运动量组成的因素应包括强度、密度、时间、数量和练功项目特性等。改变这些因素中的任何一个因素，都会使练功效果受到影响。强度是指练功过程中运动的程度，这个要求以练功者各自体质及生理适应程度而定，不可一概而论。密度是指单位时间内重复练习的次数，训练中常以密度作为一个因素来表示运动量的大小，所以密度在运动量中反映时间与次数的关系也是运

Exercise Volume

Exercise volume refers to the amount of physiological load that the human body can accomplish in the process of practicing Shaolin internal exercise. The component of the exercise volume includes intensity, density, time, quantity and characteristics of the practice items. Changing any one of these factors will affect the efficacy of Shaolin internal exercise. Intensity refers to the extent of practice, and it changes according to the different physical and physiological conditions. Density refers to the number of repetitions per unit of time. Density is often used as a factor to indicate the exercise volume, so density is also an important link in the exercise because it reflects the relationship between time

动量中一个重要的环节。时间因素是指在一次练功中应考虑练功的总时间、单一功法完成的时间、上一次练习与下一次练习之间的间歇时间以及练习中完全休息的时间等。数量是指一次练功中重复练习的量或练习的总量，练功中没有一定的数量就没有一定的质量，也就是没良好的效果。练功项目特性是指推拿练功方法对人体的影响作用不尽相同，所以在安排练功运动量时也应考虑这个因素。

练功是一种强身健体、防病治病的锻炼方法，也是一种体力活动，所以练功要适当，防止损伤，保证充沛的体力，才能有良好的效果。因此，除了科学、系统地安排练习内容外，还必须选择合适的运动量。运动量诸因素间是相互依存的，只有在全面考虑这些因素的基础上才能因人、因地制订适合自身情况的运动量，从而保证良好的效果。

and number in the exercise. The time factor refers to the total time of practice, the time of completion of a single exercise, the interval between the last exercise and the next exercise, and all the time of rest in the exercise. Quantity refers to the number of repetitive exercises or the total amount of exercises in one practice. Without a certain quantity in practice, there is no certain quality, that is, no good effect. The characteristics of practice items refer to the different effects of tuina practice on the human body, so this factor should also be considered when arranging the exercise volume.

Although practicing Shaolin internal exercise is a way to strengthen the body and prevent and cure diseases, it is also a physical activity. So, it is necessary to practice Shaolin internal exercise appropriately to prevent injuries and ensure sufficient physical strength. Therefore, in addition to the scientific and systematic arrangement of the exercise content, it is also necessary to choose the appropriate exercise volume. Only taking all these factors into fully consideration can we formulate the exercise volume suitable for different person in different places, thus delivering maximum results.

八、练功的营养卫生

Nutrition and Hygiene

营养是构成机体组织的物质基础，人进行练功等各种运动与营养的关系是非常重要的。推拿练功训练期间，可适当提高高蛋白质食物的摄入，如鸡蛋、鱼、肉等动物性蛋白食物。但需注意练功后应有适当的休息时间才能进食。因为练功时人体血液集中于运动器官，胃肠等消化系统相对处于缺血和抑制状态，消化功能减弱。如果练功结束后即进食，尤其是进食富含蛋白质

Nutrition is the material basis for the human body, and it is vital important for people to do Shaolin internal exercise. During the training period, the intake of high protein foods, such as eggs, fish, meat, and other animal protein foods, can be appropriately increased. However, it should be noted that there should be appropriate rest time before eating after practicing. Because the body's blood is concentrated in the exercise organs during practice, and the gastrointestinal system and other digestive systems are relatively in a state of ischemia and inhibition, and the digestive function is weakened. If you eat immediately

的食物，则不易消化。因此，练功结束后一般以休息30分钟以上进食为佳。合理的摄取营养和掌握适当的进食时间，才能益于身体，确保练功效果。

after practice, especially protein-rich food, it will not be easy to digest. Therefore, it is better to eat after resting for more than 30 minutes after practicing. A reasonable intake of nutrition and a proper eating time can benefit the body and ensure the efficacy of practice.

第二节 功前热身及收功

Section Two Warm-up Activities and Warm-down Activities

一、功前热身

Warm-up Activities

练功前的准备活动，是指在练功前通过各种练习进一步提高中枢神经系统的兴奋性，使其达到适宜水平，加强各器官系统的准备活动，为正式练功进一步做好功能上的准备。能使人体更快地进入练功紧张状态，以防止肌肉、韧带等损伤的发生。

练功前的准备活动往往先采用一些包括走、跑、跳、徒手操和全身各关节各方向、最大范围的放松运动。这样能普遍提高中枢神经系统的兴奋性、全身的物质代谢水平、各器官系统的功能活动以及肌肉韧带的柔韧性和弹性，并使体温略微升高，这些都将有助于练功效果的提高。准备活动持续时间的长短、强度的大小应适当，不必做得太久，防止疲劳。一般正式练功之前有2～3分钟的间隔较为适宜。

Warm-up activities refer to further improving the excitability of the central nervous system through various exercises before practicing. The purpose is to make it reach the appropriate level, strengthen the warm-up activities of all human organ systems, and further make the functional preparation for the formal practice. It can help the human body more quickly to enter the tension state of practice to prevent injuries of muscles and ligament.

Warm-up activities often include walking, running, jumping, freehand exercises and relaxation exercises for all joints of the whole body in all directions and to the maximum extent. This can generally improve the excitability of the central nervous system, the level of material metabolism of the whole body, the functional activities of all organs and systems, as well as the flexibility and elasticity of muscles and ligaments, and slightly increase the body temperature. All of these will be conductive to improving the practice efficacy. The duration and intensity of warm-up activities should be appropriate to prevent fatigue. There is usually an interval of 2 to 3 minutes before the formal practice.

通常情况下，在推拿练功前的一套准备运动由关节运动和马步冲拳两部分组成。

In normal situation, warm-up activities consist of two parts: joint movements and horse-riding step with straight.

（一）关节运动

1. 颈部运动

（1）前后屈伸运动：腿直立，稍宽于肩，两手叉腰，大拇指向后，两脚尖稍外撇，双眼平视前方。体保持正直，抬头后仰望天空，然后还原为预备姿势；低头俯视地面，再还原为原姿势；如此做4～8次。

（2）左右侧转运动：身体保持正直，头向左转至最大限度，目视左肩，然后还原成预备姿势；头向后转至最大限度，目视右肩，再还原成预备姿势；如此做4～8次。

（3）左右斜屈运动：身体保持正直，低头俯视地面，然后头向左上转至最大限度，然后还原成预备姿势；低头俯视地面，然后头向右上转至最大限度，然后还原成预备姿势；如此做4～8次。

（4）左右旋转运动：先左后右，以左为例。缓慢低头，颈部前屈，向左旋转，继而缓慢抬头，仰头颈后屈，转向右侧，然后还原成预备姿势；如此各做4～8次。

2. 肩部运动

（1）前后旋转运动：身体自然站立，双眼平视前方，两手分别置于肩前，依次作向前、后作肩部旋转运动，然后还原成预备姿势；如此各做4～8次。

（2）内外旋转运动：身体自然站立，双眼平视前方，两手分别置

Joint Movements

1. Neck movements

(1) Back and forth flexion and extension: Stand upright, the distance between the feet is wider than the shoulder-width. Bring hands to the waistline with thumb back. Toes slightly point outward with eyes looking forward. Stand upright and look up to the sky, then return to the preparatory posture. Look down at the ground and return to the original posture. Repeat it 4 ～ 8 times.

(2) Side-to-side movement: Stand upright and turn the head left at the most extent. Look at the left shoulder and return to the preparatory posture. Turn the head back at the most extent, look at the right shoulder and return to the preparatory posture. Repeat it 4 to 8 times.

(3) Left and right oblique flexion movement: Stand upright and look down at the ground. Turn the head to the upper left direction at the most extent and return to the preparatory posture; Look down at the ground, turn the head to the upper right direction at the most extent and return to the preparatory posture. Repeat it 4 to 8 times.

(4) Left and right rotation movement: First move to the left side, then the right. Bow the head slowly and flex neck forward; span it left, then lift the head slowly; flex neck backward and span it right. Then return to the preparatory posture. Repeat it 4 to 8 times respectively.

2. Shoulder movements

(1) Back and forth rotation movement: Stand naturally with eyes looking forward. Put hands before the shoulders respectively, then do back and forth rotation movement and return to the preparatory posture. Repeat it 4 to 8 times respectively.

(2) Internal and external rotation movement: Stand

于肩前，作肩部内外旋转运动。向上时尽可能向上方耸起，向前时双前臂相并，背部尽量展开，向后时胸部展开，两肩胛骨尽量向脊柱中间靠拢；如此各做4～8次。

（3）腕部和踝部运动：双手十指交叉，作腕部环绕运动。同时配合单脚踝部的环绕运动，抬起左脚跟离地10 cm左右，环绕运动，顺时针逆时针各10圈。而后换右脚；如此各做4～8次。

3. 腰部运动

（1）左右侧屈运动：分腿直立，稍宽于肩，双手叉腰，大拇指朝前。两腿伸直，两脚不动，双手用力向左、右推动骨盆，作侧屈运动。左右各做4～8次。

（2）前后伸屈运动：分腿直立，稍宽于肩，双手叉腰，大拇指朝前。两腿伸直，两脚不动，双手用力向前、后推动骨盆，作前后伸屈运动。前后各做4～8次。

4. 髋部旋转运动

自然站立，两手叉腰，手与腰部一起做扭腰画圈状运动，顺时针逆时针各做4～8圈。

5. 膝部运动

（1）左右旋转运动：两脚并拢，屈膝半蹲，两手扶膝，轻轻转动膝部，可以先从左至右转动，再从右至左转动，各自转动或交替转动4～8圈。

（2）上下屈伸运动：两脚并拢，两手扶膝，屈膝下蹲，挺膝直立，膝关节上下屈伸4～8次。

（3）抱膝压髋运动：双下肢自然并拢，双手叉指合掌抱住胫骨近

naturally with eyes looking forward. Put hands before the shoulders, do internal and external rotation movement. Raise up as far as possible and bring forearms together as you move forward. Open your back and chest. The two shoulder blades should get closer to the middle of the spine. Repeat it 4 to 8 times respectively.

(3) Wrist and ankle movement: Cross your fingers with your hands in a wrist circular motion. At the same time, with the wrap-around movement of one ankle, raise the left heel about 10cm off the ground, then rotate the ankle clockwise and counterclockwise 10 times respectively. Then change into your right foot, repeat the movement 4 to 8 times.

3. Waist movements

(1) Left and right lateral flexion movement: Step to the left, shoulder-width apart. Bring hands to the waistline with thumb forward. Stand upright and push basin left and right respectively. Repeat it 4 to 8 times respectively.

(2) Back and forth flexion and extension: Step to the left, shoulder-width apart. Bring hands to the waistline with thumb forward. Stand upright and push basin back and forth respectively. Repeat it 4 to 8 times.

4. Hip rotation movements

Stand naturally and bring hands to the waistline. Both hands and waist do the drawing circle movement clockwise and counterclockwise. Repeat it 4 to 8 circles respectively.

5. Knee movements

(1) Left and right rotation movement: Close your legs, bend the knees to the level of half squat; support knees with hands and rotate knees lightly from left to right and then from right to left. Rotate respectively or alternatively 4～8 circles.

(2) Up and down flexion and extension: Close your legs, support knees with hands, bend the knees to the level of squat, lift knee upright; make knees do up and down flexion and extension 4 to 8 times.

端前方，屈膝下蹲压髋，臀部轻击足跟 4～8 次。

（4）伸膝弯腰运动：双下肢自然并拢，屈膝下蹲，双手紧握脚踝，然后作伸膝弯腰运动，弯腰时双膝挺直，下蹲时臀部紧贴足跟，如此屈伸 4～8 次。

(3) Holding knees and pressing hips movement: Close your legs naturally, and the fingers of both hands are folded to hold the proximal front of the tibia. Squat and press the hip with knees bent, and tap the base of foot 4 to 8 times with hips.

(4) Extending knees and bending waist movement: Close your legs naturally, bend the knees to the level of squat; firmly grasp ankles and then extend knees and bend waist; stand upright when bending, and keep hips firmly close to heels. Repeat it 4 to 8 times.

（二）马步冲拳

（1）预备式：两脚并拢，两手自然放于身体两侧，身体自然站正，两眼平视，呼吸自然，思想平和。

（2）左脚向左开一大步，两脚之间距离为本人脚长的 3 倍。

（3）屈膝屈髋下蹲，膝不超过脚尖，大腿与地面的夹角大于 90°，上身端正，两手虎口反插在两膝关节上方。

（4）两手端平，两手与肩等高，与胸等宽。

（5）两手握拳，分别置于腰部两侧。

（6）冲右拳：向左拧腰，右肩松顺，伸右肘，快速旋右臂，右拳用力向前冲出，同时，左拳快速收回腰部。

（7）冲左拳：向右拧腰，左肩松顺，伸左肘，快速旋左臂，左拳用力向前冲出。同时，右拳快速收回腰部。

（8）两手端平，吸气屈肘回胸，呼气下按，伸膝起立，身体复原。

Horse-riding Step with Straight

(1) Preparatory postures: Close your legs, drop down the arms naturally, stand upright, look straight forward, breathe naturally, and keep a peaceful mind.

(2) The left foot steps largely to the left, the distance between the feet is as three times as one's feet.

(3) Bend knees and hips to the level of squat, and the knees are not surpassing the toes. The angle between legs and the ground is more than 90°. Keep the upper body upright, insert Hukou upside down above the knee joints.

(4) Keep both hands flat with hands at shoulder-height and chest-width.

(5) Place both hands in fists on both sides of the waist.

(6) Punching the right fist: Twist your waist to the left, loosen your right shoulder, stretch your right elbow, quickly rotate your right arm, and punch forward with your right fist, while your left fist quickly retracts your waist.

(7) Punching the left fist: Twist your waist to the right, loosen your left shoulder, stretch your left elbow, quickly rotate your left arm, and punch forward with your left fist. At the same time, the right fist quickly retracts the waist.

(8) Hold your hands flat, inhale and flex your elbows back to your chest, then exhale and press down. Next, stretch your knees and stand up, and the body return to the initial posture.

二、收功

"收功"也称练功后结束活动或整理活动。收功是消除疲劳，促进体力恢复的一种方法。在各种运动之后进行整理运动可使人体更好地由紧张的运动状态过渡到安静状态。练功中能量消耗较大需要供应大量氧气，如果练功结束不做整理运动而突然静止下来，身体的静止姿势首先就妨碍了强烈的呼吸动作，影响氧气的补充，同时也会影响静脉血回流，心脏血液的输出量因而减少，血压降低，造成暂时脑缺血现象而产生一系列不良感觉。因此，整理运动不是可有可无的事，而是在练功后一定要做的事。

练功结束要收功，让身心从气功态回复到平常状态，可采用自然收功或强制收功。自然收功适应于单次练功的时间足够长，练功强度逐渐趋缓直至停止，身体脏腑经络系统逐渐从练功态转变为平常态。在自然收功之前，可以做一些自发性的收功动作，如绕腹转圈、浴面理头等。强制收功适用于练功时间短，尚未达到自然收功需要停止练功。要求大脑先发出明确的停止练功的意念，动作逐渐减缓和停止。必须做些人为的收功动作，如绕腹转圈、浴面理头等。练功后放松可以选择性使用关节运动中的各部分运动。或者内功推拿常规操作。练功后身体出汗时，避免吹风着凉。也不要立刻坐下或躺下休息，建议

Warm-down Activities

Warm-down activities, also known as finishing activities or preparation activities, which is a good way to relieve fatigue and restore physical strength. Warm-down activities after various exercises can make the body better transition from a stressful exercise state to a quiet state. Exercise will consume many oxygens, so if people do not do warm-down activities after exercise, they will find it difficult to breathe. And it will affect the replenishment of oxygen, and the venous blood return, thus reducing the blood output of the heart and inevitably lowering the blood pressure, causing temporary cerebral anemia and producing a series of bad feelings. Therefore, do remember to do warm-down activities after exercise.

At the end of the exercise, it is necessary to perform warm-down activities, so that the body and mind can return from the qigong state to the normal state, and the activities could be done naturally or compulsorily. The natural warm-down activity is adapted to long-time single exercise, the intensity of the exercise gradually slows down until it stops, and the meridian system of the body organs gradually changes from the practice state to the normal state. Before the natural warm-down activity, you can do some spontaneous movements, such as circling around the abdomen, bathing the face and trimming the head, etc. Compulsory warm-down activity is suitable for the situation that the exercise should stop before natural warm-down activity. The brain is required to first send out a clear intention to stop the exercise, and the movement gradually slows down and stops. It is necessary to do some artificial warm-down movements, such as circling around the abdomen, bathing the face and trimming the head. Relax after practice and can optionally use the various movements of the joint movement or routine practice of

适当散步。练功后适当饮水，休息30分钟可以进食。

Neigong Tuina. When the body sweats after practicing, avoid catching cold in the wind. Do not immediately sit down or lie down to rest, it is recommended to walk properly. After practicing, drink water properly and have a 30-minute rest before eating.

第三节 基本裆势

Section Three Basic Stances

一、站裆势

Standing Stance

【训练方法】

（1）起式：两脚并拢，头如顶物，两目平视，口微开，舌顶上腭，下颌微向内收，含胸舒背，蓄腹收臀直腰，两手臂自然下垂于身体两侧，五指并拢微屈，中指贴近裤缝，身体正直，心平气静（图4–1）。

（2）功式：左脚向左平跨一步，两脚距离略宽于肩部，足尖略收成内八字，足跟踏实，十趾抓地，两腿用力内夹，运用霸力，劲由上贯下注足。两手叉腰，两拇指按在肾俞穴上，两肘夹紧，前胸微挺，后臀要蓄。两手后伸，挺肘伸腕，肩腋莫松，四指并拢，拇指外展，两上肢与上身夹角大于30°。两目平视，头勿左右盼顾，精神贯注（图4–2）。

（3）收式：两手叉腰，下肢放松，上肢放松放下，身体复原至起式。

【Training methods】

(1) Preparation form: Stand upright with feet together, make the head erect like supporting something, look straight ahead; open mouth slightly, make the tip of the tongue on the palate and withdraw mandible slightly inward; relax chest and extend the back; hold in the abdomen, draw buttocks in and erect waist; drop down the arms naturally, put five fingers together and bend them slightly with the middle finger close to the seam. Make the trunk upright and calm down the mind. (Figure 4–1)

(2) Exercise form: Move the left foot one step to the left, the distance between the feet is wider than the shoulder-width; the toes should be slightly inward to form a pigeon toe pose; grasp the ground forcefully with the toes, make the power radiate from the torso to feet. Bring hands to the waistline, press Shenshu (BL 23) point with two fingers, and keep the elbows tucked in. Slightly protrude the chest, hold the buttocks in, stretch the hands backward; extend the elbows and the wrists; do not relax shoulders; close the four fingers with the thumb apart. The angle between two upper limbs and upper body is more

than 30°. Look straight ahead, do not move the head and concentrate the mind. (Figure 4–2)

(3) Closing form: Bring hands to the waistline, relax lower limbs, put upper limbs down and return to the preparation form.

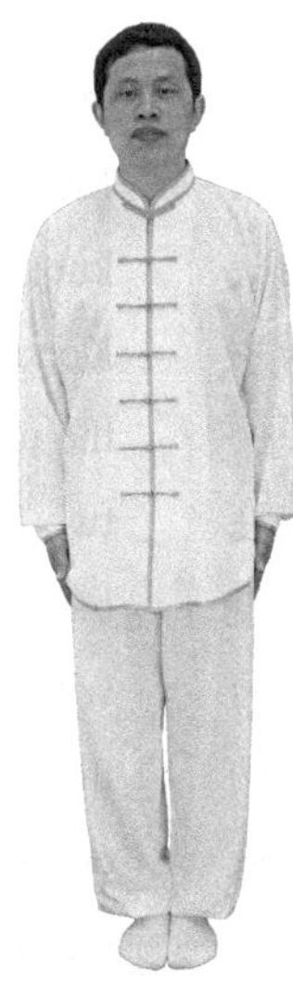

Figure 4–1

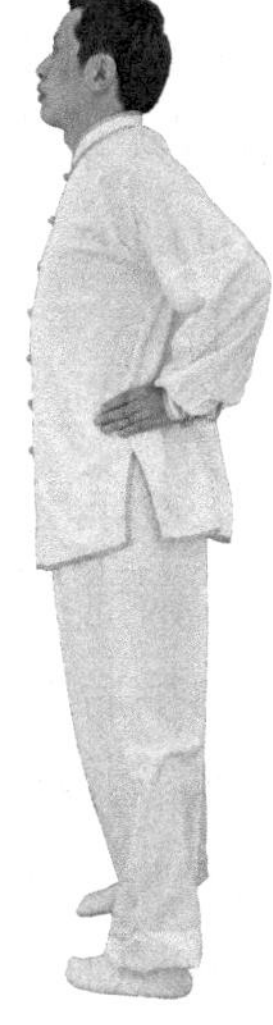

Figure 4–2

【动作要领】

（1）三直四平：三直即臂直、腰直、腿直；四平即头平、肩平、掌平、脚平。

（2）运用霸力。夹肩、挺肘、伸腕、翻掌、立指。

（3）挺胸收腹，舌抵上腭，两目平视，呼吸自然。

【Key points】

(1) Keep arms, waist, and legs straight and keep head, shoulder, palms and feet flat.

(2) Keep the body stable. Tighten shoulders, extend the elbows and the wrists, make the palm and fingers upward.

(3) Throw out the chest, hold in the abdomen; make the tongue against the palate; look straight ahead and breath naturally.

【主要作用】

站裆势是少林内功中最基本的下肢桩功。具有扶助正气、行气活血的作用，久练以意运气，以气生劲，劲循经络达于四肢，增强指、臂、腰、腿部的功力。同时具有调整内脏功能和祛病延寿的作用。

【Main functions】

As one of the most fundamental exercises of lower limbs in Shaolin internal exercise, standing stance has the function of reinforcing healthy qi, circulating qi and blood. Long-time exercise can let the will lead qi to four limbs, thus increasing the strength of fingers, limbs, waist and legs. Standing stance also has the functions of internal organs and eliminating diseases and prolonging life.

二、马裆势

【训练方法】

（1）起式：同站裆势起式。

（2）功式：左脚向左开一大步，两脚之间距离为本人脚长的3倍，足尖略收成内八字。屈膝屈髋下蹲，膝盖不超过脚尖，大腿与地面的夹角尽量保持45°，上身端正，两手虎口反插在两膝关节上方。头顶平，两目平视。双手叉腰，两拇指按在肾俞穴上，两肘夹紧，收腹敛臀直腰挺胸。两手后伸，挺肘伸腕，肩腋莫松，四指并拢，拇指外展，两上肢与上身夹角大于30°。裆势稳定，精神饱满（图4-3）。

（3）收式：两手叉腰。两手从后划圆到胸前，屈肘双掌下按，伸膝伸髋，身体恢复至起式。

Horse Stance

【Training methods】

(1) Preparation form: as the same as the standing stance.

(2) Exercise form: Move the left foot largely to the left, the distance between is as three times as one's own foot and the shape of feet is like pigeon toe pose. Bend the knees and hips down, the knees do not surpass the tiptoe. Keep the angle between the thigh and the ground 45°, keep the upper body upright, and insert Hu Kou opposite above two knees. Raise the head up, look straight ahead, bring hands to the waistline, press the Shenshu (BL 23) point with two fingers, and keep the elbows tucked in. Hold in the abdomen, draw buttocks in, straighten waist and erect chest. Stretch the hands backward, extend the elbows and the wrists and do not relax shoulders; close the four fingers with the thumb apart; keep the angle between the two upper limbs and the upper body over 30°. Make the stance stable and be in good spirits. (Figure 4–3)

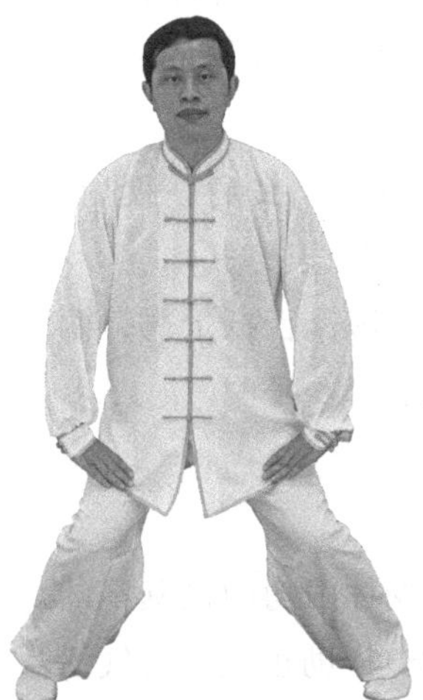

Figure 4–3

(3) Closing form: Bring hands to the waistline, make two hands draw a circle from back to the chest, extend knees and hips and return to the preparation form.

【动作要领】

（1）屈膝屈髋，马步下蹲，角度大于45°。

（2）足尖内扣或平行，不得外展。

（3）头顶平，两目平视，挺胸直腰，呼吸自然。

【Key points】

(1) Bend the knees and hips down, squat with a horse-riding step and the angle is over 45°.

(2) Make toes point inward or parallel with each other. And do not make toes point outward.

(3) Raise head up, look straight ahead, erect chest, straighten waist and breathe naturally.

【主要作用】

马裆势是少林内功中锻炼下肢的基础功法。能调内脏、固神元，是气血循经络贯于四肢末端。久练能增强腿、足、臂等力，使筋骨强健，脏腑坚固。

【Main functions】

As one of the fundamental exercises in Shaolin internal exercise to exercise lower limbs, horse stance has the function of regulating internal organs, consolidating Yuan-Primordial Spirit, promoting qi, blood, meridians and collaterals to four extremities. Long-time exercise can improve the strength of legs, feet and arms, and strengthen sinews, bones and internal organs.

三、弓箭裆势

Bow Stance

【训练方法】

（1）起式：同站裆势起式。

（2）功式：左脚向左开一大步，两脚之间距离为本人脚长的4倍，身体左转，左脚尖向左外旋转，脚尖内扣。左腿屈膝屈髋前弓，膝盖不超过脚尖，不落后于后脚跟。右脚脚尖向内旋转，右腿膝关节伸直。双手叉腰，两拇指按在肾俞穴上，两肘夹紧，收腹敛臀，上身端正，略前倾。两手后撑，挺肘伸腕，肩腋莫松，四指并拢，拇指外展，两上肢与上身夹角大于30°。两腿呈前弓后绷势，左小腿垂直地面，大腿尽量保持水平位（图4-4）。

【Training methods】

(1) Preparation form: as the same as the standing stance.

(2) Exercise form: Move the left foot largely to the left, the distance between is as four times as one's own foot. Turn the body left and rotate the left tiptoe left with the toes inward. Bend the left knees and hips to bow stance; the knees do not surpass the tiptoes and behind the back heels. Rotate the right tiptoes inward and extend the right knee. Bring hands to the waistline, press the Shenshu (BL 23) point with two fingers, and keep the elbows tucked in. Hold in the abdomen and draw buttocks in; keep the trunk upright with the upper part of the body slightly forward. Stretch the hands backward, extend the elbows and the wrists and do not relax shoulders; close the four

（3）收式：两手叉腰。两手放松垂下，身体转身起立，复原至起式。右弓箭裆势同上。

fingers with the thumb apart; keep the angle between the two upper limbs and the upper body over 30°. Make two legs in bow stance and keep the left shank vertical with the ground and the thigh in high position. (Figure 4–4)

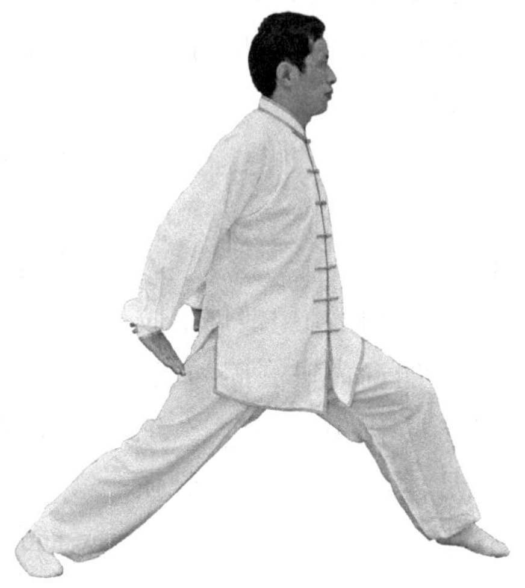

Figure 4–4

(3) Closing form: Bring hands to the waistline, drop down the arms naturally, keep the body erect and return to the preparation form.

【动作要领】

（1）前弓后箭，重心下沉，臀须微收。

（2）挺胸收腹，上身正直，挺肘伸腕，蓄势待发。

（3）前腿屈膝屈髋 45° 以下，小腿垂直地面，膝不过脚尖。

（4）全神贯注，呼吸自然。

【Key points】

(1) Extend the knee of the back leg with the heel touching the ground to form a bow stance, sink the body, hold in the buttocks.

(2) Throw out the chest, hold in the abdomen, keep the trunk upright, extend the elbows and the wrists, and store up strength.

(3) Bend the knees and hips of the front leg down to below 45°, keep the left shank vertical with the ground, and the knees do not surpass the tiptoes.

(4) Concentrate the mind and breathe naturally.

【主要作用】

弓箭裆势是少林内功中锻炼下肢的基础功法。能提神顺气、活血

【Main functions】

Bow stance is the fundamental exercise in Shaolin internal exercise, which has the function of lifting mind

通络，使内外坚固。练习弓箭裆势可以提升下肢的稳定性和相互协调。

and smoothing the flow of qi, activating the blood and freeing the collateral vessels. Bow stance can improve the stability and coordination of lower limbs.

四、磨裆势

Mill Stance

【训练方法】

（1）起式：同站裆势起式。

（2）功式：左脚向左开一大步，两脚之间距离为本人脚长的 4 倍，身体左转，左脚尖向左外旋转，脚尖内扣。左腿屈膝屈髋前弓，膝盖不超过脚尖，不落后于后脚跟。右脚脚尖向内旋转，右腿膝关节伸直。双手叉腰，两拇指按在肾俞穴上，两肘夹紧，收腹敛臀。上身略向前俯，重心下沉，右手仰掌护腰，左手俯掌屈肘向右上方推出，掌根及臂外侧运劲徐徐向左方磨转，同时身体随之向左旋转，右弓步演变成左弓步。得全势由右转左后，即左俯掌变仰掌收回护腰，右仰掌变俯掌屈肘向左上方推出（两掌在一收一出之际于胸口处交会）。

（3）收式：两手叉腰。两手放松垂下，身体转身起立，复原至起式。

【Training methods】

(1) Preparation form: as the same as the standing stance.

(2) Exercise form: Move the left foot largely to the left, the distance between is as four times as one's own foot. Turn the body left and rotate the left tiptoe left with the toes inward. Bend the left knees and hips; the knees do not surpass the tiptoes and behind the back heels. Rotate the right tiptoes inward and extend the right knee. Bring hands to the waistline, press Shenshu (BL 23) point with two fingers, and keep the elbows tucked in. Hold in the abdomen and draw buttocks in; keep the trunk upright with the upper part of the body slightly forward. Sink the body, bring the right hand to the waistline with palm upward, and push the left-hand top front right with palm downward. Turn palm, arm and body left, and change bow stance from right leg to left leg. Withdraw the left hand to the waistline with palm upward and push the right-hand top front left with palm downward.

(3) Closing form: Bring hands to the waistline, drop down the arms naturally, keep the body erect and return to the preparation form.

【动作要领】

（1）前弓后箭，重心下沉。

（2）仰掌化俯掌，屈肘推出，两掌在胸前交会。

（3）上肢蓄力，徐徐磨转，磨转时掌根及臂外侧运力。

【Key points】

(1) Extend the knee of the back leg with the heel touching the ground to form a bow stance, sink the body.

(2) Change the palms from the erect position to downward position. Bend the elbow to push hands and make two hands meeting at the chest.

(3) Store up strength in upper limbs and move with strength in palm and arms.

【主要作用】

与弓箭裆势相似。能提神顺气、活血通络，使内外坚固。久练能提升下肢的稳定性和相互协调。

【Main functions】

It has the function of lifting spirit and smoothing qi, promoting blood circulation for removing obstruction in collaterals, so as to strengthen body constitution. Long-time exercise can improve the stability and coordination of upper limbs.

五、亮裆势

Flash Stance

【训练方法】

（1）起式：同站裆势起式。

（2）功式：左脚向左开一大步，两脚之间距离为本人脚长的4倍，身体左转，左脚尖向左外旋转，脚尖内扣。左腿屈膝屈髋前弓，膝盖不超过脚尖，不落后于后脚跟。右脚脚尖向内旋转，右腿膝关节伸直。双手叉腰，两拇指按在肾俞穴上，两肘夹紧，收腹敛臀。两手由后向上亮掌，指端相对，掌心朝上，目视掌背，上身略向前俯，重心下沉（图4-5）。

（3）收式：两手叉腰。两手放松垂下，身体转身起立，复原至起式。

【Training methods】

(1) Preparation form: as the same as the standing stance.

(2) Exercise form: Move the left foot largely to the left, the distance between is as four times as one's own foot. Turn the body left and rotate the left tiptoe left with the toes inward. Bend the left knees and hips; the knees do not surpass the tiptoes and behind the back heels. Rotate the right tiptoe inward and extend the right knee. Bring hands to the waistline, press Shenshu (BL 23) point with two fingers, and keep the elbows tucked in. Hold in the abdomen and draw buttocks in. Flash two palms from backward with fingertips facing with each other. Turn the palms upward and look at the back of the palms; stand with the upper part of the body slightly forward and sink the body. (Figure 4–5)

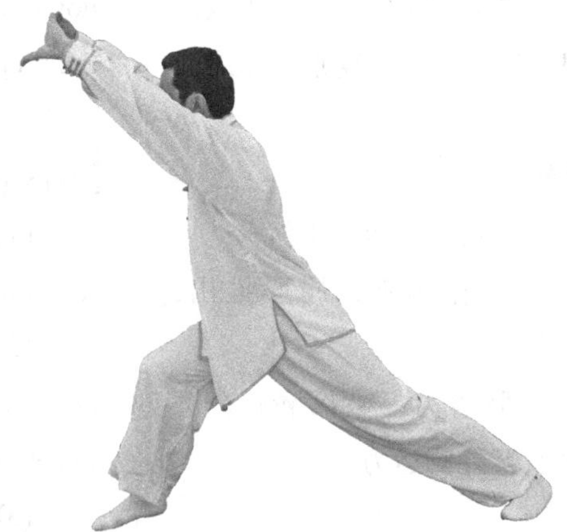

Figure 4–5

(3) Closing form: Bring hands to the waistline, drop down the arms naturally, keep the body erect and return to the preparation form.

【动作要领】

（1）上举亮掌，须高过头，目注掌背。

（2）上身前倾，并于下肢成一线。

（3）换步后转，转身变换，自然协调。

【Key points】

(1) Put palms up over the head and look at the back of the palms.

(2) Stand with the upper part of the body forward, being the same line with the lower limbs.

(3) The change of stances and movements should be coordinated.

【主要作用】

亮裆势久练能使气血周流，百脉通畅，劲贯全身，以达强筋壮骨，内外坚实的目的。

【Main functions】

Long-time exercise has the function of circulating qi and blood, promoting meridians and collaterals, and strengthening tendons and bones.

六、并裆势

Folding Stance

【训练方法】

（1）起式：同站裆势起式。

（2）功式：两脚跟向外旋转，脚尖相靠拢呈内八字形。两脚踏实，十趾抓地，两膝伸直，两腿内收夹紧。两手叉腰，两拇指按在肾俞穴上，两肘夹紧，收腹敛臀，上身端正，略前倾。两手后撑，挺肘伸腕，肩腋莫松，四指并拢，拇指外展，两上肢与上身夹角大于30°（图4-6）。

（3）收式：两手叉腰，下肢放松，上肢放松放下，身体复原至起式。

【Training methods】

(1) Preparation form: as the same as the standing stance.

(2) Exercise form: Rotate the heels outward, and the shape of feet is like pigeon toe pose. Grasp the ground forcefully with the toes, extend the knees and tighten two legs; bring hands to the waistline, press Shenshu (BL 23) point with two fingers, and keep the elbows tucked in. Hold in the abdomen and draw buttocks in; keep the trunk upright with the upper part of the body slightly forward. Stretch the hands backward, extend the elbows and wrists and do not relax shoulders; close the four fingers with the thumb apart; keep the angle between the two upper limbs and the upper body over 30°. (Figure 4–6)

(3) Closing form: Bring hands to the waistline, relax lower limbs, put down upper limbs and return to the preparation form.

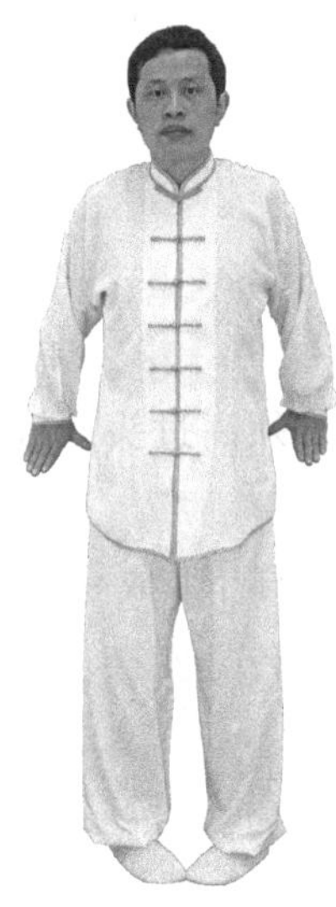

Figure 4–6

【动作要领】

（1）头如顶物，挺胸收腹，上身正直。

（2）两肩向背靠拢，两臂尽量后伸。

（3）下肢用劲内夹，膝关节不可弯曲，足跟尽量外展，两足间夹角不得小于90°。

【Key points】

(1) Keep the head erect like supporting something, erect chest, hold in the abdomen and keep the trunk upright.

(2) Make shoulders back and extend two arms back.

(3) Do not bend knees, keep the toe heel outward and the angle between two toes over 90°.

【主要作用】

并裆势是少林内功功法中的基础裆势之一，主要增强两下肢的平衡功力。

【Main functions】

As one of the basic stances in Shaolin internal exercise, it aims to strengthen the balanced power of lower limbs.

七、大裆势

Splitting Stance with Hands Backward

【训练方法】

（1）起式：同站裆势起式。

（2）功式：左脚向左开一大步，两脚之间距离为本人脚长的5倍。脚趾抓地，脚尖内扣，脚跟外蹬，膝直腿收，两手自然放于身侧。两手

【Training methods】

(1) Preparation form: as the same as the standing stance.

(2) Exercise form: Move the left foot largely to the left, the distance between is as five times as one's own foot. Grasp the ground forcefully and make the toes inward and the heels outward; keep the knees erect and withdraw

叉腰，两拇指按在肾俞穴上，两肘夹紧，收腹敛臀，上身端正，略前倾。两手后撑，挺肘伸腕，肩腋莫松，四指并拢，拇指外展，两上肢与上身夹角大于30°（图4–7）。

（3）收式：两手叉腰。两手放松下垂，收脚身体起立，复原至起式。

the legs; drop down the arms naturally. Bring hands to the waistline, press Shenshu (BL 23) point with two fingers, and keep the elbows tucked in. Hold in the abdomen, draw buttocks in, and stand upright with the upper part of the body slightly forward. Stretch hands backward, extend the elbows and wrists and do not relax shoulders; close the four fingers with the thumb apart; keep the angle between the two upper limbs and the upper body over 30°. (Figure 4–7)

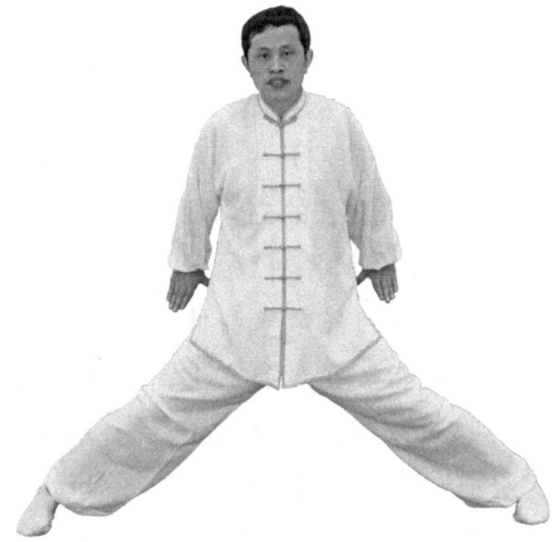

Figure 4–7

(3) Closing form: Bring hands to the waistline. Drop down the arms naturally, withdraw feet, keep the body upright and return to the preparation form.

【动作要领】

（1）三直四平，挺胸直腰，头顶平直，目须前视。

（2）下肢伸直，膝勿屈曲。

（3）两足跟间距不小于本人5～6足的长度。

（4）两足尖不得外撇。

【Key points】

(1) Erect chest, straighten waist, raise head up and look straight ahead.

(2) Extend lower limbs, and do not bend knees.

(3) The distance between two feet should be more than 5 to 6 times of the length of one's own feet.

(4) Do not make tiptoes point outward.

【主要作用】

大裆势是少林内功中的主要裆势之一，可锻炼两下肢在外展动作下的霸力，促进气血充盈。

【Main functions】

Splitting stance is the main stance in Shaolin internal exercise, which can strengthen the stability of lower limbs and make qi and blood abundant.

八、悬裆势

悬裆势要求两脚之间距离为本人脚长的4倍，其余练习方法和要领与马裆势相同，故又称为大马裆势。

Squatting-splitting Stance with Hands on the Waist

Squatting-splitting stance with hands on the waist requires that the distance between two feet is as four times as one's own foot. So, it is also called the large horse stance.

【训练方法】

（1）起式：同站裆势起式。

（2）功式：左脚向左开一大步，两脚之间距离为本人脚长的5倍。脚趾抓地，脚尖内扣，脚跟外蹬。屈髋屈膝下蹲，两手自然放于身侧。两手叉腰，两拇指按在肾俞穴上，两肘夹紧，收腹敛臀，上身端正，略前倾。两手后撑，挺肘伸腕，肩腋莫松，四指并拢，拇指外展，两上肢与上身夹角大于30°（图4-8）。

（3）收式：两手叉腰。两手放松下垂，收脚身体起立，复原至起式。

【Training methods】

(1) Preparation form: as the same as the standing stance.

(2) Exercise form: Move the left foot largely to the left, the distance between is as five times as one's own foot. Grasp the ground forcefully with the toes, and make the tiptoes inward and the heels outward. Bend hips and knees to the level of squat. Drop down the arms naturally, bring hands to the waistline, press Shenshu (BL 23) point with two fingers, and keep the elbows tucked in. Hold in the abdomen, draw buttocks in, stand upright with the upper part of the body slightly forward. Stretch the hands backward, extend the elbows and wrists and do not relax shoulders; close the four fingers with the thumb apart; keep the angle between the two upper limbs and the upper body over 30°. (Figure 4–8)

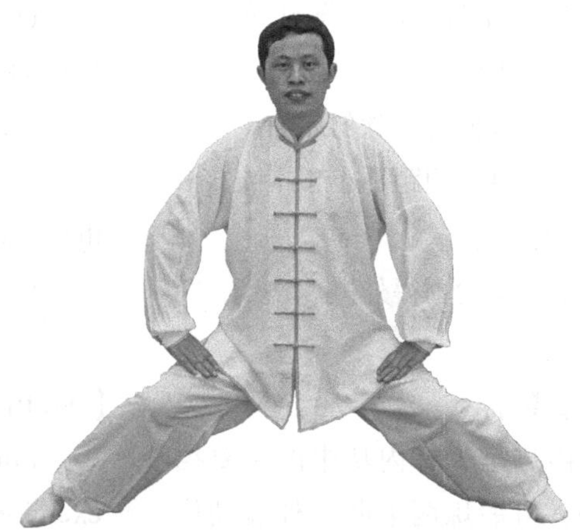

Figure 4–8

(3) Closing form: Bring hands to the waistline. Drop down the arms naturally, withdraw feet, keep the body upright and return to the preparation form.

【动作要领】

（1）上身挺直，直腰收腹，重心在两腿间。

（2）屈髋屈膝45°以下，使大腿平行地面。

（3）下蹲时两膝不得超过足尖。

【Key points】

(1) Keep the upper body erect, straighten waist, and hold in the abdomen. The center of gravity of the body is between two legs.

(2) Bend hips and knees below 45°, making legs parallel with the ground.

(3) Two knees do not surpass the tiptoes when squatting.

【主要作用】

悬裆势是少林内功中的主要裆势之一，可锻炼两下肢在外展动作下的霸力，促进气血充盈。

【Main functions】

Squatting-splitting stance with hands on the waist is the main stance in Shaolin internal exercise, which can strengthen the stability of lower limbs and make qi and blood abundant.

九、低裆势

Lower Stance

（1）起式：同站裆势起式。

（2）功式：两手握拳，两臂前上举至头顶。十趾抓地，脚尖内扣，脚跟外蹬，膝直腿收，两手自然放于身侧。两手叉腰，两拇指按在肾俞穴上，两肘夹紧，收腹敛臀，上身端正，略前倾。两手后撑，挺肘伸腕，肩腋莫松，四指并拢，拇指外展，两上肢与上身夹角大于30°（图4–9）。

（3）收式：两手放松落臂，身体缓慢起立复原至起式。

(1) Preparation form: as the same as the standing stance.

(2) Exercise form: Make fists with two hands and raise them up over the head. Grasp the ground forcefully with the toes, and make the tiptoes inward and the heels outward. Keep the knees erect and withdraw the legs; drop down the arms naturally. Bring hands to the waistline, press Shenshu (BL 23) point with two fingers, and keep the elbows tucked in. Hold in the abdomen, draw buttocks in, and stand upright with the upper part of the body slightly forward. Stretch hands backward, extend the elbows and wrists and do not relax shoulders; close the four fingers with the thumb apart; keep the angle between the two upper limbs and the upper body over 30°. (Figure 4–9)

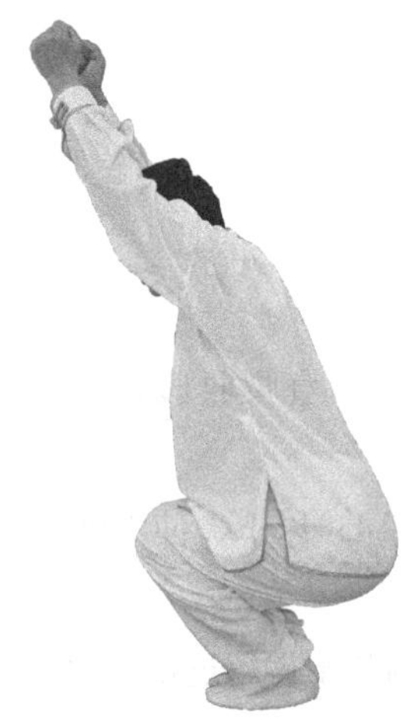

Figure 4–9

(3) Closing form: Drop down the arms naturally, stand up slowly and return to the preparation form.

【动作要领】

（1）屈膝下蹲，上身下沉，臀部紧贴足跟。

（2）握拳上举过头，拳心相对。

（3）两足踏实，五趾抓地，足跟不可提起。

【Key points】

(1) Bend the knees to squat down, sink the torso, and make the buttocks touch the heels.

(2) Make the hands into fists above the head with the palms facing each other.

(3) Make two feet grasp the ground forcefully with the toes.

【主要作用】

低裆势是少林内功中锻炼下肢屈伸功力的姿势，可以促进全身气血运行，增进消化功能。

【Main functions】

Lower stance aims to exercise the flexion and extension of lower limbs, which has the functions of promoting the circulation of qi and blood and promoting the digestion of food.

十、坐裆势

Sitting Stance

【训练方法】

坐裆势要求两脚交叉，盘膝而坐，脚外侧着地，臀部坐于足跟。其余动作同站裆势（图4–10）。

【Training methods】

Cross the feet, sit with the crossed legs, make the lateral sides of the feet touch the ground and the buttocks on heel. The other stances are the same with standing stance. (Figure 4–10)

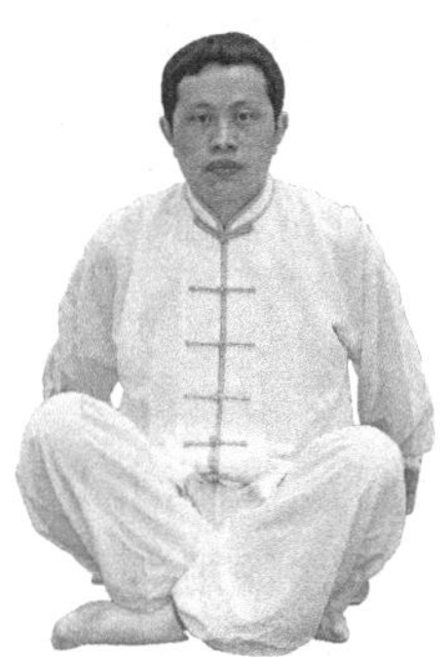

Figure 4–10

【动作要领】

（1）盘膝而坐，足侧着地，上身微前俯，保持身体平衡。

（2）头如顶物，两眼平视，全神贯注。

【Key points】

(1) Sit with the crossed legs, the lateral sides of the feet touching the ground. Slightly lean the torso forward and keep the balance of body.

(2) Make the head erect like supporting something, look straight ahead and concentrate the mind.

【主要作用】

坐裆势是少林内功中坐盘功架，主要锻炼身法内功。

【Main functions】

Sitting stance is crossed-legged sitting stance in Shaolin internal exercise, which is aimed to exercise body techniques and strengthen internal force.

第四节 上肢动作

Section Four Movement in Upper Limbs

一、前推八匹马

Qian Tui Ba Pi Ma (Pushing Eight Horses Forward)

【训练方法】

（1）起式：站裆势或指定裆势。两手屈肘，立掌于两胁，拇指向上，四肢向前，虎口分开。

（2）功式：出声发力，蓄劲于肩臂指端，拇指伸直，四指并拢，

【Training methods】

(1) Preparation form: Take standing stance or the appointed stance. Bend the elbows and put the palm at the rib-sides. Keep the thumbs tilted and limbs forward with Hu Kou (the web between the thumb and index finger) apart.

虎口用力撑开；使两臂徐徐运力前推至肘直，两掌心相对，与肩等高，与胸等宽。两目有神，意念集中，呼吸自然（图4-11）。

（3）收式：出声发力，蓄劲于肩臂指端，拇指伸直，四指并拢，虎口用力撑开；两臂徐徐用力，慢慢屈肘，立掌收回于两胁。两手后撑挺肘伸腕，回复至原裆势。

(2) Exercise form: Speak loudly, focus the strength on the shoulders, arms and fingertips, keep the thumbs apart and four fingers closed and upright, and keep Hu Kou apart. Slowly push the arms forward forcefully until the shoulders and palms are on the same lever, keep two palms facing each other, make two arms in the same height of shoulders and the same width of the chest. Concentrate the mind and breathe naturally. (Figure 4–11)

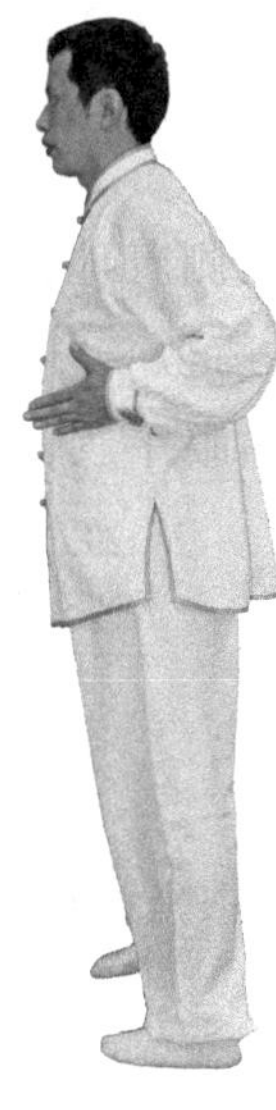

Figure 4–11

(3) Closing form: Speak loudly, focus the strength on the shoulders, arms and fingertips, keep the thumbs apart and four fingers closed and upright, and keep Hu Kou apart. Slowly bend the elbows and draw them back to the rib-sides. Stretch the hands backward, extend the elbows and the wrists, and return to the original stance.

【动作要领】

（1）两目平视，呼吸自然，胸须微挺，头勿顾盼。

（2）蓄劲于腰，运劲于肩臂，贯于掌、达于指，所谓"蓄劲于腰，发力于指"。

（3）两手动作一致，两臂肩平，

【Key points】

(1) Look straight ahead, breathe naturally, slightly straighten up the chest and do not move the head.

(2) Store up strength in the waist, shoulders arms and palms and exert strength at fingers.

(3) Both hands do the same movements. And make two arms in the same height and the same width of

与肩等宽。

shoulders.

【主要作用】

前推八匹马是少林内功中锻炼手臂、指端功力的功法，能增强两臂蓄劲和指端功夫，久练则能宽胸理气，通三焦，疏腠理，活关节，壮骨骼，并能健运脾胃，使百脉流通，以达到精力充沛、正气旺盛的目的。

【Main functions】

Pushing eight horses forward aims to exercise arms and fingers. Long-time exercise has the function of soothing the chest to regulate qi, unblocking triple energizer, freeing interstice, invigorating joints, fortifying bones, strengthening the transporting functions of the spleen and the stomach, and unlocking all vessels. The goal is to make people full of energy and the healthy qi abundant.

二、倒拉九头牛

Dao La Jiu Tou Niu (Pulling Nine Oxen Backward)

【训练方法】

（1）起式：站裆势或指定裆势。两手屈肘，立掌于两胁，拇指向上，四肢向前，虎口分开。

（2）功式：出声发力，蓄劲于肩臂指端，拇指伸直，四指并拢，虎口用力撑开；两掌缓缓向前推，两臂换向内旋，边旋边推，两肘伸直后，四指向前，拇指向下，手背相对。两目有神，意念集中，呼吸自然（图4-12）。

（3）收式：出声发力，蓄劲于肩臂指端，五指用力屈收握拳，劲注拳心，手臂缓缓外旋，屈肘收手臂，边旋边收，两拳回收到两胁，拳心向上。缓缓松手变掌，立掌扶胁。两手后撑，挺肘伸腕，回复至原裆势。

【Training methods】

(1) Preparation form: Choose standing stance or the appointed stance. Bend the elbows and put the palm at the rib-sides. Keep the thumbs tilted and limbs forward with Hu Kou apart.

(2) Exercise form: Speak loudly, focus the strength on the shoulders, arms and fingertips, keep the thumbs apart and four fingers closed and upright, and keep Hu Kou apart. Rotate two arms inward while slowly pushing them forward. After extending elbows, keep four fingers forward and the thumb downward with the back of hand facing with each other. Have bright eyes, concentrate the mind, and breathe naturally. (Figure 4–12)

(3) Closing form: Speak loudly, focus the strength on the shoulders, arms and fingertips, flex five fingers to form fists, focus the strength on the palms, slowly rotate arms outward, constrict arms while bending elbows. Withdraw fists to the rib-sides with fists upward. Slowly change fists into palms and support ribs with upward palms. Stretch the hands backward, extend the elbows and the wrists, and return to the original stance.

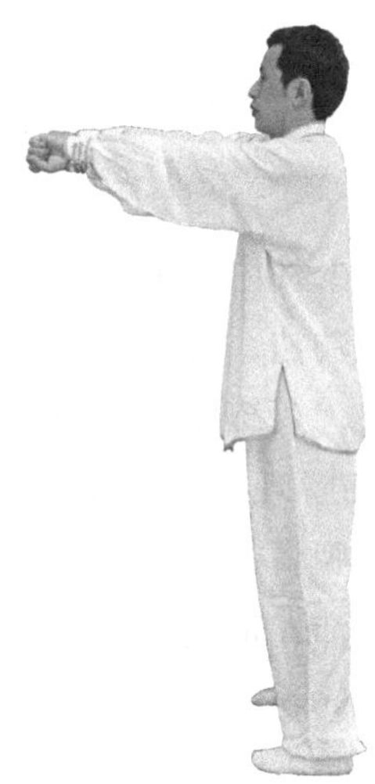

Figure 4–12

【动作要领】

（1）两手动作一致，两臂与肩平，与肩等宽。

（2）前推时，肘腕伸直与肩平，勿抬肩。

（3）两臂前推、后拉与前臂内旋、外旋动作要协调。两臂收回后拉时，两拳握紧，不可松劲。

【Key points】

(1) Make two arms in the same height and the same width of shoulders.

(2) The wrist and elbows should be straight at the shoulder-levels. Do not lift shoulders.

(3) The movements of two arms should be coordinated. When pushing two arms backward, clench fists and do not relax.

【主要作用】

倒拉九头牛是少林内功中锻炼两臂的悬劲于手掌握力的主要姿势。久练则能疏通经络、调和气血，使阴阳相对平衡，达到健肺益肾、内外坚固、扶正祛邪的目的。

【Main functions】

Pulling nine oxen backward aims to improve the strength of two arms. Long-time exercise can free meridians and collaterals, harmonize qi and blood, and balance yin and yang, which can achieve the goal of fortifying the lung and replenishing the kidney, reinforcing the healthy qi, and dispelling pathogenic factors.

三、单掌拉金环

Dan Zhang La Jin Huan (Pulling Golden Ring with One Hand)

【训练方法】

（1）起式：站裆势或指定裆势。两手屈肘，立掌于两胁，拇指向上，

【Training methods】

(1) Preparation form: Choose standing stance or the

四肢向前，虎口分开。

（2）功式：出声发力，蓄劲于肩臂指端。右手前推边推拇指缓缓向下，渐渐内战，待虎口正朝下时，掌心朝外，四肢并拢向前，拇指外分，臂蓄劲掌侧着力时，腕伸直，松肩，身体勿随之偏斜。两目平视，意念集中，呼吸自然。五指内收，握拳使劲注拳心，旋腕，拳眼朝上，紧紧内收，立掌于两胁。出声发力，蓄劲于肩臂指端，拇指伸直，四指并拢，虎口用力撑开；两掌缓缓向前推，两臂换换向内旋，边旋边推，两肘伸直后，四指向前，拇指向下，手背相对。两目有神，意念集中，呼吸自然（图4–13）。

（3）收式：出声发力，蓄劲于肩臂指端，五指用力屈收握拳，劲注拳心，手臂缓缓外旋，屈肘收手臂，边旋边收，两拳回收到两胁，拳心向上。缓缓松手变掌，立掌扶胁。两手后撑，挺肘伸腕，回复至原裆势。

appointed stance. Bend the elbows and put the palm at the rib-sides. Keep the thumbs tilted and limbs forward with Hu Kou apart.

(2) Exercise form: Speak loudly, and focus the strength on the shoulders, arms and fingertips. Push the right hand forward and move the thumb slowly downward. After Hu kou facing downward, make the palm outward. Close four fingers with the thumb apart. Extend the wrists, relax shoulders and do not tilt the body. Look straight ahead, concentrate the mind and breathe naturally. Close five fingers, make fists and focus the strength on the palms. Rotate the wrists, keep palms at the rib-sides with fists facing upward. Speak loudly, focus the strength on the shoulders, arms and fingertips, keep the thumbs apart and four fingers closed and upright, and keep Hu Kou apart. Rotate two arms inward while slowly pushing them forward. After extending two elbows, keep four fingers forward and the thumb downward with the back of hand facing with each other. Have bright eyes, concentrate the mind, and breathe naturally. (Figure 4–13)

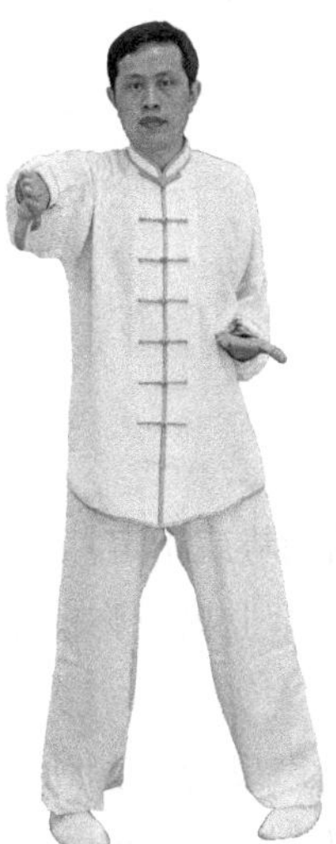

Figure 4–13

(3) Closing form: Speak loudly, focus the strength on the shoulders, arms and fingertips, flex the fingers to form fists, focus the strength on the palms, slowly rotate arms outward, constrict arms while bending elbows. Withdraw

fists to the rib-sides with fists upward. Slowly change fists into palms and support ribs with upward palms. Stretch the hands backward, extend the elbows and the wrists, and return to the original stance.

【动作要领】

（1）身体勿偏斜，头勿顾盼，两目平视，呼吸自然。

（2）前推至肘、腕伸直与肩平，勿抬肩。

（3）臂前推后拉与前臂内外旋动作要协调，臂收回后拉时拳握紧，不可松劲。

【Key points】

(1) Do not tilt the body and move the head. Look straight ahead and breathe naturally.

(2) The wrist and elbows should be straight at the shoulder-levels. Do not lift shoulders.

(3) The movements of two arms should be coordinated. When pushing hips backward, clench fists and do not relax.

【主要作用】

与倒拉九头牛相似，久练则能疏通经络，调和气血，使阴阳相对平衡，达到健肺益肾、扶正祛邪的目的。

【Main functions】

Similar with pulling nine oxen backward, long-time exercise of pulling golden ring with one hand can free meridians and collaterals, harmonize qi and blood, and balance yin and yang, which can achieve the goal of fortifying the lung and replenishing the kidney, reinforcing the healthy qi, and dispelling pathogenic factors.

四、凤凰展翅

Feng Huang Zhan Chi (Chinese Phoenix Spreading its Wings)

【训练方法】

（1）起式：站裆势或指定裆势。两手屈肘，两手徐徐上提至胸前呈立掌交叉。

（2）功式：出声发力，蓄劲于肩臂指端，拇指伸直，四指并拢，虎口用力撑开；使两臂徐徐运力，两掌缓缓向两侧用力分开，形同展翅，劲如开弓，至两上肢与身体成一直线，腕关节与肩等高。两目有神，意念集中，呼吸自然（图4-14）。

【Training methods】

(1) Preparation form: Take a standing stance or the appointed stance. Bend the elbows and move the hands upward slowly to the chest, and then cross the erect palms in front of the chest.

(2) Exercise form: Speak loudly, focus the strength on the shoulders, arms and fingertips, keep the thumbs apart and four fingers closed and upright, and keep Hu Kou apart. Slowly push the arms forward and separate the palms and extend the arms forcefully to the sides like flying wings.

（3）收式：出声发力，蓄劲于肩臂指端，拇指伸直，四指并拢，虎口用力撑开；使两臂徐徐运力，两掌缓缓由左右向前向内合拢，于胸前立掌交叉。由上胸前之立掌化俯掌下按，两臂后撑，回复原裆势。

Make two upper limbs and the body in the same level and keep the wrists in the same height of the shoulder. Have bright eyes, concentrate the mind, and breathe naturally. (Figure 4–14)

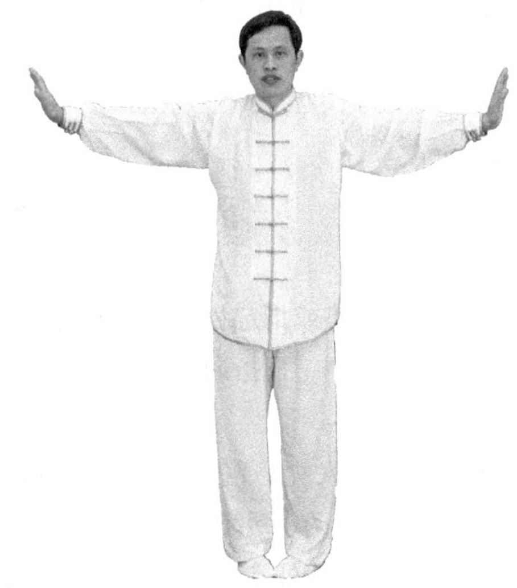

Figure 4–14

(3) Closing form: Speak loudly, focus the strength on the shoulders, arms and fingertips, keep the thumbs apart and four fingers closed and upright, keep Hu Kou apart. Slowly push the arms forward, move the arms inward until the palms facing with each other, and then cross the erect palms in front of the chest. Change the palms from the erect position to downward position and press down. Stretch the arms backward and return to the original stance.

【动作要领】

（1）身体勿偏斜，头如顶物，两目平视。

（2）两臂动作一致，优美有力，如凤凰展翅，神态飘逸。

（3）以气发劲，劲由肩循臂贯于腕、达于指，所谓“蓄劲如开弓，发劲如发箭”。

【Key points】

(1) Make the head erect like supporting something and look straight ahead. Do not skew the body.

(2) Both arms move in the same gestures, graceful and powerful, like a Chinese phoenix spreading its wings.

(3) Squat to pool your strength and give full rein to it quickly.

【主要作用】

凤凰展翅是少林内功中锻炼肩、

【Main functions】

Chinese Phoenix spreading its wings is the basic

臂、肘、腕、指端的基本姿势。它对腕、指功夫大有助益，久练则能调和内脏，舒展胸廓，增加气劲和悬力，具有宽胸理气、平肝健肺的作用。

stance to exercise shoulders, arms, elbows, wrist and fingertips. Long-time exercise can harmonize internal organs, relax thorax, increase strength, soothe the chest to regulate qi, calm the liver and fortify the spleen.

五、霸王举鼎

【训练方法】

（1）起式：站裆势或指定裆势。两手屈肘，仰掌于腰间，拇指向前，四指并拢，虎口分开。

（2）功式：出声发力，蓄劲于指掌，虎口用力撑开。两掌缓缓向上托起，至胸前伸腕、手臂外旋，边旋边上举，推至头顶后，四指相对，掌心向上，肘关节伸直。两目有神，意念集中，呼吸自然（图4-15）。

（3）收式：出声发力，虎口用力撑开。两臂内旋屈腕，屈肘回收，两臂缓缓用力内旋，肘尖下沉，两掌回收，仰掌收腰。两手后撑，回复原裆势。

Ba Wang Ju Ding (Hegemonic King Supporting Tripot)

【Training methods】

(1) Preparation form: Take a standing stance or the appointed stance. Bend the elbows and set the hands against the waist with palms facing upward. Close four fingers with the thumb forward and Hu Kou apart.

(2) Exercise form: Speak loudly, focus the strength on the fingers and palms, and keep Hu Kou apart. Raise hands slowly to the chest and then extend the wrist while rotating arms outward. After raising the hands above the head, extend the elbows with four fingers facing with each other and palms upward. Have bright eyes, concentrate the mind and breathe naturally. (Figure 4–15)

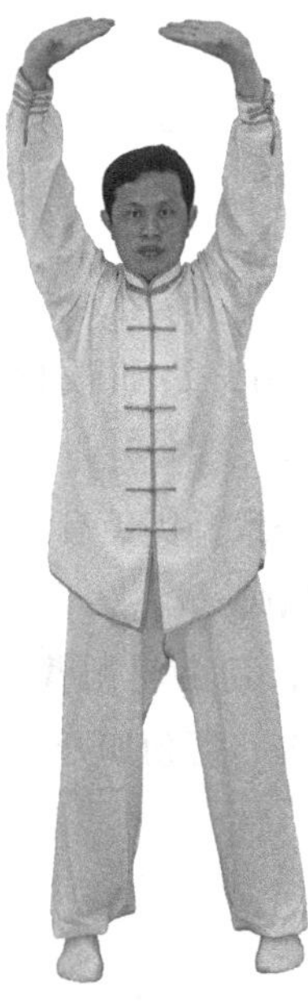

Figure 4–15

(3) Closing form: Speak loudly and keep Hu Kou apart. Rotate arms inward, bend wrists and withdraw the hands. Sink the tip of the elbows, withdraw two palms, and protect the waist with upward palms. Stretch the hands backward and return to the original stance.

【动作要领】

（1）上身勿偏斜，两目平视，头勿盼顾，呼吸自然。

（2）仰掌上托，两膝勿松，劲欲含蓄。

（3）上举收回，动作一致有力。

【Key points】

(1) Look straight ahead and breathe naturally. Do not skew the upper body or move the head.

(2) Raise the hands with the palm upward and do not relax knees.

(3) The movements must be consistent and forceful.

【主要作用】

霸王举鼎是少林内功中锻炼两臂上托、下沉的姿势，通过通调三焦气机以调和脾胃。

【Main functions】

Hegemonic king supporting tripot aims to exercise the up and down movements of two arms. It can harmonize the spleen and the stomach through regulating the qi mechanism of the triple energizer.

六、两手托天

Holding the Sky with Two Hands

【训练方法】

（1）起式：站裆势或指定裆势。两手屈肘，立掌于两胁，拇指向上，四肢向前，虎口分开。

（2）功式：出声发力，蓄劲于指掌，虎口用力撑开。两掌上托掌心朝上，缓缓上举，指端着力，肩欲松开，肘欲伸直。两目平视，头如顶物，意念集中，呼吸自然。（图4–16）

（3）收式：出声发力，拇指向外侧运动倾斜，四指并拢，掌根蓄力，屈肘徐徐而下，收回护腰。两手后撑，回复原裆势。

【Training methods】

(1) Preparation form: Take a standing stance or the appointed stance. Bend the elbows and put the upward palms at the ribs. Keep fingers upward with four limbs forward and Hu Kou apart.

(2) Exercise form: Speak loudly, focus the strength on the fingers and palms, and keep Hu Kou apart. Slowly raise the palms up, the palms centers facing upward, accumulate the strength in the fingertips, relax the shoulders, extend the elbows. Look straight ahead, erect the head like supporting something. Concentrate the mind and breathe naturally. (Figure 4–16)

(3) Closing form: Speak loudly and keep Hu Kou apart. Make the thumb point outward, close four fingers

and focus strength on the heel of the hand. Bend the elbows and withdraw them to protect the waist. Stretch the hands backward and return to the original stance.

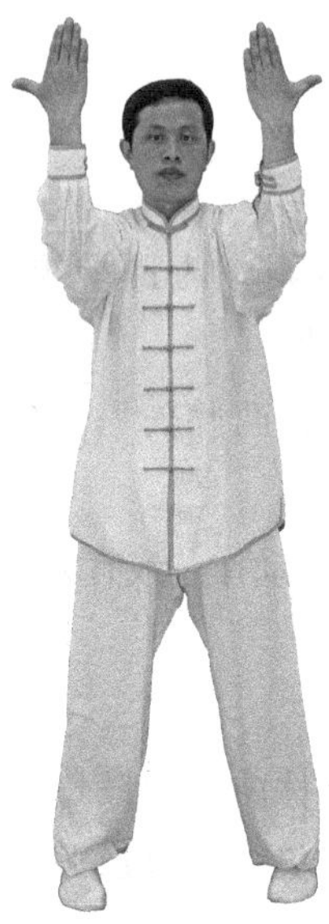

Figure 4–16

【动作要领】

（1）上身勿偏斜，两目平视，头勿盼顾。

（2）仰掌上托，四指并拢，拇指用力外展，掌心朝上。

（3）回收时前臂外旋，使手背向前。

【Key points】

(1) Do not skew the upper body, look straight ahead, and do not move the head.

(2) Raise the palms up, keep the four fingers closed and the thumb outward with palms' center facing upward.

(3) Rotate forearms outward and keep the back of the hands forward.

【主要作用】

与霸王举鼎相似，可锻炼两臂上托、下沉的姿势，通过通调三焦气机以调和脾胃。

【Main functions】

Like hegemonic king supporting tripot, holding the sky with two hands aims to exercise the up and down movements of two arms. It can harmonize the spleen and the stomach through regulating triple energizer and qi mechanism.

七、顺水推舟

【训练方法】

（1）起式：站裆势或指定裆势。两手屈肘，立掌于两胁，拇指向上，四肢向前，虎口分开。

（2）功式：出声发力，蓄劲于指掌。两掌运劲徐徐向前推出，边推边背伸腕关节，至腕关节背伸90°后，手臂旋内前推，四指并拢，拇指外分，前推至肘直，指尖相对。两目有神，意念集中，呼吸自然。（图4–17）

（3）收式：出声发力，蓄劲于指掌。虎口用力撑开，前臂外旋屈腕，至腕平后，两臂徐徐运力，屈肘回收，立掌扶于两胁。两手后撑，回复原裆势。

Shun Shui Tui Zhou (Pushing Boat along Water-Flowing)

【Training methods】

(1) Preparation form: Take a standing stance or the appointed stance. Bend the elbows and put the upward palms at the ribs. Keep fingers upward with four limbs forward and Hu Kou apart.

(2) Exercise form: Focus the strength on the fingers and palms. Push palms forward slowly, and at the same time, extend the wrists backward. When the wrists extending to 90°, rotate arms inward and push them forward with four fingers closed and the thumb abduct. Push arms until the elbows become erect and keep fingertips facing with each other. Have bright eyes, concentrate the mind and breathe naturally. (Figure 4–17)

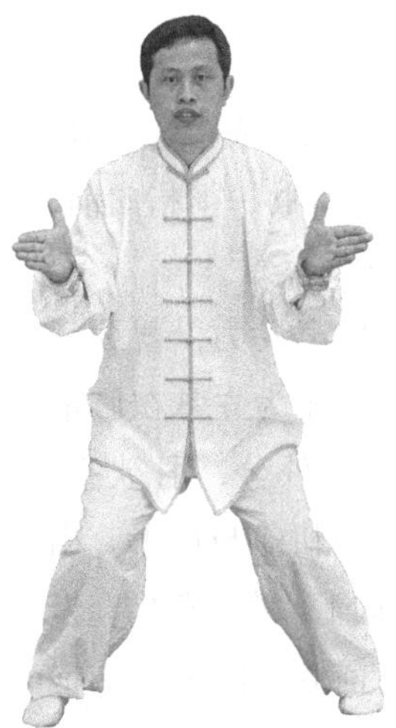

Figure 4–17

(3) Closing form: Speak loudly and focus the strength on the fingers and palms. Keep Hu Kou apart, rotate forearms outward and bend the wrists. Bend the elbows and withdraw them to protect the ribs with upward palms. Stretch the hands backward and return to the original stance.

【动作要领】

（1）头勿低，身勿斜，呼吸自然，勿屏气。

（2）两肩下沉，勿抬肩，肘直与肩平，腕尽量背屈，似推舟。

【Key points】

(1) Keep the head and body erect. Breathe naturally and stop breath-holding.

(2) Sink shoulders, do not lift the shoulders. Keep the elbows extended, making them on the same lever with the shoulders, and extend the wrists backward to form a ring-shaped between the arms.

【主要作用】

顺水推舟是少林内功中锻炼手臂前推旋劲的姿势，具有宽胸理气、健脾和胃的作用。

【Main functions】

Pushing boat along water-flowing aims to exercise the pushing movement and the rotating force of arms, which has the function of soothing the chest to regulate qi and invigorating spleen and harmonizing stomach.

八、怀中抱月

Huai Zhong Bao Yue (Embracing the Moon)

【训练方法】

（1）起式：悬裆势或指定裆势。两手屈肘，仰掌于两胁，拇指向前，四肢并拢，虎口分开。

（2）功式：出声发力，蓄劲于指掌。两掌上提，化为立掌在胸前交叉，缓缓向左右外分，肘欲直，指端朝左右，掌心朝前与肩平。出声发力，两指端向下，掌心朝内，慢慢蓄劲，上身略前倾，两手势如抱物。由上而下，由下而上徐徐抄起，立掌收回于胸前交叉。两目有神，意念集中，呼吸自然（图4-18）。

（3）收式：由胸前立掌化俯掌下按，两手后撑，回复原裆势。

【Training methods】

(1) Preparation form: Take a squatting-splitting stance with hands on the waist or the appointed stance. Bend the elbows and put the upward palms at the ribs. Keep the thumb forward with four fingers closed and Hu Kou apart.

(2) Exercise form: Speak loudly and focus the strength on the fingers and palms. Raise the palms upward; then change the upward palms into the erect palms and cross them in front of the chest. Then, slowly separate the hands to the sides, extend the elbows with the fingers pointing to the sides and the palms facing forward; keep the palms and the shoulders at the same lever. Speak loudly and turn the fingertips downward and the palms inward; slightly lean the torso forward, focus the strength on the palms and arms and raise them like embracing something. Finally cross the hands with erect palms in front of the chest. Have bright eyes, concentrate the mind and breathe naturally. (Figure 4–18)

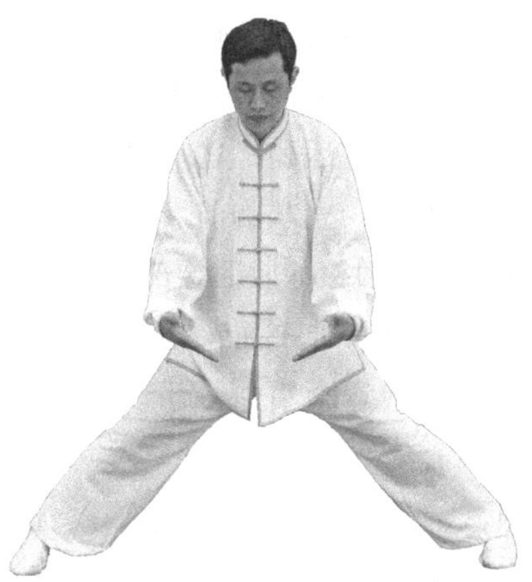

Figure 4–18

(3) Closing form: Change the palms from erect position to downward position and press down. Stretch the arms backward and return to the original stance.

【动作要领】

（1）两臂徐徐抱拢，势如抱月。

（2）上身正直，松肩使气下沉。

【Key points】

(1) Make two arms like embracing the moon.

(2) Keep the trunk upright and relax shoulders to sink qi.

【主要作用】

怀中抱月式能调和内脏，舒展胸廓，增加气劲和悬力，具有宽胸理气、平肝健肺的作用。

【Main functions】

Embracing the moon can harmonize internal organs, extend thorax, strengthen forces, soothe the chest to regulate qi and calm the liver and fortify the spleen.

九、仙人指路

Xian Ren Zhi Lu (Immortal Guiding Way)

【训练方法】

（1）起式：大裆势或指定裆势。两手屈肘，仰掌于两胁，拇指向前，四肢并拢，虎口分开。

（2）功式：出声发力，蓄劲于指掌。右仰掌上提至胸立掌而出，四指并拢，拇指伸直，手心内凹成瓦楞掌，肘臂运劲，立掌着力徐徐推出至肘直，立掌胸前。出声发力，

【Training methods】

(1) Preparation form: Take a splitting stance with hands backward or the appointed stance. Bend the elbows and put the upward palms at the ribs. Keep the thumb forward with four fingers closed and Hu Kou apart.

(2) Exercise form: Speak out loudly, focus the strength on the fingers and palms. Light the right palm to the chest and change to an erect palm; then push the palm forward with the four fingers closed and the thumb apart, the center

蓄劲于指掌。左仰掌上提至胸立掌而出，四指并拢，拇指伸直，手心内凹成瓦楞掌，肘臂运劲，立掌着力徐徐推出至肘直，立掌胸前。同时，右掌握拳，屈肘徐徐收回腰部，变仰掌扶腰。两手一伸一屈，动作协调。两目有神，意念集中，呼吸自然（图4–19）。

（3）收式：出声发力，左掌握拳，屈肘徐徐收回腰部，变仰掌扶腰。两手后撑，回复原裆势。

of the palm is hollow; focus the strength on the elbow and arm, push the erect palm forward until the elbow becomes erect and make the erect palm in front of the chest. Speak out loudly, focus the strength on the fingers and palms. Light the left palm to the chest and change to an erect palm; then push the palm forward with the four fingers closed and the thumb apart, the center of the palm is hollow; focus the strength on the elbow and arm, push the erect palm forward until the elbow becomes erect and make the erect palm in front of the chest. At the same time, make the right hand into a fist, bend the elbow to the waist and support the waist with the upward palm. Have bright eyes, concentrate the mind and breathe naturally. (Figure 4–19)

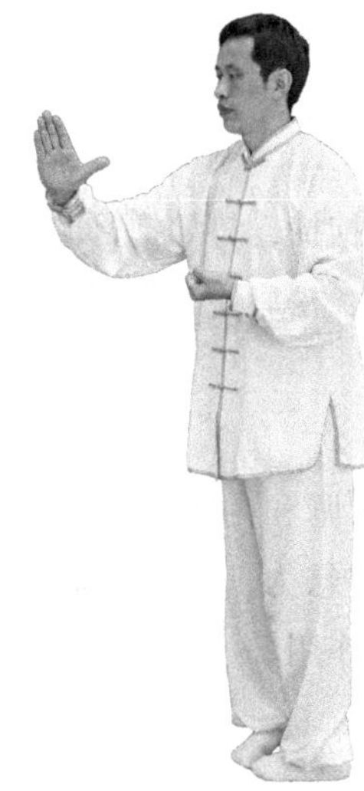

Figure 4–19

(3) Closing form: Speak out loudly, make the left hand into a fist, bend the elbow to the waist and support the waist with the upward palm. Stretch the arms backward and return to the original stance.

【动作要领】

（1）四指并拢，拇指伸直，手心内凹，呈瓦楞状。

（2）肘臂运力，向前推出肘欲直，握拳回收拳须紧。

【Key points】

(1) Keep the four fingers closed and the thumb apart and make the center of the palm hollow.

(2) Focus strength on the elbows and arms, extend the elbows when pushing forward and clench fists when

（3）一手收拳，一手推掌，动作协调。

withdrawing the fists.

(3) The movements of two arms should be coordinated.

【主要作用】

仙人指路是少林内功中左右臂交替运劲锻炼的姿势，可以增强习练者双手交替操作技能的协调能力，具有平和阴阳、行气活血的作用。

【Main functions】

Immortal guiding way can strengthen the coordination of two hands and has the function of balancing yin and yang, and circulating qi and blood.

十、平手托塔

Ping Shou Tuo Ta (Holding Tower with Flat Hand)

【训练方法】

（1）起式：站裆势或指定裆势。两手屈肘，仰掌于两胁，拇指向前，四肢并拢，虎口分开。

（2）功式：出声发力，蓄劲于指掌。两掌犹如托物前推，两前臂运力外旋，至肘直，两掌与肩等高等宽。两目有神，意念集中，呼吸自然（图4-20）。

（3）收式：出声发力，蓄劲于指掌。两掌犹如托物回收，前臂运力外旋屈肘，至仰掌扶腰。两手后撑，回复原裆势。

【Training methods】

(1) Preparation form: Take a standing stance or the appointed stance. Bend the elbows and put the upward palms at the ribs. Keep the thumb forward with four fingers closed and Hu Kou apart.

(2) Exercise form: Speak out loudly, focus the strength on the fingers and palms. Push the upward palms forward forcefully like supporting something in the hands, revolve the forearms outward until the elbows become erect, and keep the palms in the same width and height of the shoulder. Have bright eyes, concentrate the mind and breathe naturally. (Figure 4–20)

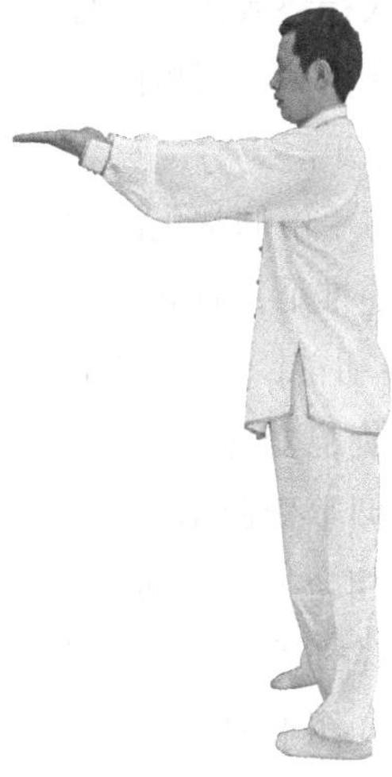

Figure 4–20

(3) Closing form: Speak out loudly and focus the strength on the fingers and palms. Withdraw the upward palms forward forcefully like supporting something in the hands; revolve the forearms outward, bend the elbow to support the waist with upward palms. Stretch the hands backward and return to the original stance.

【动作要领】

（1）用劲平推，拇指左右倾斜，犹如托物在手。

（2）手与肩平，两掌距离与肩同宽，两掌直线来回运行。

【Key points】

(1) Push the upward palms forward forcefully with the thumbs separated from the other fingers like supporting something in the hands.

(2) Keep the hands in the same height of the shoulder. And make the distance between the two hands in the same width of the shoulder.

【主要作用】

平手托塔是少林内功中仰掌前推旋劲锻炼的姿势，具有通畅气机、调和气血的作用。

【Main functions】

Holding tower with flat hand has the function of freeing qi movement and harmonizing qi and blood.

十一、运掌合瓦

Yun Zhang He Wa (Turning Palm to Fold Tile)

【训练方法】

（1）起式：大裆势或指定裆势。两手屈肘，仰掌于两胁，拇指向前，四肢并拢，虎口分开。

（2）功式：右手由仰掌化俯掌，运劲于臂贯指向前推足，肩欲松开，肘欲伸直，指端朝前，掌心向下，蓄劲待发。右手旋腕变仰掌徐徐收回，待近胸时左仰掌变俯掌在右仰掌上交叉，掌心相合。慢慢向前推出，掌心向下，右仰掌收回胁部，左仰掌收回腰间。（图4-21）

（3）收式：将腰间仰掌化俯掌

【Training methods】

(1) Preparation form: Take a splitting stance with hands backward or the appointed stance. Bend the elbows and put the upward palms at the ribs. Keep the thumb forward with four fingers closed and Hu Kou apart.

(2) Exercise form: Change the right palm from upward position to downward position, push the hand forward forcefully with the strength released from the arm to the fingers, relax the shoulder and the elbow, the fingers pointing forward and the palm downward. Hold the strength for next movement. Rotate the right wrist to make the palm upward and slowly withdraw the hand, then change the left upward palm into downward position when

下按。两手后撑，回复原裆势。

the right palm is close to the chest; cross the hands, the left downward palm over the right upward palm, the palms thus face each other, then the left palm slowly pushes forward with the palm downward. Withdraw the right upward palm to the ribs and the left upward palm to the waist. (Figure 4–21)

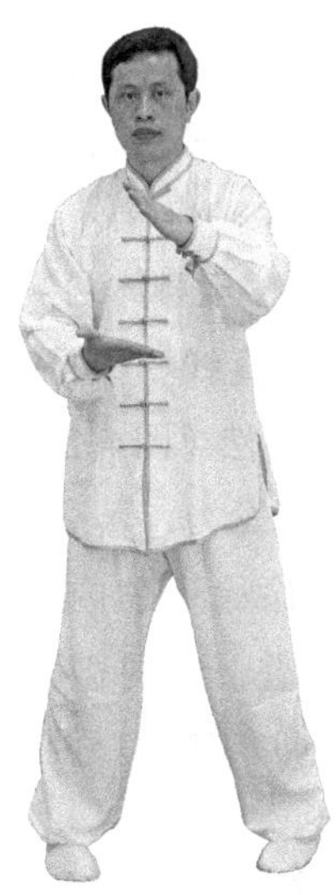

Figure 4–21

(3) Closing form: Change the palm form upward position to downward position and press down. Stretch the hands backward and return to the original stance.

【动作要领】

（1）运劲于臂，向前推出，肘欲伸直。

（2）两掌于胸前交合，掌心相合，用劲勿松。

（3）两掌缓慢有力配合协调。

【Key points】

(1) Push the hand forward forcefully with the strength released from the arm and relax the elbow.

(2) Cross the hands in front of the chest, the palms thus face each other. Hold on and do not relax.

(3) The two palms slowly coordinate with each other.

【主要作用】

与仙人指路相似，可以增强习练者双手交替操作技能的协调能力，具有平和阴阳、行气活血的作用。

【Main functions】

Similar to immortal guiding way, it can strengthen the coordination of two hands and has the function of balancing yin and yang, circulating qi and activating blood.

十二、风摆荷叶

【训练方法】

（1）起式：站裆势或指定裆势。两手屈肘，仰掌于两胁，拇指向前，四肢并拢，虎口分开。

（2）功式：两掌徐徐前推，至前胸两掌上下相叠，两肘微屈。出声发力，蓄劲于指掌。前臂外旋，分掌向两侧徐徐分开，至身体两侧，两掌与肩等高，成一直线。两目有神，意念集中，呼吸自然（图4–22）。

（3）收式：出声发力，蓄劲于指掌。两掌由两侧徐徐运劲内合，至前胸两掌上下相叠，两肘微屈。两掌回收至腰部，仰掌扶腰。两手后撑，回复原裆势。

Feng Bai He Ye (Wind Blowing Lotus Leaf)

【Training methods】

(1) Preparation form: Take a standing stance or the appointed stance. Bend the elbows and put the upward palms at the ribs. Keep the thumb forward with four fingers closed and Hu Kou apart.

(2) Exercise form: Push hands slowly forward to the chest, then make the left palm over the right palm and slightly bend the elbows. Speak out loudly and focus strength on the fingers and palms. Revolve the forearm outward, then slowly separate the arms to both sides of the body. Keep the palms in the same height of the shoulder. Have bright eyes, concentrate the mind, and breathe naturally. (Figure 4–22)

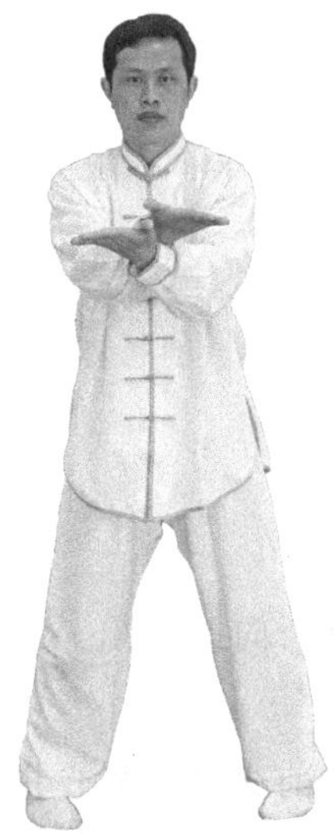

Figure 4–22

(3) Closing form: Speak out loudly, focus the strength on the fingers and palms. Slowly close the palms, and when it comes to the chest, make the left hand over the right hand. Bend the elbows slowly. Withdraw the hands to the waist, keeping the palms upward and supporting the waist. Stretch the hands backward and return to the original stance.

【动作要领】

（1）头身正直，两目平视，呼吸自然。

（2）肩、肘、掌平成一直线。

（3）仰掌交叉前推，外旋挺肘拉开，肩、肘、腕、掌平齐。

【Key points】

(1) Keep the head erect and the trunk upright. Look straight ahead and breathe naturally.

(2) Keep the waist, elbows, and palms in the same line.

(3) Push the crossed upward palms forward, revolve them outward and erect the elbows. Keep the shoulders, elbows, wrists, and palms in the same line.

【主要作用】

风摆荷叶是少林内功中锻炼内合和外分内劲的姿势，久练能强筋健骨，使气血顺利，元气充固。

【Main functions】

Wind blowing lotus leaf has the function of strengthening tendons and bones, advancing the circulation of qi and blood and promoting primordial qi.

十三、顶天抱地

Ding Tian Bao Di (Supporting the Sky and Embracing the Earth)

【训练方法】

（1）起式：并裆势或指定裆势。两手屈肘，仰掌于两腰，拇指向前，四肢并拢，虎口分开。

（2）功式：出声发力，蓄劲于指掌，虎口用力撑开。两掌缓缓向上托起，至胸前伸腕、手臂外旋，边旋边上举，推至头顶后，四指相对，掌心向上，肘关节伸直。两目有神，意念集中，呼吸自然。出声发力，蓄劲于指掌，虎口撑开。两掌用力，两手臂向两侧缓缓外展，至与肩平后，腰同时前屈。两手中指相叠后，腰部缓缓直起，两掌用力如同抱重物，屈肘分掌，仰掌扶腰（图4-23）。

（3）收式：两手后撑，回复原裆势。

【Training methods】

(1) Preparation form: Take a folding stance or the appointed stance. Bend the elbows and put the upward palms at the ribs. Keep the thumb outward with four fingers closed and Hu Kou apart.

(2) Exercise form: Speak out loudly, focus the strength on the palms and fingers, and keep Hu Kou apart. Raise the hands up to the chest and extend wrists and revolve the arms. When raising hands above the head, keep the four fingers facing with each other and palms upward and extend the elbows. Have bright eyes, concentrate the mind, and breathe naturally. Speak out loudly, focus the strength on the palms and fingers, and keep Hu Kou apart. Focus strength on the palms, revolve arms outward to the same height of the shoulder, and bend the waist forward. Cross the middle fingers of the two hands, erect the waist slowly. Bend

elbows and keep the palms upward and support waist. (Figure 4–23)

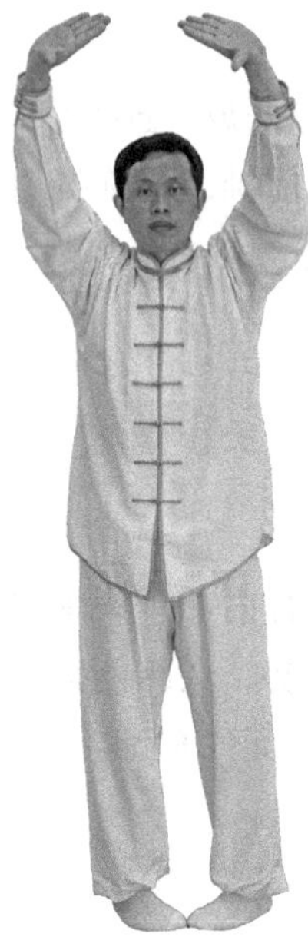

Figure 4–23

(3) Closing form: Stretch the hands backward and return to the original stance.

【动作要领】

（1）上举四指并拢，拇指外分，蓄劲于指端。

（2）旋腕翻掌，徐徐上举，指端相对。

（3）上身前俯，掌背着地，蓄劲待发。

（4）下肢挺直，不可屈膝。

【Key points】

(1) Close four fingers with the thumb apart and focus the strength on the palms and fingers.

(2) Revolve the wrists and palms, slowly raise them up with fingertips facing with each other.

(3) Bend the upper part of the body, keep the back of the hands facing the ground, and hold the strength for next movement.

(4) Erect the lower limbs and do not bend knees.

【主要作用】

顶天抱地具有调畅气机、调和任督二脉的作用。

【Main functions】

Supporting the sky and embracing the earth has the function of regulating the qi movement and harmonizing the Ren meridian and the Du meridian.

十四、海底捞月

【训练方法】

（1）起式：悬裆势或指定裆势。两手屈肘，仰掌于两腰，拇指向前，四肢并拢，虎口分开。

（2）功式：出声发力，蓄劲于指掌，虎口用力撑开。两掌缓缓向上托起，至胸前伸腕、手臂外旋，边旋边上举，推至头顶后，四指相对，掌心斜向上，肘关节伸直。两目有神，意念集中，呼吸自然。出声发力，蓄劲于指掌，虎口撑开。两手臂徐徐运劲向两侧外展，腰部前屈，屈髋伸膝。前臂内旋，于掌尺侧乏力，至两掌相叠。伸腰屈膝，两掌慢慢抄起，分掌仰掌于腰（图4–24）。

（3）收式：两手后撑，回复原裆势。

Hai Di Lao Yue (Scooping the Moon from Sea Bottom)

【Training methods】

(1) Preparation form: Take a squatting-splitting stance with hands on the waist or the appointed stance. Bend the elbows and put the upward palms at the waist. Keep the thumb forward with four fingers closed and Hu Kou apart.

(2) Exercise form: Speak out loudly, focus the strength on the palms and fingers, and keep Hu Kou apart. Raise hands up to the chest and extend the wrist and revolve the arms. When raising hands above the head, keep the four fingers facing with each other and palms upward and extend the elbows. Have bright eyes, concentrate the mind and breathe naturally. Speak out loudly, focus the strength on the palms and fingers, and keep Hu Kou apart. Extend two arms outward, bend the waist forward, bend hips and extend knees. Revolve forearms inward and make one palm cover the other. Extend the waist and bend the knees and keep upward palms at the waist. (Figure 4–24)

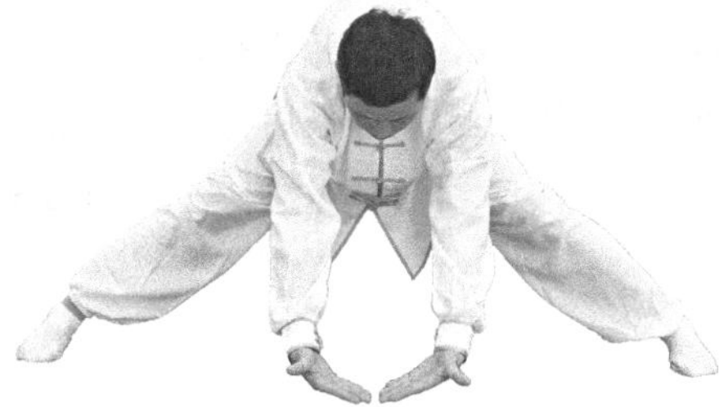

Figure 4–24

(3) Closing form: Stretch the hands backward and return to the original stance.

【动作要领】

（1）腰向前俯，腿不可屈，脚用霸力。

（2）蓄劲待发，两臂运劲，指

【Key points】

(1) Bend the waist forward, do not bend the legs and keep the stability of legs.

(2) Hold the strength for the next movement and focus

端着力，慢慢抄起。

（3）上举与弯腰配合要协调。

strength on two arms and fingertips.

(3) Raising and bending should be coordinated.

【主要作用】

海底捞月是少林内功中锻炼两臂蓄力的姿势，具有调畅三焦、调和任督二脉的作用。

【Main functions】

Hai Di Lao Yue (Scooping the moon from sea bottom) aims to exercise the strength of the arms and has the function of regulating the triple energizer and harmonizing the Ren meridian and the Du meridian.

十五、饿虎扑食

E Hu Pu Shi (Hunger Tiger Pouncing on its Prey)

【训练方法】

（1）起式：弓箭裆势。两手屈肘，仰掌于两腰，拇指向前，四肢并拢，虎口分开。

（2）功式：出声发力，蓄劲于指掌。指掌前推，边伸腕边前臂内旋，腰随势前俯，前腿待势似冲，后腿使劲勿放松，至肘直腰平。两目有神，意念集中，呼吸自然（图4–25）。

（3）收式：出声发力，蓄劲于指掌。握拳屈肘内收，腰随势上抬，拳到腰间变立掌扶腰。两手后撑，回复原裆势。

【Training methods】

(1) Preparation form: Take a squatting-splitting stance with hands on the waist stance or the appointed stance. Bend the elbows and put the upward palms at the waist. Keep the thumb forward with four fingers closed and Hu Kou apart.

(2) Exercise form: Speak out loudly, focus the strength on the palms and fingers. Push the hands forward. At the same time, revolve the forearms inward to make the dorsum sides of wrists facing each other. The torso leans forward along with the movement of the arms. When the front leg steps firmly, the back leg should be ended forcefully. Erect the elbows and the waist. Have bright eyes, concentrate the mind and breathe naturally. (Figure 4–25)

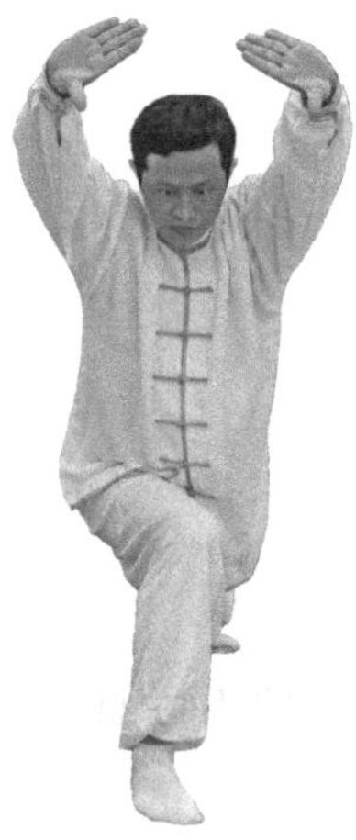

Figure 4–25

(3) Closing form: Speak out loudly, focus the strength on the palms and fingers. Bend five fingers to clench fists, bend the elbows, lift the waist, and move the hands back to the waist sides and protect the waist with upward palms. Stretch the hands backward and return to the original stance.

【动作要领】

（1）直掌旋推，腰向前俯，劲注拳心，两拳紧握，屈肘紧收。

（2）前推内旋与上身前倾配合协调，屈肘收拳和直腰动作配合协调。

【Key points】

(1) Push the upward palms forward. The torso leans forward along with the movement of the arms. Clench fists and bend the elbows.

(2) The movements of arms and the upper body should be coordinated.

【主要作用】

饿虎扑食可增强腰腿内功，提高手法内劲。

【Main functions】

Hunger tiger pouncing on its prey has the function of improving the strength of waist and legs and improving the force of manipulations.

十六、力劈华山

【训练方法】

（1）起式：取马裆势或指定裆势，两手屈肘，在胸前交叉。

（2）功式：出声发力，蓄劲于指掌。两立掌缓缓向左右分推，两肩松开，肘部微屈，四指并拢，拇指后翘，掌心向前，力求成水平线。两手同时用力，上下劈动，头勿转侧俯仰摇动，两目有神，意念集中，呼吸自然。最后一次劈动后成仰掌收回腰间（图4–26）。

（3）收式：仰掌变俯掌下按。两手后撑，回复原裆势。

Li Pi Hua Shan (Splitting Huashan Mountain with Vigorous Efforts)

【Training methods】

(1) Preparation form: Take a horse stance or the appointed stance. Bend the elbows and cross the erect palms in the chest.

(2) Exercise form: Speak out loudly, focus the strength on the palms and fingers. Slowly separate the arms and push the erect palms to the sides, relax the shoulders, flex the elbows slightly, make the fingers closed and the thumb tilted backward, keep the palm center outward, and keep the arms at the same lever. Do chopping movement up and down while not moving the head. Have bright eyes, concentrate the mind, and breathe naturally. Put the upward palms at the waist sides after the lasting chopping movement. (Figure 4–26)

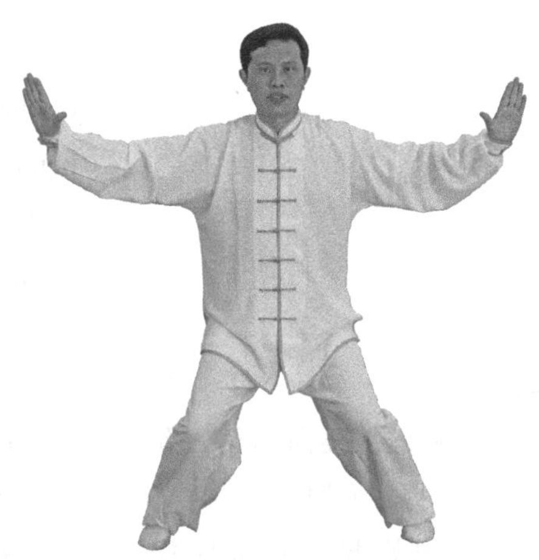

Figure 4–26

(3) Closing form: Change the palm from upward position to downward position and press down. Stretch the arms backward and return to the original stance.

【动作要领】

（1）上身正直，头勿摇动，两目平视，呼吸自然。

（2）两臂蓄劲，四指并拢伸直，用力下劈。

【Key points】

(1) Keep the trunk upright, do not move the head, look straight ahead, and breathe naturally.

(2) Focus strength on two arms, keep four fingers closed and extended, and do chopping movement.

【主要作用】

锻炼肩、臂、肘、腕、指端的重要姿势。对上肢锻炼大有助益，久练则能调和内脏，舒展胸廓，增加气劲和悬力，具有宽胸理气、平肝健肺的作用。

【Main functions】

Splitting Huashan Mountain aims to exercise the upper limbs, including shoulders, arms, elbows, wrists and fingertips. Long-time exercise has the function of regulating and harmonizing internal organs, extending the thorax, increasing forces and strength, soothing the chest and regulating qi as well as calming the liver and fortifying the spleen.

十七、乌龙钻洞

Wu Long Zuan Dong (Black Chinese Dragon Crawling into Cave)

【训练方法】

（1）起式：大裆势或指定裆势。两手屈肘，立掌于两胁，拇指向上，四肢向前，虎口分开。

【Training methods】

(1) Preparation form: Take a splitting stance with hands backward or the appointed stance. Bend the elbows

（2）功式：出声发力，蓄劲于指掌。两立掌掌心相对，缓缓前推，边推边掌心向下逐渐变成俯掌，指端朝前，上身随势前俯，下部两足尖内扣，用霸力而蓄（图4-27）。

（3）收式：出声发力，蓄劲于指掌。推足后旋腕，指端外展，蓄力而收，边收边掌心慢慢朝上，俯掌变仰掌护腰。仰掌变俯掌下按，两手后撑，回复原裆势。

and put the upward palms at the ribs. Keep the thumb upward with four fingers forward and Hu Kou apart.

(2) Exercise form: Speak out loudly, focus the strength on the palms and fingers. Push the erect palms forward slowly with the palms facing each other, turn the palms downward. The torso bends forward along with the movement of the arms. Stand firmly with the toe tips slightly inward. (Figure 4–27)

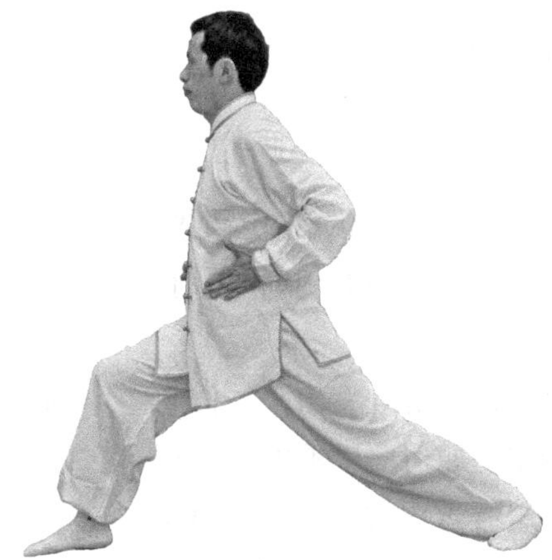

Figure 4–27

(3) Closing form: Speak out loudly, focus the strength on the palms and fingers. When the arms are fully extended, rotate the wrist, make the fingertips abduct, turn the palms upward and move them back forcefully to the waist side. Turn the palms downward and press down. Stretch the arms backward and return to the original stance.

【动作要领】

（1）直掌并行，掌心相对，徐徐前推。

（2）上身随势前俯，推尽后蓄力而收。

（3）两足尖内扣，五趾抓地，霸力而蓄。

（4）上肢运劲与腰部运动要协调。

【Key points】

(1) Push the erect palms forward slowly with the palms facing each other.

(2) Make the torso bend forward along with the movement of the arms, and then move them back forcefully to the waist side.

(3) Stand firmly with the toe tips slightly inward, keeping five toes firmly grasping the ground.

(4) The movement of the upper limbs should be

coordinated with the waist movement.

【主要作用】

乌龙钻洞与饿虎扑食相似，可增强腰腿内功，提高手法内劲。

【Main functions】

Like hunger tiger pouncing on its prey, black Chinese dragon crawling into cave has the function of enhancing the strength of waist and legs and improving the force of manipulations.

十八、单凤朝阳

Dan Feng Chao Yang (Single Phoenix Facing the Sun)

【训练方法】

（1）起式：马裆势或指定裆势。两手屈肘，仰掌于两腰，拇指向前，四肢并拢，虎口分开。

（2）功式：出声发力，右仰掌旋腕变俯掌，屈肘向胸前左上方运力外展，缓缓运向右下方，屈肘运劲上抄作半圆形，收回护腰。两目有神，意念集中，呼吸自然。左手动作仅方向相反，余同（图4-28）。

（3）收式：仰掌变俯掌下按，两手后撑，回复原裆势。

【Training methods】

(1) Preparation form: Take a horse stance or the appointed stance. Bend the elbows and put the upward palms at the waist. Keep the thumb forward with four fingers closed and Hu Kou apart.

(2) Exercise form: Speak out loudly, change the right palms from upward position to downward position, move the right elbow forcefully leftward, then to the left lower direction, finally move the hand upward to draw a half-circle back to the waist sides. Have bright eyes, concentrate the mind, and breathe naturally. The left hand does the opposite direction. (Figure 4–28)

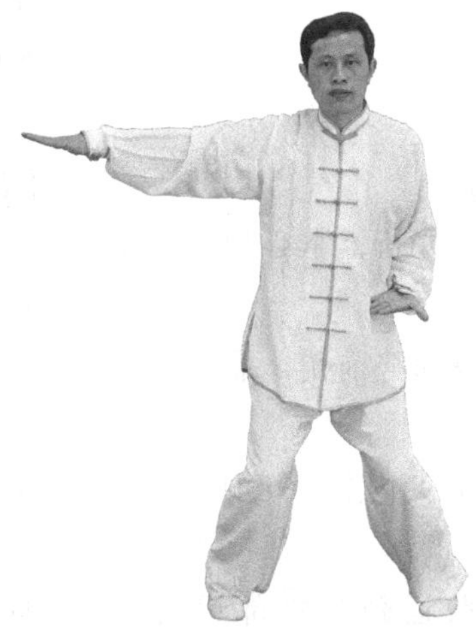

Figure 4–28

(3) Closing form: Change the palms from the erect position to downward position and press down. Stretch the hands backward and return to the original stance.

【动作要领】

（1）旋腕化掌，蓄力外展，缓缓下运，形似半圆。

（2）外展有力缓慢，运劲勿松。

【Key points】

(1) Revolve the wrists and move palms slowly downward, like drawing a half-circle.

(2) Abduct movements should be forceful and slow, and do not relax.

【主要作用】

单凤朝阳具有强筋健骨，使气血顺利，元气充固的作用。

【Main functions】

Single phoenix facing the sun has the function of strengthening tendons and bones, promoting the flow of qi and blood and consolidating the primordial qi.

十九、三起三落

San Qi San Luo (Three Ups and Three Downs)

【训练方法】

（1）起式：低裆势。两手屈肘，立掌于两胁，拇指向上，四肢向前，虎口分开，屈髋屈膝，大腿与地面平行。

（2）功式：出声发力，蓄劲于指掌，拇指上翘，四指并拢，虎口用力撑开。两臂徐徐运力前推至肘直，两掌心相对，与肩等高，与胸等宽。同时屈髋屈膝下蹲，臀部下落。两目有神，意念集中，呼吸自然，上肢动作和下肢屈蹲协调（图4–29a）。出声发力，蓄劲于指掌，拇指上翘，四指并拢，虎口用力撑开。两臂徐徐运力回收，立掌扶于两胁。同时臀部上抬，屈髋屈膝，大腿与地面平行。上述动作重复3次。两手屈肘，立掌于两胁，屈髋

【Training methods】

(1) Preparation form: Take a lower stance. Bend the elbows and put the upward palms at the ribs. Keep the thumb upward with four fingers forward and Hu Kou apart. Bend hips and knees, making legs parallel with the ground.

(2) Exercise form: Speak out loudly, focus strength on the palms and fingers, make the thumbs upward with four fingers closed and Hu Kou apart. Slowly push arms forward until the elbows become erect. Keep two palms facing each other and in the same height of the shoulder and the same width of the chest. At the same time, bend hips and knees to the level of squat. Have bright eyes, concentrate the mind, and breathe naturally. Make the movements of the upper limbs coordinate with the squat of the lower limbs (Figure 4–29a).Speak out loudly, focus strength on the palms and fingers, make the thumbs upward, close four fingers and open the Hu Kou forcefully. Withdraw two arms forcefully and protect ribs with upward palms. Lift buttocks, bend hips

屈膝，大腿与地面平行（图4–29b）。出声发力，蓄劲于指掌，拇指上翘，四指并拢，虎口用力撑开。两臂徐徐运力前推至肘直，两掌心相对，与肩等高，与胸等宽，同时伸膝伸髋。两目有神，意念集中，呼吸自然，上肢动作和下肢伸屈协调。出声发力，蓄劲于指掌，拇指上翘，四指并拢，虎口用力撑开。两臂徐徐运力回收，立掌扶于两胁。同时臀部上抬，屈髋屈膝，大腿与地面平行。上述动作重复3次。

（3）收式：两手后撑，回复原裆势。

and knees, making legs parallel with the ground. Repeat it for 3 times. Bend the elbows and put the upward palms at the ribs. Bend hips and knees, making legs parallel with the ground (Figure 4–29b). Speak out loudly, focus strength on the palms and fingers, make the thumbs upward with four fingers closed and Hu Kou apart. Slowly push arms forward until the elbows become erect. Keep two palms facing each other and in the same height of the shoulder and the same width of the chest. At the same time, extend hips and knees. Have bright eyes, concentrate the mind, and breathe naturally. Make the movements of the upper limbs coordinate with the extension of the lower limbs. Speak out loudly, focus strength on the palms and fingers, make the thumbs upward, close four fingers and open the Hu Kou forcefully. Withdraw two arms forcefully and protect ribs with upward palms. Lift buttocks, bend hips and knees, making legs parallel with the ground. Repeat it for 3 times.

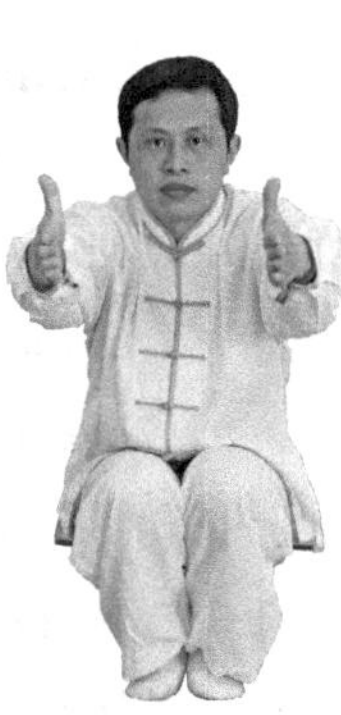
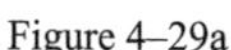
Figure 4–29a

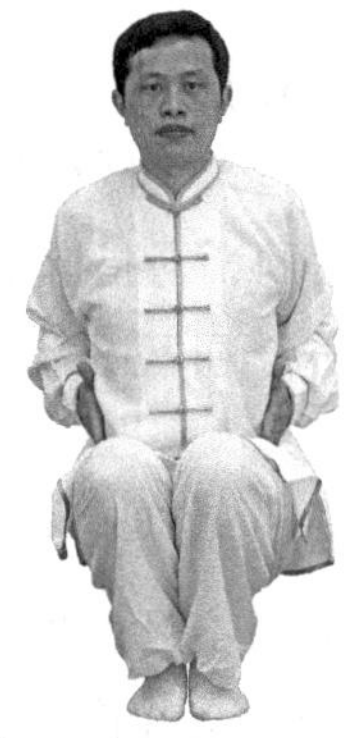
Figure 4–29b

(3) Closing form: Stretch the hands backward and return to the original stance.

【动作要领】

（1）上身正直，头勿摇动。

（2）指臂蓄力，前推下蹲，用劲后收，随之而起。

（3）上肢运劲与下肢伸屈运动须配合协调。

【Key points】

(1) Keep the trunk upright and do not move the head.

(2) Focus strength on the fingers and arms, and do not relax when squatting.

(3) Make the movements of the upper limbs coordinate with the extension of the lower limbs.

【主要作用】

三起三落是少林内功中以两臂向前后运动，同时配合下肢下蹲与站立锻炼的姿势，具有健脾和胃、强心畅肺的作用。

【Main functions】

Three ups and three downs has the function of strengthening the spleen and harmonizing the stomach, and tonifying the heart and dispersing the lung.

第五节 双人锻炼

Section Five Exercise in Pairs

一、推把上桥

Tui Ba Shang Qiao

【训练方法】

（1）甲乙双方同时左足向前一步各成左弓右箭步，各自两手屈肘成直掌护腰。

（2）甲方取主动，两手掌心相对，四指并拢，拇指用力上翘，两臂运劲；乙方两手亦主动去接按甲方两手，以两拇指在甲方虎口向内扣，示指按于腕之桡侧，余指由尺侧下内屈，虎口相咬，蓄劲待发（图4–30）。

（3）甲方（可“嗨”一声）两臂运劲，用足力气前推，乙方亦蓄劲用力前推，各不相让甲乙双方争推时间量力而行，甲乙双方的上身略前俯，下部姿势均需踏实。由乙方逐渐蓄劲让势，甲方占优势，两臂运劲前推。

（4）甲方推足时，主动（可“嗨”一声）由前推变为用力后拉，乙方即用拇指、示指与其他三指用

【Training methods】

(1) Both A and B take one step forward with their left feet, with bow stance in left leg and arrow stance in right leg. Both bend the elbows and support the waist with the palms upward.

(2) A takes the initiative, keeps two palms facing with each other, closes the four fingers, keeps the thumb up with strong force and stores up strength in arms. B takes the initiative to press the hands of A, holds A’s Hu Kou with his two thumbs and the radial side with his index finger. (Figure 4–30)

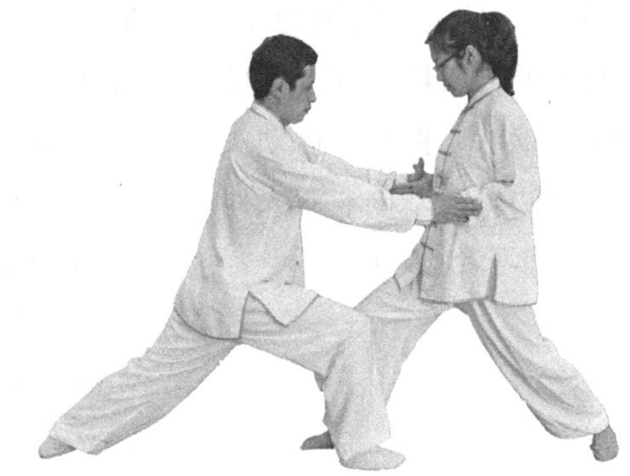

Figure 4–30

力紧握，由前推变为后拉，不让甲方收回，双方争拉时间酌情而定。再由乙方逐渐蓄劲让势，使甲方占优势收回。

（5）等甲方两手屈肘收回，乙方即主动（可“嗨”一声）五指用力内扣收回，甲方即用力向后争拉，双方争拉时间酌情而定；甲方逐渐蓄劲让势，由乙方占优势后拉。

(3) A stores force in two arms, and pushes them forward with full force, so does B. Both A and B slightly lean the upper body forward, and the stances of their lower limbs should be stable. B gradually steps back, and A takes the dominant position, pushing two arms forward with strength.

(4) A pulls the feet and draws backward (speaks “Hi” loudly). While B grasps A firmly with thumbs, index fingers and the other fingers, pulls backward and prevents A from drawing back. Then B gradually stores strength and steps back, so A can take the dominant position and draw back.

(5) After A bends the elbow, B takes the initiative to hold five fingers inwardly with strong force and A scratches backward forcefully. Then A gradually steps backs and B takes the dominant position to pull backward.

【动作要领】

（1）双方上身略前俯，下肢姿势均须平稳踏实。

（2）相持争推时，应量力而行，切忌在推拉中突然使力。

（3）双方运劲前推后拉用力变换须自然。

【Key points】

(1) Both slightly leans his upper body forward, and the stance of lower limbs should be stable.

(2) When scratching and pushing, both should exercise according to their personal heath conditions, so as not to move suddenly and abruptly.

(3) The changes of stances should be natural.

【主要作用】

推把上桥在练习中，上、下肢动作同时变化，而上肢以推为主，使肱三头肌等臂伸肌群得到全面的锻炼，为练习擦法、推法、运动关节类等推拿手法打下基础；双人对练，可以激发练习者的兴趣。

【Main functions】

In the exercise of Tui Ba Shang Qiao, the upper and lower limbs of A and B move at the same time. It focuses on the pulling gesture of upper limbs, which provides a comprehensive workout for the triceps muscle of arm and other extensors and lays the foundation for the exercise of linear rubbing manipulation, pushing manipulation and the manipulation on joints. Double workouts can also help to spark people’s interest in Shaolin internal exercise.

二、双龙搅水

【训练方法】

（1）甲乙双方左（右）脚同时向前方跨出一步成左（右）弓步，两足相距约 20 cm，左（右）肩与左（右）肩相对。双方下部的姿势成菱形。

（2）甲乙双方左（右）手握拳，拳面向下，两臂相拢，脉门（间使穴）相对，臂欲伸直，不可弯曲。甲乙双方右手各自撑腰，双目均向前看，待势。

（3）甲方采取主动，以左手腕向上搅起（可“嗨”一声），乙方握紧拳用力向下按，按重心力点在于两腕，各不相让，上身姿势要求不变，下部保持原状。

（4）乙方逐渐让势，手臂仍欲蓄力相搅，由甲方先胜（切忌突然相让）。甲方占优势向上，动成车轮形。待第二圈时，在乙方向上搅时，双方两拳均已上举，甲方的脉门转为腕背交叉与乙方手腕相搅并向下压，再次成为脉门相对的姿势。

（5）乙方采取主动（可“嗨”一声）向上搅，甲方动作同步骤三乙方的动作。

（6）甲方逐渐让势，手臂仍欲蓄劲相搅（切忌突然相让），由乙方获胜，乙方动作同步骤四甲方的动作。

Shuang Long Jiao Shui (Two Chinese Dragons Stirring the Water)

【Training methods】

(1) Both A and B step forward, with the left leg or right leg in bow stance. The two feet are about 20 cm apart, with the left (right) shoulder opposites with the left (right) shoulder. The lower limbs of both are in a diamond shape.

(2) Both A and B make a fist with the left (right) hand and keep the fist facing downward. Close two arms and make Jianshi (PC 5) point face with each other. Extend arms and do not bend. Both A and B support the waistline with their hands and look straight ahead.

(3) A takes the initiative to stir his left wrist upward, and B clenches the fist and presses down firmly, with the focus on the two wrists. Keep the gestures of upper and lower limbs unchanged.

(4) B gradually steps back, but still stirs with the arm forcefully. A take the dominate position, moving like a wheel. In the second circle, both put fists up.

(5) A takes the initiative to stir upward. A repeats B's action in step 3.

(6) B gradually steps back, but still stirs with the arm forcefully. B repeats A's action in step 4.

【动作要领】

（1）双方用力相搅时，力点在两腕。

（2）双方上身正直勿偏斜，下肢姿势均须平稳踏实。

【Key points】

(1) When stirring forcefully, both should focus the force on the wrists.

(2) Both should keep their upper body straight and do not lean. The stance of the lower limbs should be stable

（3）双方须逐渐协调用力。

（4）双方两目前视，呼吸自然。

and forceful.

(3) The exercise of both A and B should be coordinated with strong force.

(4) Both A and B look straight ahead and breathe naturally.

【主要作用】

双龙搅水是少林内功中环转运劲的双人锻炼之法，可以增强肩部摇法等手法的内劲。

【Main functions】

Two dragons stirring the water is conducive to increasing the internal force of shaking manipulation on the shoulder.

三、双虎夺食

【训练方法】

（1）甲乙双方左足同时向前半步，右腿后伸成左弓右箭步。左脚交叉，脚凹相对，相距约10 cm。

（2）甲方右手（掌心向下）与乙方右手（掌心向上）相合，双方四指内扣相握，拇指均向内屈收，各自左手虎口朝上叉腰。

（3）甲方取主动向内拉（即向后拉，可“嗨”一声）动，前腿勿跪，后腿劲欲蹬足。乙方以全力相争（向后拉），互相争拉用力不可松，下部姿势扎实不可移，重心踏平，用力均匀，争夺时间量力而行。

（4）乙方逐渐让势，四指仍向内扣紧，由甲方取胜。甲方占优势身向后迎。下部姿势由弓步变为伏虎势（左腿由屈变直，右腿由直变屈），力在后腿，乙方上身略前俯，下部姿势含蓄不移。

（5）乙方采取主动（可“嗨”一声），前腿运力，上身蓄劲，四指

Shuang Hu Duo Shi (Two Tigers Fighting over Food)

【Training methods】

(1) Both A and B take half a step forward of the left foot and stretch the right leg backward, with the left leg in bow stance and the right leg in arrow stance. Cross the left leg to make toe tips facing with each other and the distance between 10 cm.

(2) The palm of A faces the palm of B, with A’s palm downward and B’s palm upward. Both hold each other’s four fingers inwardly with both thumbs bending inward and support the waist with the left hand with the Hu Kou upward.

(3) A takes the initiative to pull inward, and do not kneel the front leg and stores strength in the back leg and stomps the foot. B pulls backwards with full force. When scratching, both keep the balance of the body, and do not relax force or change the stance of upper limbs. The exercise should be based on personal healthy conditions with the appropriate force.

(4) B gradually steps back and holds his four fingers inwardly. While B changes his stance of lower limbs from bow stance to the stance like a crouching tiger (erect his

用力内扣向后争拉，甲方即用力向后争夺，时间酌情而定。

（6）甲方逐渐让势，四指仍欲运劲内扣，上身略前倾，下部由伏虎势变为弓步，乙方上身略后仰，下部由弓步变为伏虎势。

left leg and bend his right leg), with strength in the back leg. B slightly leans his upper body forward and keeps the stance of lower limbs unchanged.

(5) B takes the initiative and speaks "Hi" loudly, raises strength in the front leg and the upper body, holds his four fingers inwardly and pulls back. And A uses full force to scratch backward according to the specific conditions.

(6) A gradually steps back, holds his four fingers inwardly, and slightly leans his upper body forward, changing the stance of lower limbs from the stance like a crouching tiger to bow stance.

【动作要领】

（1）争拉时劲勿松，下肢姿势勿移，重心平稳。用力均匀，争夺时间量力而行。

（2）弓步、伏虎势变换须平稳有力，双方用力须逐渐增减，以免动作猛烈突然。

（3）双方两目前视，呼吸自然。

【Key points】

(1) When scratching, keep the balance of the body, and do not relax force and change the stance of upper limbs. The force should be appropriate.

(2) The changes between bow stance and stance like a crouching tiger should be stable and forceful. Both must gradually increase or decrease the force, so as not to move suddenly and abruptly.

(3) Both look straight ahead and breathe naturally.

【主要作用】

双虎夺食是少林内功功法中对拉运劲双人锻炼之势。在练习中，甲乙双方上、下肢动作同时变化，而上肢以拉为主，使肱二头肌等前臂屈肌群得到全面的锻炼，为练习擦法、推法、运动关节类法等推拿手法打下基础。

【Main functions】

In the exercise of two tigers fighting over food, the upper and lower limbs of A and B move at the same time. It focuses on the pulling gesture of upper limbs, which provides a comprehensive workout for the biceps and other forearm flexors and lays the foundation for the exercise of linear rubbing manipulation, pushing manipulation and the manipulation on joints.

四、箭腿压法

Jian Tui Ya Fa

【训练方法】

（1）甲乙双方同时左脚向前一

【Training methods】

(1) Both A and B move the left foot forward and stand

步并半蹲，后腿伸直成左弓右箭步，左腿交叉，脚凹相对并相靠。

（2）甲乙双方各自两手撑腰，待势。

（3）甲方采取主动，先以左腿外侧向下压，乙方亦以左腿外侧蓄力相抵（勿使双方胫骨相碰）。

（4）乙方逐渐让势，由甲方先压，使左腿由屈变直，右腿由直变屈，成伏虎势。甲方左腿前冲侧逐渐压下，身略前俯，右腿要蓄力。

（5）乙方采取主动，运用全力在左腿外侧，向上相抵，甲方亦以全力控制上压之力。

（6）由甲方逐渐蓄力让势，将左弓裆变为伏虎势，乙方占优势由伏虎势转为左弓裆，向下慢压。

（7）甲方再次采取主动，仍运全力于左腿外侧，着力下压。乙方动作同（3）。

in a half-crouch. Stretch the back leg, with the left leg in bow stance and the right leg in arrow stance. Cross the left leg, making the foot face with and press against each other.

(2) Both A and B support the waist with their hands.

(3) A moves first and presses the peripheral side of the left leg down. And B presses against the left leg of A with the peripheral side of his left leg.

(4) B gradually steps back and lets B press down, erecting his left leg first and then bending the right leg. A presses his left leg down, slightly bents forward and stores strengthen on the right leg.

(5) B takes an action firstly and gives his full strength on the peripheral side of the left leg, pressing upward, while B also controls the strength upward.

(6) B gradually stores up force and steps back, changing from the bow stance of the left leg to the stance like a crouching tiger. A takes an action firstly, changing from the stance like a crouching tiger to the bow stance of the left leg and slowly pressing down.

(7) A takes an action firstly and presses the peripheral side of the left leg down. So does B.

【动作要领】

（1）双方两腿蓄力压抵时，使髌骨前内侧相碰。

（2）双方用力须逐渐增减，以免动作猛然突兀。

（3）双方两目前视，呼吸自然。

【Key points】

(1) When the two legs are pressed against each other, both A and B should make sure that their anterior medial sides of the patella touch each other.

(2) Both must gradually increase or decrease the force, so as not to move suddenly and abruptly.

(3) Both look straight ahead and breathe naturally.

【主要作用】

箭腿压法是少林内功中膝关节对压的双人锻炼之法，可增强胸椎扳法等手法的内劲，提高膝关节参与手法运用的综合技能。

【Main functions】

This exercise is conducive to strengthening the internal force of pulling manipulations on thoracic vertebrae and increasing the comprehensive manipulation skills on the knee joints.

五、八走势

【训练方法】

（1）甲乙双方同时先提右脚成箭步，后提左腿向左成左弓右箭步，同时两右手臂向上提起，由右后方向左，握拳轻击手臂内侧脉门（间使穴）与手臂外侧支沟穴，两左手臂同时随势撑腰。

（2）甲乙双方同时转身箭步转换，向右转侧，右腿上前成右弓左箭步，上部右手握拳，轻击手臂内侧脉门（间使穴）与手臂外侧支沟穴。

（3）甲乙双方同时右箭步上势，后提左腿向左成左弓右箭步，双方各将胸脯挺起前冲，轻撞左侧，同时两手臂握拳后伸，肘伸直，上身挺直。

（4）甲乙双方同时左箭步上势，即成右弓左箭步，双方各将胸脯挺起前冲，轻撞右侧，同时两手臂握拳后伸。

（5）甲乙双方同时先提右脚成箭步，后提左腿向左成左弓右箭步，同时两左手握拳上举。

（6）甲乙双方同时左箭步上势，即成右弓左箭步，同时两右手握拳上举，两左手握拳后伸，舒展胁肋，双方的左侧胁肋相互轻撞。

（7）甲乙双方同时先提右脚成箭步，后提左腿向左成左弓右箭步（或半马步），双方各用左侧臀部相互轻撞，相撞的同时，双方击掌，各将右拳上举，左拳收于下部左侧，类似打虎势。

Ba Zou Shi

【Training methods】

(1) Both A and B first lift the right foot into an arrow stance at the same time, then lift the left foot towards the left direction. Both A and B lift the right arms, moving from the right backward to the left. Then both make a fist and lightly strike Jianshi (PC 5) on the medial side of the arm and Zhigou (SJ 6) on the peripheral side of the arm, with two left arms supporting the waist.

(2) Both A and B turn right at the same time, and step forward with the right leg, with the right leg in bow stance and the left leg in arrow stance. Then both hold a fist with the right hand, and lightly strike Jianshi (PC 5) on the medial side of the arm and Zhigou (SJ 6) on the peripheral side of the arm.

(3) Both A and B make arrow stances with the right leg, then lift the left leg left, with the left leg in bow stance and the right leg in arrow stance. Both raise the chest forward and lightly hit the left side. At the same time, both hold a fist and stretch two arms backward, erect elbows and straighten the upper body.

(4) Both A and B make arrow stance with the left leg, with the right leg in bow stance and the left leg in arrow stance. Both raise the chest forward and lightly hit the right side. At the same time, both hold a fist and stretch two arms backward.

(5) Both A and B make arrow stance with the right leg, then lift the left leg left, with the left leg in bow stance and the right leg in arrow stance. At the same time, both make a fist with left hands and hold them up.

(6) Both A and B make arrow stance with the left leg, with the right leg in bow stance and the left leg in arrow stance. At the same time, both make a fist with right hands and hold them up and make a fist with left hands and

（8）甲乙双方同时左箭步上势，即成右弓左箭步（或半马步），双方各用右侧臀部相互轻撞，相撞的同时，双方击掌，各将左拳上举，右拳收于下部右侧。

stretch them backward. Both hit each other lightly on the left side of the rib cage.

(7) Both A and B make arrow stance with the right leg, then lift the left leg left, with the left leg in bow stance and the right leg in arrow stance. Both hit each other lightly on the left side of the hips. At the same time, both do high fives, raise the right fist up, and withdraw the left fist to the lower left side, like posture of fighting a tiger.

(8) Both A and B make arrow stance with the left leg, with the right leg in bow stance and the left leg in arrow stance. Both hit each other lightly on the right side of the hips. At the same time, both do high fives, raise the right fist up, and withdraw the left fist to the lower left side.

【动作要领】

（1）双方相互撞击之力须有控制，切勿猛力撞击。

（2）双方裆势变换须自然协调。

【Key points】

(1) Make a control of the force when hitting with each other.

(2) The changes of stances should be natural and coordinated.

【主要作用】

八走势可以促进周身气血流通、经脉舒畅。

【Main functions】

This exercise is conducive to promoting the circulation of qi and blood, regulating meridians and collaterals.

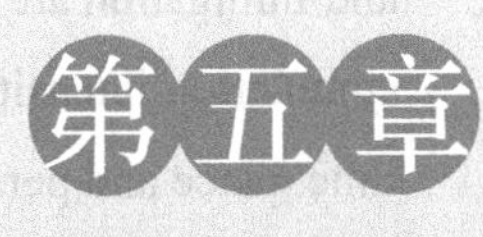

Chapter Five
Clinical Application

第一节 总论

Section One Introduction

内功推拿流派防治手段以手法治疗和功法训练为主，尤其注重手法治疗时的辨证论治和功法治疗的针对性。手法一般要求功法锻炼和手法治疗有机结合。临床治疗时根据具体情况，选择棒击、膏摩、热敷和熏蒸等方法和技术，操作时因时、因地、因人制宜，灵活掌握治疗方法和刺激强度。

推拿疗法是以力为主要特征，兼具调气和调意的功效。推拿手法或功法之所以能发挥治疗作用，并不单纯依靠手法或功法本身扶正祛邪的功效，还应包括适当的刺激能够激发机体自身调节功能，使人体生命活动恢复到平衡状态。因此，手法的作用有赖于机体自身正气的强弱。临床治疗时应当根据中医学理论或现代医学知识辨证论治或辨病治疗，寻求安全有效的推拿方法。

内功推拿具有治疗范围广的特点，在临床上不仅适用于骨伤科疾病，对于内科虚劳杂病、妇科经带胎产也有一定优势。内功推拿作为一种治疗方法，尚未形成完整的理论体系，具有多元性的特点。如治疗运动系统疾病时，基本上是采用现代解剖学、生理学、病理学等理论；治疗内科、妇科疾病时，是采用中医脏腑理论、经络学说。

The prevention and therapeutic methods of the Neigong Tuina are based on manipulation treatment and Shaolin internal exercise, with particular emphasis on the treatment based on pattern identification. In general, the manipulation requires the organic combination of Shaolin internal exercise and manipulation treatment. In clinical treatment, according to the specific situation, methods and manipulation such as stick-knocking manipulation, Gao Mo (Tuina combined with herbal ointment), hot compress and fumigation are selected, and the treatment methods and stimulation intensity are flexibly changed according to the time, place and person.

Tuina therapy is mainly characterized by force and has the efficacy of regulating both qi and intention. Tuina manipulations or Shaolin internal exercise can not only reinforce healthy qi to eliminate pathogenic factors, but also stimulate the body's own regulatory function and restore the body's vital activities to a state of balance, to achieve good therapeutic efficacy. Therefore, the efficacy of manipulations depends on the body's own healthy qi. Clinical treatment should be based on the theory of traditional Chinese medicine or modern medical knowledge to treat the disease, and to find a safe and effective method of tuina.

Neigong Tuina has a wide therapeutic scope and are clinically applicable not only to orthopedic and traumatic diseases, but also to internal deficiency and miscellaneous diseases, gynecology, menstruation and fetal birth. As a treatment method, Neigong Tuina has not yet formed a complete theoretical system. Its theoretical

内功推拿秉承《黄帝内经》"杂合以治，各得其所宜"的指导思想，依据病邪的特异性、中病层次、体质特异性及推拿治法的特异性选择适当的治疗方法，综合功法、手法、膏摩、熏蒸、热敷、药物等要素，达到良好的临床疗效。内功推拿治疗范围虽然广，但是并不等于包治百病。要客观地认识内功推拿的作用，熟悉手法、功法治疗的宜忌，临床医生应根据疾病的种类和发展阶段，选择合适的综合治疗方法，而不仅仅是推拿方法。

system is characterized by pluralism. For example, when treating diseases of the motor system, modern theories of anatomy, physiology and pathology are used; when treating diseases of internal medicine and gynecology, the theory of internal organs and meridians and the theory of meridians and collaterals of traditional Chinese medicine are used.

Neigong Tuina adheres to the guiding principles of the *Yellow Emperor's Canon of Medicine*, which states that "the sages brought various patterns together in treatment; each case received what was appropriate for it." According to the features and severity of diseases, personal health conditions and the specialty of manipulations, people can integrate Shaolin internal exercise, manipulations, Gao Mo, fumigation, hot compress and medicine to achieve good clinical efficacy. Although the scope of Neigong Tuina is wide, it does not mean it can cure all the diseases. We should objectively understand the role of Neigong Tuina and be familiar with the contraindications of manipulations and Shaolin internal exercise. Clinical physicians should choose appropriate treatment methods according to the type and development of diseases, not just tuina methods.

一、内功推拿治疗骨伤科疾病的指导思想

Guiding Principles of Neigong Tuina to Treat Orthopedic Disease

骨伤科疾病是推拿临床上的常见病之一，多因急性或慢性损伤（疲劳、劳损和退变）导致骨、软组织和关节病变，产生一系列的临床症状和体征。运用内功推拿治疗骨伤科疾病可减轻病痛，恢复身体健康、感受轻松舒适。

临诊时，注意正确认识骨伤疾

Orthopedic disease is one of the common diseases in tuina clinics, mostly due to acute or chronic injuries (fatigue, strain and degeneration) resulting in bone, soft tissue and joint lesions, producing a series of clinical symptoms and signs. The application of Neigong Tuina to treat orthopedic and traumatic diseases can alleviate pain, restore health, and make patients feel relaxed and comfortable.

病病理变化，不能过于强调骨质增生、关节软骨面破坏及脊柱椎间盘退变等形态学改变在疾病发病过程中的作用，忽视肌肉、韧带、肌腱和筋膜等功能损伤在疾病发展过程中的作用；不能过于强调影像学检查，忽视体征检查；不能过于强调骨结构变化，忽视软组织病变造成的脊柱与四肢骨关节整体动态功能改变。一些疾病，如常见的颈椎病不仅是形态结构的异常，更多的是功能性紊乱，或许也可以称为功能性颈椎病，这可能是手法、功法治疗颈椎病及其他骨伤科疾病的部分理论基础。因此，调整类手法运用需要明确的指征。脊柱和四肢骨关节运动类手法不可滥用，以免因反复使用而进一步损害其稳定性。

合理的运用推拿手法或练功解决脊柱和四肢骨组织结构、软组织及关节的稳定性问题，是推拿治疗干预骨伤科疾病的切入点。在临床上运用推拿疗法治疗骨伤科疾患，应建立整体观念及“筋骨整体观”的指导思想，恰当地运用脊柱和四肢骨关节推拿手法和功法，符合安全、有效、简单、省力、规范的标准。

In the clinical treatment, we should have a correct understanding of the pathological changes of orthopedic diseases and should not overemphasize the role of morphological changes such as osteophytes, destruction of articular cartilage surfaces and spinal disc degeneration in the pathogenesis of the disease and ignore the role of functional injuries such as muscles, ligaments, tendons and fascia in the development of the disease. We should not overemphasize imaging examinations and ignore physical examinations; we should not overemphasize structural changes of bone and ignore the overall dynamic functional changes of the spine and limb bones and joints caused by lesions. Some diseases, such as common cervical spondylosis, are not only abnormalities of morphological structure, but more functional disorders. Perhaps it can be called functional cervical spondylosis. When we apply manipulations and Shaolin internal exercise to treat cervical spondylosis and other orthopedic diseases, we should know this. Therefore, the application of adjustment-type manipulation requires clear indications. Spinal and extremity bone and joint movement-type manipulations should not be abused to avoid further damage to their stability through repeated use.

Reasonable use of Tuina manipulations or Shaolin internal exercise to solve the problems of bone structure, soft tissue and joint stability of the spine and extremities is the entry point for tuina therapy to intervene in orthopedic diseases. In the clinical treatment of orthopedic disorders with Tuina therapy, a holistic concept and the guiding idea of “holistic view of tendons and bones” should be established. And tuina manipulations and Shaolin internal exercise for the spine and limbs should be appropriately applied to meet the criteria that is safe, effective, simple, labor-saving and standard.

二、内功推拿治疗内科、妇科、五官科疾病的指导思想

Guiding Principles of Neigong Tuina to Treat Internal, Gynecological, and Other Miscellaneous Diseases

应用推拿方法治疗内、妇、五官科疾病已有数千年的历史。中医经络学说和脏腑理论是内功推拿治疗内、妇、五官科疾病的主要理论基础。按照传统中医学理论的认识，推拿具有疏通经络、调节脏腑、行气活血的作用。经络内属脏腑、外联肢节，是人体内信息、物质和能量传递的通道，经气运行于经络之内，穴位是经气汇聚之所。推拿手法作用于经穴，通过激发经气的运行，从而起到疏通经络的作用。《素问·血气形志》载："形数惊恐，经络不通，病生于不仁，治之以按摩醪药。"

To apply tuina therapy to treat internal, gynecological, and other miscellaneous has a history of over thousands of years. It is based on the theory of meridians and collaterals and the theory of internal organs. In TCM, tuina has the function of promoting meridians and collaterals, regulating internal organs, circulating qi and blood. Meridians and collaterals belong to internal organs and connect the four limbs, which are the passage to transport information, materials and energy inside the body. Meridian qi moves in the meridians, and gathering into the acupoints. Do tuina manipulations on the acupoints can activate the circulation of qi, thus regulating meridians and collaterals. It is recorded in *Plain Question* that "The disease of those with frequent fright is marked by numbness due to stagnation of the meridians and collaterals and can be cured by tuina manipulations and medicated liquor."

推拿手法调节脏腑主要通过以下三个途径来实现：一是通过对经络的刺激，直接调节与之相连的脏腑功能；二是通过对背俞穴和腹募穴的刺激，调节对应脏腑的功能；三是通过对特定穴的作用，综合调节内在脏腑的功能。总之，推拿手法疏通经络、行气活血、调节脏腑三方面的作用是相互联系的。经络疏通是基础，气血畅达是关键，脏腑功能协调一致是根本。以上三方面的作用是推拿手法用于治疗内、妇、五官科疾病的理论基础。

The tuina manipulation on regulating internal organs are realized by the following three ways: regulating the functions of internal organs by the stimulation on meridians and collaterals; regulating the functions of internal organs by the stimulation on back Shu point and front Mu point; regulating the functions of internal organs by the stimulation on the specific points. Generally speaking, promoting meridians and collaterals is important, circulating qi and blood is the critical and harmonizing internal organs is fundamental. They are the theoretical basis for treating internal, gynecological, and other miscellaneous diseases.

近些年"脊柱病因学"的提出，为我们进一步认识推拿方法治疗内、妇、五官科疾病的机制开辟了一个更为广阔的空间。此外，一些新的理论假说也被不断引入，如"生物

The proposal of "Etiology of Spine" in recent years has opened a wider space for us to understand the mechanism of internal, gynecological, and other

全息律学说”“反射区学说”等。随着研究的深入，将进一步阐明推拿方法对内、妇、五官科疾病确切的治疗作用和临床价值，不断丰富内、妇、五官科疾病的推拿理论与实践，使古老的推拿疗法更好地造福于人类。

应用内功推拿方法治疗疾病时，应注意掌握以下施治原则。

（1）根据中医辨证论治结果，选择一种或多种推拿治疗方法，确定适宜的推拿治疗方案或推拿处方。

（2）明确推拿治疗方案确切的临床作用和地位，手法或功法是作为主要的治疗措施，还是辅助性治疗方法，必要时配合其他治疗手段。

（3）在进行某些特殊手法或功法治疗之前，应向患者详细说明情况，必须征得患者同意后方可进行。

（4）施行调整脊椎关节类手法之前，应进行必要的影像学检查，在排除禁忌证之后方可进行，以确保手法的安全性。

miscellaneous diseases. In addition, with the introduction of some new theories and hypothesis and the progress of research, we will have a deeper understanding of the treatment efficacy and clinical value of tuina manipulations on internal, gynecological, and other miscellaneous diseases. Then we will improve and enrich tuina theories and practice to make it better benefit people.

We should grasp the following therapeutic principles when applying Shaolin internal exercise in treating diseases.

(1) Choose tuina manipulation methods or prescriptions based on pattern identification.

(2) Make sure the role of tuina manipulations in treatment. If necessary, combine tuina manipulations with other treatment methods.

(3) Ask patients' permission before doing some special tuina manipulation or exercise and tell them about the situation in detail.

(4) Before operating the manipulation of adjusting spines and joints, imaging examinations are required to exclude contradictions to ensure the safety of manipulations.

第二节 常见疾病应用

Section Two Application of Common Diseases

一、虚劳

Deficiency

虚劳又称虚损，是由多种原因所致的脏腑、阴阳、气血严重亏损，久虚不复的多种慢性衰弱病证的总

Deficiency, also known as chronic consumptive conditions, is a general term for a variety of chronic and debilitating illnesses. They are hard to recover and

称。现代医学的许多慢性疾病出现各种虚损证候与状态等，可参考本证辨证论治。

manifested as the severe consumption of yin and yang, internal organs and qi and blood. In modern medicine, various deficiency symptoms and states of many chronic diseases can be treated based on pattern identification of it.

【诊断要点】

病史存在生活失节、调摄不当等因素，或大病、久病，产后或手术后失血过多等。临床症状可见面色无华、发白或黯黑，消瘦，气短声低，心悸，健忘，头晕眼花，自汗、盗汗，形寒肢冷或五心烦热，倦怠乏力，食欲不振，腹胀，便溏，遗精滑泄，月经不调或停经、闭经等。可见多个脏腑气血阴阳虚损，呈慢性、难复性、进行性的演变过程。

（1）气虚：面色萎黄，气短懒言，语声低微，体倦乏力，动则汗出，易感冒，腹胀，纳差，便溏。舌质淡胖、苔薄白，脉虚大无力。

（2）血虚：面色、唇甲淡白，头晕眼花，心悸、心慌，形体消瘦，肌肤粗糙，月经量少或闭经。舌质淡，脉细弱。

（3）阴虚：两颧潮红，唇红口干，午后低热，手足烦热，失眠，遗精，盗汗。舌质红苔少，脉细数。

（4）阳虚：面色苍白，畏寒肢冷，自汗，喜卧懒动，口淡吐清涎。舌质淡胖嫩，苔白润，脉沉细。

【Diagnoses】

Patients with this disease have the medical history of a bad living lifestyle, improper food intake, or serious and prolonged illness or excessive blood loss after childbirth or surgery, etc. For clinical symptoms, patients may have a dark, pale or dull complexion. They may be very thin. And they may have the shortness of breath and a low voice. Besides, they may also have the symptoms of palpitations, forgetfulness, dizzy head and vision, spontaneous sweating, night sweating, physical cold and cold limbs, or vexing heat in the chest, palms and soles, fatigue and lack of strength, loss of appetite, abdominal distention, sloppy stools, seminal emission and efflux diarrhea, menstrual irregularities or block, etc. The deficiency of qi, blood, yin and yang in several zang-fu organs can be seen in a chronic, irreversible and progressive evolutionary process.

(1) Qi deficiency: Patients may have the symptoms of sallow complexion, shortness of breath, laconic speech, faint low voice, lack of strength, sweating easily brought on by exertion, having a cold, abdominal distention, poor appetite and sloppy stools. In addition, they may have pale and fat tongue with thin white coating, and weak and deficient pulse.

(2) Blood deficiency: Patients may have the symptoms of pale complexion, lips and nails, dizzy head and vision, palpitations and flusteredness, emaciation, pachylosis, scant menstrual flow or menstrual block. They may have pale tongue and thin and weak pulse.

(3) Yin deficiency: Patients may have the symptoms of tidal reddening of cheeks, reddish lips and dry mouth, low-grade fever in the afternoon, vexing heat in the extremities,

insomnia, seminal emission and night sweating. They may have red tongue with little coating and thin and rapid pulse.

(4) Yang deficiency: Patients may have the symptoms of pale complexion, intolerance of cold and cold extremities, spontaneous sweating, preferring lying to walking, bland taste in the mouth, spitting drivel. They may have pale tender-soft enlarged tongue with white and moist coating and sunken and thin pulse.

【治则】

对于虚劳的治疗，当以“虚者补之”“损者益之”，即扶正为主。根据病理属性的不同，分别采取益气、养血、滋阴、温阳的原则。遵循辨证施治原则，以加强治疗的针对性。

【Therapeutic principles】

For the treatment of deficiency, we should obey the principle of treating deficiency with tonification and treating impairment with benefiting, which is reinforcing the healthy qi. According to the different pathological properties, the principles of benefiting qi, nourishing blood, enriching the yin and warming the yang are adopted respectively. And follow the principle of syndrome differentiation can help to make the treatment more targeted.

【手法】

擦法、拿法、按揉法、扫散法等。

【Manipulations】

Linear rubbing manipulation, grasping manipulation, pressing-kneading manipulation and sweeping manipulation.

【取穴】

以任、督二脉经穴及背俞穴为主。

【Selection of points】

The points on the Ren meridian, the Du meridian and Back Shu points.

【操作】

以头面、躯干及上肢常规操作为主。

【Operations】

It focuses on the head, face, and upper limbs.

【辨证加减】

（1）气虚

1）肺气虚者，加强对胸背擦法，以温热为度。按揉膻中、中府、云门，提拿风池、风府。

【Modification based on pattern identification】

(1) Qi deficiency

1) For patients with lung qi deficiency, scrubbing manipulation should be given on the chest and back until they feel warm. Press Danzhong (CV 17), Zhongfu (LU)

2）脾气虚者，加强腹部擦法，温热为度。按揉气海、中脘、上脘、期门、章门、脾俞、胃俞。大便溏薄，加强对少腹平推，并配合横擦八髎，透热为度。

（2）血虚

1）心血虚者，加强头面部手法的操作，尤其推桥弓，拿脑空穴，擦中脘，揉心俞。

2）肝血虚者，加强头面部手法操作，以扫散法为主，拿脑空穴，推桥弓，揉脾俞、胃俞。

3）如见胁痛，加强推两胁，以温热为度。如见妇人月经不调，多擦少腹，以温热为度，并按揉血海、三阴交。

（3）阳虚：加强少腹平推，以见热为度，加腰部肾俞、命门横推，以透热为度。宜推脊柱两侧膀胱经，以透热为度。

（4）阴虚：加强头面部常规手法操作，尤以推桥弓，提拿胸锁乳突肌，并加强胸背擦法，以透热为度。

and Yunmen (LU 2), and lift Fengchi (GB 20) and Fengfu (GV16).

2) For patients with spleen qi deficiency, scrubbing manipulation should be given on the abdomen until they feel warm. Press Qihai (CV 6), Zhongwan (CV 12), Shangwan (13), Qimen (LR 14), Zhangmen (LR 13), Pishu (BL 20) and Weishu (BL 21). For patients suffering from loose stool, push the lower abdomen and transversely scrub Baliao (BL 31–34) to the penetration of heat.

(2) Blood deficiency

1) For patients with heart and blood deficiency, manipulation should be given on the head and face, especially pushing Bridge Arch[1], grasping Naokong (GB 19) and scrubbing Zhongwan (CV 12) and kneading Xinshu (BL 15).

2) For patients with liver and blood deficiency, sweeping manipulation should be given on the head and face. Grasp Naokong (GB 19), push Bridge Arch, knead Pishu (BL 20) and Weishu (BL 21).

3) If there is thoracic pain, strengthen pushing manipulation on the two hypochondriacs to the penetration of warmness. Rub the lower abdominal part to the warmness and press and knead Xuehai (SP 10) and Sanyinjiao (SP 6) for women with irregular menstruation.

(3) Yang deficiency: Strengthen the flat-pushing manipulation on the lower abdominal part to the warmness and the transverse-pushing manipulation on Shenshu (BL 23) and Mingmen (DU 4) to the penetration of heat. It is advisable to push the bladder meridian on two side of the spine to the penetration of heat.

(4) Yin deficiency: For patients with yin deficiency, manipulation should be given on the head and face, especially pushing Bridge Arch, grasping sternocleidomastoid muscle and rubbing the chest and back to the penetration of heat.

[1] Bridge Arch: the arch from Yifeng (SJ 17) point to Quepen (ST 12) point.

1）肺阴虚者，可按揉膻中、中府、云门、璇玑。

2）心阴虚者，加强头部五指拿法，按揉脑空及项后两侧，按揉心俞、合谷、少商。

3）脾胃阴虚者，加强对上腹部擦法，按揉中脘、脾俞、胃俞，直擦八髎，以透热为度。

4）肝阴虚者，加强头面部常规手法操作，尤以扫散法、推桥弓为主。

5）肾阴虚者，加强少腹擦法操作，按揉气海、关元、中极，擦法，以温热为度。并配合横擦腰部，按揉命门、肾俞、腰阳关，以透热为度。

1) For patients with lung yin deficiency, press and knead Danzhong (CV 17), Zhongfu (LU 1), Yunmen (LU 2) and Xuanji (RN 21).

2) For patients with heart yin deficiency, strengthen the grasping manipulation on the head with five fingers, pressing and kneading Naokong (GB 19), both sides of the back of the neck, Xinshu (BL 15), Hegu (LI 4) and Shaoshang (LU 11).

3) For patients with spleen and stomach yin deficiency, strengthen the linear rubbing manipulation on the upper abdomen, press and knead. Zhongwan (CV 12), Pishu (BL 20), Weishu (BL 21), and rub Baliao (BL–31–34) to the penetration of heat.

4) For patients with liver yin deficiency, manipulation should be given on the head and face, with the focus on sweeping manipulation and pushing Bridge Arch.

5) For patients with kidney yin deficiency, strengthen the linear rubbing manipulation on the lower abdomen, press and knead Qihai (CV 6), Guanyuan (CV 4) and Zhongji (CV 3) to the penetration of warmness. And rub the waist, press and knead Mingmen (DU 4), Shenshu (BL 23) and Yaoyangguan (GV 3) to the penetration of heat.

【功法处方】

练功是内功推拿治疗虚劳的重要方法。可先选择站裆式结合前推八匹马、倒拉九头牛的动作进行锻炼，以后逐渐加强马裆、弓箭裆、大裆锻炼，并可选择两手托天、霸王举鼎的动作进行练习。每天早晚各锻炼1次，每次30分钟左右，以汗出或舒适为度。也可辨证施治，对相应经络、穴位进行拍击敲打，使经络畅通，气血旺盛，以达“诸脉皆通，通则疾除”的效果。可在腰背部，配合强身健体熏蒸方熏蒸

【Exercise treatments】

Exercise is an important method of Neigong Tuina to treat deficiency. Patients can first choose the standing stance combined with the exercise of Qian Tui Ba Pi Ma (Pushing Eight Horses Forward) and Dao La Jiu Tou Niu (Pulling Nine Oxen Backward). And then gradually strengthen the exercise of horse stance, bow stance and splitting stance with hands backward, and choose the actions of Liang Shou Tuo Tian (Supporting the Sky with Two Hands) and Ba Wang Ju Ding (Hegemonic King Supporting Tripot). Exercise once a day in the morning and evening, for about 30 minutes each time, to sweat or feel comfortable. You can also identify and treat the

或者热敷治疗。

corresponding meridians and acupuncture points by tapping, so that the meridians are smooth, and the blood and qi are flourish, so as to achieve the effect of "all the meridians are smooth, and the disease is dispelled". In the lower back, it can be treated by fumigation or hot compressing with the formula for strengthening the body.

【注意事项】

（1）避风寒，适寒温。虚劳过程中，感受外邪，耗伤正气，通常是病情恶化的重要原因；而虚劳患者由于正气不足，卫外不固，又容易招致外邪入侵，故应注意冷暖，避风寒，适寒温，尽量减少伤风感冒。

（2）调饮食，戒烟酒。人体气血全赖水谷以资生，故调理饮食对虚劳至关重要。一般以富于营养，易于消化，不伤脾胃为原则。对辛辣厚味，过分滋腻、生冷不洁之物，则应少食甚至禁食。吸烟、嗜酒均有损正气，应该戒除。

（3）慎起居，适劳逸。生活起居要有规律，做到动静结合，劳逸适度。根据自己体力的情况，可适当参加户外散步、功法锻炼等活动。病情轻者，可适当安排工作和学习。适当节制房事。

（4）舒情志，少烦忧。过分的情志刺激，易使气阴伤耗，是使病情加重的重要原因之一。而保持情绪稳定，舒畅乐观，则有利于虚劳的康复。

【Attentions】

(1) Avoid wind cold, make the body adapt to cold and warmth. In the process of deficiency overwork, feeling external evil and depletion of healthy qi are usually the important cause for the deterioration of the disease; and due to the insufficiency of healthy qi and protective qi failing its external assignment, patients are easy to attract the invasion of external evil, so patients should pay attention to cold and warmth, so as to avoid wind cold and catching cold.

(2) Regulate diet and quit smoking and drinking. The human body relies on water and grain to feed the body, so regulating the diet is vital to deficiency overwork. The general principle is to be rich in nutrition, easy to digest, not to hurt the spleen and stomach. It is advisable to eat little spicy, greasy, cold and unclean food or even avoid them. Smoking and drinking should be banned, as they are detrimental to the healthy qi.

(3) Having a regular lifestyle and maintaining a balance between work and rest. Life and living should be regular, so as to achieve the combination of work and rest. Go on a walk outside and do Shaolin internal exercise according to the personal physical condition. For patients with mild symptoms, work and study can be arranged appropriately and frequent sexual intercourse should be avoided.

(4) Relax your emotions and worry less. Excessive emotional stimulation makes it easy to deplete qi and yin, which is one of the important reasons for aggravation

of the disease. Keeping emotions stable, relaxed and optimistic is conducive to the recovery of deficiency overwork.

二、失眠

失眠又称不寐，是指以经常不能获得正常睡眠为特征的一种病症，轻者难以入寐，或睡中易醒，醒后不能再寐，或时寐时醒；重者彻夜不能入寐。本病可单独出现，也可以与头痛、健忘、眩晕、心悸等症同时出现。

Insomnia

Insomnia, also known as sleeplessness, refers to a disease that patients have trouble sleeping. In mild cases, patients have difficulty to sleep, or it is easy for them to wake up in the middle of sleep, and after waking up, it is impossible for them to sleep again, or they wake up at times; in severe cases, it is impossible for them to sleep all night. The disease can occur alone or occur with headache, amnesia, vertigo, and palpitations, etc.

【诊断要点】

（1）心脾两虚：多梦易醒，面色不华，头晕目眩，心悸健忘，神疲肢倦，饮食无味。舌质淡苔薄，脉细弱。

（2）阴虚火旺：心烦不寐，头晕耳鸣，心悸健忘，颧红潮热，口干少津，手足心热，腰膝酸软。舌质红少苔，脉细数。

（3）痰热内扰：不寐多梦，头重心烦，头晕目眩，口苦痰多，胸闷脘痞，不思饮食。舌质红苔黄腻，脉滑或滑数。

（4）肝郁化火：心烦不能入寐，急躁易怒，头痛面红，目赤口苦，胸闷胁痛，不思饮食，口渴喜饮，便秘尿黄。舌质红、苔黄，脉弦数。

【Diagnoses】

(1) Deficiency of both heart and spleen: Patients may have the symptoms of profuse dreams, susceptibility to wake, pale complexion, dizzy head and vision, palpitations, forgetfulness, lassitude of spirit, fatigued limbs, inability to taste food. They may have pale tongue with thin coating and thin and weak pulse.

(2) Yin deficiency with effulgent fire: Patients may have the symptoms of vexation, insomnia, dizziness, tinnitus, palpitations, forgetfulness, tidal fever in the check, dry mouth, feverish sensation in palms and soles, aching lumbus and knees. They may have red tongue with little coating and thin and rapid pulse.

(3) Internal harassment of phlegm-heat: Patients may have the symptoms of insomnia, profuse dreams, heavy headedness, vexation, dizzy head and vision, bitter taste in mouth, profuse sputum, oppression in chest and stomach stuffiness, loss of appetite. They may have red tongue with yellow and greasy coating and slippery or slippery and rapid pulse.

(4) Depressed liver qi transforming into fire: Patients may have the symptoms of insomnia due to vexation, rashness, impatience, irascibility, headache, reddened complexion, red eyes, bitter taste in mouth, oppression in chest and pain in the subcostal region, loss of appetite, desire to drink, constipation and yellow urination. They may have red tongue with yellow coating and wiry and rapid pulse.

【治则】

养心安神，滋阴降火，清热化痰，疏肝解郁。

【Therapeutic principles】

Nourishing the heart to tranquilize, nourishing yin and reducing fire, clearing heat and eliminating phlegm, and soothing liver and relieving depression.

【手法】

擦法、拿法、按揉法、搓法等。

【Manipulations】

Linear rubbing manipulation, grasping manipulation, pressing-kneading manipulation and palm-twisting manipulation.

【取穴】

脑空、缺盆、脾胃区、桥弓、心俞、肺俞、通里、神门、膻中、璇玑、中府、云门。

【Selection of points】

Naokong (GB 19), Quepen (ST 12), Pishu (BL 20), Weishu (BL 21), Bridge Arch, Xinshu (BL 15), Feishu (BL 13), Tongli (HT 15), Shenmen (HT), Danzhong (CV 17), Xuanji (CV 21), Zhongfu (LU 1) and Yunmen (LU 2).

【操作】

以头面、躯干及上肢部常规操作为主。

【Operations】

The manipulation is focused on the head, trunk and upper limbs.

【辨证加减】

（1）心脾两亏：以补养心脾、生气血为主，用常规手法操作。若见多梦易醒、心悸健忘者，头部五指拿法配合拿脑空、按揉缺盆穴，擦脾胃区，背部擦法配合按揉心俞。心脾两虚者，指按、指揉神门、天

【Modification based on pattern identification】

(1) Insufficiency of both heart and spleen: Treatment should be based on tonifying and nourishing heart and spleen and generating qi and blood with regulate manipulation. For patients with excessive dreams, palpitations and forgetfulness and are easy to wake up, do the grasping manipulation on the head with five fingers, grasp Naokong (GB 19), press

枢、足三里、三阴交，每穴1～2分钟；擦背部督脉，以透热为度。

（2）阴亏火旺：宜滋补肾阴、清心降火。在常规手法操作中加强头面部操作，尤以扫散法为要，推桥弓，重拿脑空，按揉心俞、肺俞、通里、神门，擦手三阴经。阴虚火旺推桥弓，左右各20次；擦两侧涌泉穴，以透热为度。

（3）痰热内扰：以化痰清热为主。指按、指揉神门、内关、丰隆、足三里，每穴1～2分钟；横擦脾俞、胃俞、八髎，以透热为度。失眠者重拿脑空穴；胸闷多擦前胸两胁，按揉膻中、璇玑、中府、云门穴；头重者加重扫散法刺激。

（4）肝郁化火：以疏肝解郁、安抚情绪为主。在常规手法操作中加强胁肋部操作。如按揉肝俞、胆俞、期门、章门、太冲，每穴1～2分钟；搓两胁，约1分钟。

and knead Quepen (ST 12) and rub Pishu (BL 20), Weishu (BL 21). And do the linear rubbing manipulation on the back and press and knead Xinshu (BL 15). For patients with dual deficiency of heart and spleen, press and knead Shenmen (HT 7), Tianshu (ST 25), Zusanli (ST 36) and Sanyinjiao (SP 6) for 1 to 2 minutes each with fingers; rub the Du meridian on the back to the penetration of heat.

(2) Yin deficiency leading to fire hyperactivity: Treatment should be based on enriching and supplementing kidney yin and clearing heart and reducing fire. Strengthen the manipulation on the head and face, especially the sweeping manipulation. Push Bridge Arch, grasp Naokong (GB 19) with strong force, press and knead Xinshu (BL 15), Feishu (BL 13), Tongli (HT 4) and Shenmen (HT 6) and rub three hand-yin meridians. For patients with yin deficiency leading to fire hyperactivity, push Bridge Arch for 20 times and rub Yongquan (KI 1) to the penetration of heat in both sides.

(3) Phlegm-heart attacking internally: Treatment should be based on resolving phlegm and clearing heat. Press and knead Shenmen (HT 6), Neiguan (PC 6), Fenglong (ST 40) and Zusanli (ST 36) for 1 to 2 minutes each with fingers; transversely rub Pishu (BL 20), Weishu (BL 21) and Baliao (BL 31–34) to the penetration of heat. For patients with insomnia, grasp Naokong (GB 19) with strong force; and for patients with chest oppression, rub hypochondrium, press and knead Danzhong (CV 17), Xuanji (RN 21), Zhongfu (LU 1) and Yunmen (LU 2). Do sweeping manipulation on patients with heavy headache.

(4) Liver depression transforming into fire: Treatment should be based on soothing liver and relieving depression. Based on the regular treatment, manipulation should pay more attention to ribs. Press and knead Ganshu (BL 18), Danshu (BL 19), Qimen (LR 14), Zhangmen (LR 13) and Taichong (LR 3) for 1 to 2 minutes respectively and twist two ribs for 1 minutes.

【功法处方】

练功是内功推拿治疗失眠的重要手段之一。患者可选择少林内功站裆式结合前推八匹马、倒拉九头牛等动作锻炼，也可选择坐裆势并配合意念导引。每天早晚各锻炼1次，每次30分钟左右，以汗出或略感疲劳为度。睡前可配合强身健体或活血祛瘀熏蒸方熏蒸足部。

【Exercise treatments】

Shaolin internal exercise is one of the most important methods of internal exercise and tuina to treat insomnia. Patients can choose standing stance combined with the exercise of Qian Tui Ba Pi Ma (Pushing Eight Horses Forward) and Dao La Jiu Tou Niu (Pulling Nine Oxen Backward). Or they can choose sitting stance combined with the guidance of thought. Exercise twice a day in the morning and evening, about 30 minutes each time, to sweat or feel slightly fatigue as degree. Before sleep, patients can fumigate their feet, which can strengthen the body or activate blood and remove stasis.

【注意事项】

（1）失眠者在晚饭后应忌服刺激性和兴奋性食物和药物。

（2）手法应轻柔缓和，以诱导大脑皮层逐渐进入抑制状态。

（3）养成良好的作息习惯。

【Attentions】

(1) Patients with insomnia should not have stimulating and excitatory foods and medications after dinner.

(2) The manipulation should be mild and soft to induce the cerebral cortex gradually into the state of inhibition.

(3) Develop a good habit of rest and work.

三、头痛

Headache

头痛是临床常见症状之一，通常指局限于头颅上半部，包括眉弓、耳轮上缘和枕外隆突连线上的疼痛。病因较复杂，可由颅内病变、颅外头颈部病变、躯体疾病及神经官能症、精神病引起。头痛是临床常见症状之一，可因多种原因引起。外感头痛、颈源性头痛、偏头痛、内伤头痛等适宜手法治疗。本节所讨论的头痛，乃属内科疾病之范畴，以头痛为主要症状者。若属外伤及

Headache, also known as cephalalgia, is a common clinical symptom. It usually refers to pain confined to the upper part of the skull, including the arch of the eyebrow, the superior margin of pinnae and the line of the external occipital protuberance. The etiology is complex and can be caused by intracranial lesions, extracranial head and neck lesions, somatic diseases, and neurosis and psychosis. The headache discussed in this chapter belongs to the category of internal medicine diseases with headache as the main symptom. It is not our main content to discuss the headache caused by trauma or some other concurrent

一些疾病过程中所出现的兼证，则主病去，头痛亦自除，不在本节讨论范围之内。

symptoms which can be removed with the recovery of diseases.

【诊断要点】

头痛的诊断应以经络辨证为主，结合脏腑辨证，同时，注意检查是否存在颈部“筋出槽”或“骨错缝”的病理变化，综合分析，才能做出正确判断。

（1）颈源性头痛：起病或急或缓，有长时间低头伏案工作或失枕史，头痛连及颈项，伴颈椎活动不利，或头晕、恶心、畏光、目胀等，在患侧风池周围及上位颈椎关节突关节附近可触及明显压痛和结节状物。疼痛也可出现在前额眉棱骨及眼窝附近。

（2）外感头痛：起病较急，有明显感受外邪史，或头痛连及项背，或胀痛欲裂，或头痛如裹；可伴有发热、恶寒或恶风、身困、鼻塞、流涕、咽痛、咳嗽等症状。

（3）偏头痛：反复发作的一侧或双侧头痛，女性多于男性，发作前多有先兆，常因紧张、忧郁等诱发。麦角胺治疗可缓解症状。

（4）内伤头痛：可因肝阳上亢、气血不足、肾虚失充、瘀血阻络等引起，表现各异。

【Diagnoses】

The diagnosis of headache should be based on meridian syndrome differentiation and combined with visceral pattern identification. To make correct adjustment, physicians also need to check if there are pathological changes in the neck, such as tendon dislocation or bone dislocation.

(1) Cervicogenic headache: The onset of the disease may be acute or slow, with a history of prolonged head-down work or loss of pillow. The pain sprawls to cervical spine leading to its unfavorable movement, or dizziness, nausea, photophobia, eye swelling, etc. There are obvious pressure pain and nodularity around the Fengchi (GB 20) and the superior cervical synovial joints. Pain may also be present in the forehead near the brow bones and eye sockets.

(2) Exogenous headache: The onset of the disease is urgent, with a clear history of feeling external evil. The headache may even reach the back of the neck, or swelling and pain, or headache like a wrap. The headache may be accompanied by fever, aversion to cold or wind, body sleepiness, nasal congestion, runny nose, sore throat, cough and other symptoms.

(3) Migraine: It is a primary headache disorder characterized by recurrent one or two sides headaches that are caused by tension and melancholy with auras The morbidity of women is higher than men's. Treatment with ergotamine may relieve symptoms.

(4) Headache due to internal dysfunctions: It may be caused by the hyperactivity of liver yang, deficiency of qi and blood, kidney deficiency due to the loss of nourishment, obstruction of phlegm and blood with various manifestations.

【治则】

疏经，通络，止痛。

【Therapeutic principles】

Dredging meridians, freeing the collateral vessels and relieving pain.

【手法】

擦法、滚法、按揉法、一指禅推法、叩击法、拿法、分推法、摩法、抹法、扫散法。

【Manipulations】

Linear rubbing manipulation, rolling manipulation, press-kneading manipulation, Yi Zhi Chan pushing, tapping manipulation, grasping manipulation, pushing manipulation with two hands parting from each other, circular rubbing manipulation, wiping manipulation and sweeping manipulation.

【取穴】

风池、天鼎、印堂、神庭、鱼腰、攒竹、头维、太阳、百会、四神聪、桥弓，头面部六阳经及督脉循行部位。

【Selection of points】

Fengchi (GB 20), Tianding (LI 17), Yintang (EX–HN 3), Shenting (GV 24), Yuyao (EX–HN 4), Cuanzhu (BL 2), Touwei (ST 8), Taiyang (EX–HN 5), Baihui (GV 20), Sishencong (EX–HN 1), Bridge Arch, the point on the Six yang meridian, the Du meridian and the Ren meridian on the head and face.

【操作】

按照头面部、躯干部、上肢部、下肢部的顺序实施内功推拿常规操作。

【Operations】

Operation is performed in the order of head and face, trunk, upper limbs and lower limbs.

【辨证加减】

（1）颈源性头痛：宜滚项肩部、上背部主要肌群，一指禅推项部两侧、按揉风池、天鼎及肩部穴位。必要时行颈椎调整手法，以提拿或叩击肩部肌肉结束。

（2）外感头痛：外感风寒头痛，可重用捏拿巅顶，按压风池、风门、肺俞等穴，以祛风散寒，通络止痛。外感风热头痛，可重用推抹额颞部，

【Modification based on pattern identification】

(1) Cervicogenic headache: The treatment should be focused on neck and shoulders as well as major muscles in the upper back. Push two sides of the neck with Yi Zhi Chan pushing, press and knead Fengchi (GB 20), Tianding (LI 17) and other points in the shoulders. If necessary, change manipulation operated on the cervical spine and end at lifting or tapping muscles in the shoulder.

(2) Exogenous headache: For the headache due to exogenous wind-cold, pinch and grasp parietal bone with

按压曲池、合谷等穴，宜清泄风热止头痛。外感风湿头痛，可用重力揉抹头顶，按压止痛配合两手捏拿肩井，单手多指拍击项背部，亦可头顶、前额以祛风胜湿止痛。

（3）偏头痛：可用重力重推抹前额，拨揉两颞及推抹桥弓，以祛风平肝，配合按压角孙、率谷等穴。

（4）内伤头痛：内伤头痛需辨证治疗。肝阳头痛，可左右交替推桥弓，扫散和拨揉两颞，按揉太冲、行间等，重用掌心击百会及擦足底涌泉穴。血虚头痛可重用擦上背部及督脉，以透热为度，结合摩腹操作，以气海、关元、中脘为重点，按揉心俞、膈俞、足三里、三阴交等穴。肾虚头痛可用擦督脉及背部膀胱经，结合摩腹操作，以气海、关元为重点。瘀阻头痛可按揉太阳、攒竹及前额、头侧部。重用擦前额及两侧太阳穴部位。

strong force, press Fengchi (GB 20), Fengmen (BL 12) and Feishu (BL 13) to dispel wind and dissipate cold and dredge collaterals and relieve pain; for the headache due to exogenous wind-heat, push and wipe frontal-temporal area strongly, press Quchi (LI 11) and Hegu (LI 4) to clear wind-heat that relieves pain; for the headache due to exogenous wind-dampness, forcefully knead and wipe the vertex and press the vertex to alleviate pain combined with pinch and grasp Jianjing (GB 21) with both hands, rap neck and back with fingers of one hand, which can be operated at the vertex and forehead to dispel wind and eliminate dampness to relieve pain.

(3) Migraine: Forcefully push and wipe forehead, fiddle and knead two temporal and push Bridge Arch to dispel wind and calm the liver combined with pressing Jiaosun (TE 20) and Shuaigu (GB 8).

(4) Endogenous headache: Endogenous headache should be treated on the basis of syndrome differentiation. For live yang headache, push Bridge Arch, sweep, fiddle and knead two temporal, press and knead Taichong (LR 3) and Xingjian (LR 2), strike Baihui (GV 20) forcefully with palms and scrub Yongquan (KI 1) ; for blood vacuity headache, forcefully scrub back and the Du meridian to the penetration of heat combined with circular manipulation on the abdomen, with a focus on the manipulation of Qihai (CV 6), Guanyuan (CV 4) and Zhongwan (CV 12), rub Xinshu (BL 15), Geshu (BL 17), Zusanli (ST 36) and Sanyinjiao (SP 6) ; for kidney vacuity headache, scrub the Du meridian and baldder meridian on the back. Do circular rubbing manipulation on the abdomen with a focus on Qihai (CV 6) and Guanyuan (CV 4) ; for headache due to stasis, press and rub Temples (EX–HN 5), Cuanzhu (BL 2), forehead and cephalic regions. Forcefully rub forehead and temples.

【功法处方】

练功是内功推拿治疗头痛的重

【Exercise treatments】

Shaolin internal exercise is one of the most important

要手段之一。患者须加强练习少林内功，可选择站裆势结合前推八匹马、倒拉九头牛等动作锻炼，以后逐渐加强马裆势、弓箭裆势的锻炼，并可选择凤凰展翅的动作进行锻炼。每天早晚各锻炼1次，每次30分钟左右，以汗出或略感疲劳为度。

methods to treat headache. Patients need to strengthen Shaolin Internal Exercise, taking standing stance combined with Qian Tui Ba Pi Ma (Pushing Eight Horses Forward) and Dao La Jiu Tou Niu (Pulling Nine Oxen Backward). And then patients can gradually take horse stance and bow stance combined with Feng Huang Zhan Chi (Chinese Phoenix Spreading its Wings). Exercise once every morning and evening, about 30 minutes each time, with sweating or slight fatigue as the degree.

【注意事项】

（1）推拿治疗前，须注意排除蛛网膜下腔出血、腔隙性脑梗死、脑膜炎、颅内肿瘤等常见的急慢性头痛的颅脑疾病；必要时，做头颅CT或MRI检查。

（2）头痛者应保持安静，心情愉快，保证充足的睡眠和休息，避免用脑过度、精神紧张，宜清淡饮食，适当进行散步、气功、太极拳等活动。

（3）头痛由颈椎病引起者，睡眠时要选用合适的枕头，仰卧时宜低，侧卧时与肩等宽，避免工作中长时间低头，注意颈部保暖。

（4）头痛由高血压、动脉硬化引起者，要经常测量血压，保持血压稳定，控制饮食及血脂，饮食宜清淡，情绪宜稳定。

【Attentions】

(1) Before treatment, doctors should pay attention to exclude the common brain diseases of acute and chronic headache such as subarachnoid hemorrhage, lacunar cerebral infarction, meningitis and intracranial tumors; if necessary, do CT or MRI examination of the head.

(2) Headache sufferers should keep quiet, be in a happy mood, ensure adequate sleep and rest, avoid overuse of brain and mental tension, have light diet, and properly carry out activities such as walking, doing qigong and taijiquan.

(3) Patients with headache caused by cervical spondylosis should choose a suitable pillow during sleep. It should be low when lying on the bed and keep shoulder width when lying on your side. Avoid lowering your head for a long time during work and pay attention to keeping your neck warm.

(4) Patients with headache caused by hypertension and arteriosclerosis should be measured frequently to keep the blood pressure stable. In addition, they should control their blood lipids, have light diet and keep a stable mood.

四、高血压

Hypertension

高血压是一种常见的慢性疾病，又称“原发性高血压病”，以动脉血压持续性增高为主要临床表现。成

Hypertension (HTN or HT), also known as a kind of common disease with high blood pressure, is a long term medical condition in which the blood pressure in the

年人正常血压在安静状态下，收缩压＞140 mmHg 和（或）舒张压＞90 mmHg，即称为高血压。其临床表现以头目眩晕、头痛头昏、耳鸣、健忘、失眠、乏力等为特征，后期可有心、脑、肾等多脏器损害。

arteries is persistently elevated. High blood pressure is present if the resting blood pressure is persistently at or systolic blood pressure above 140 mmHg and diastolic blood pressure is above 90 mmHg for adults. Its clinical manifestations are characterized by dizziness, headache, tinnitus, forgetfulness, insomnia and fatigue. In the later stage, there may be damage to multiple organs such as heart, brain, and kidney.

【诊断要点】

高血压的诊断应以血压值为主，中医治疗时应结合脏腑理论辨证论治，同时，注意检查是否存在颈部“筋出槽”或“骨错缝”的病理变化，综合分析，才能做出正确判断。

（1）肝阳上亢：头晕目眩，头痛且胀，耳鸣、面赤，急躁易怒，夜寐不宁，每因烦劳、恼怒而诱发或加剧，伴胁胀、口苦。舌苔薄黄，脉弦有力。

（2）痰浊壅盛：头昏头痛，沉重如蒙，胸闷脘痞，呕恶痰涎，食少多寐。舌苔白腻，脉濡滑或弦滑。

（3）阴虚阳亢：以眩晕、耳鸣、腰酸膝软、五心烦热为主症，兼见头重脚轻、口燥咽干、两目干涩等症。舌红少苔，脉细数。

（4）阴阳两虚：血压升高兼见头晕目眩、心悸失眠、腰腿酸软、畏寒肢冷、小便清长。舌淡，脉沉细。

【Diagnoses】

Hypertension should be diagnosed based on a persistently high blood pressure. Treatment should be based on pattern identification combined with viscera theory. Besides, doctors should pay attention to examination whether there are pathological changes of “tendon dislocation” or “bone dislocation” in the neck. Comprehensive analysis is the prerequisite of the right judgment.

(1) Hyperactivity of liver yang: Patients may have the symptoms of dizziness, headache and heavy headedness, tinnitus, red countenance, rashness, impatience, irascibility, failure to sleep soundly. And it will be intensified with fatigue and irascibility and accompanied with rib-side distention and pain, bitter taste in mouth. They may have thin and yellow tongue fur, wiry and forceful pulse.

(2) Phlegm turbidity stasis: Patients may have the symptoms of dizziness, headache, head heaviness as if being wrapped up, oppression in the chest and stomach stuffiness, nausea and vomiting of phlegm and saliva, reduced eating and profuse sleeping; they may have slimy white tongue fur and slippery and soggy or string-like pulse.

(3) Yin deficiency with yang hyperactivity: Patients may have the symptoms of dizziness, tinnitus, aching lumbus and limp knees, and vexing heat in the chest, palms and soles and accompanied with heavy head and light feet, dry mouth sore throat and dry eyes. They may have red tongue with little coating and thin and rapid pulse.

(4) Dual deficiency of yin and yang: Patients may have the symptoms of the elevated blood pressure accompanied with dizziness, palpitations, insomnia, aching lumbus and leg intolerance of cold, cold extremities, clear urine in large amounts, pale tongue, sunken and thin pulse.

【治则】

根据本病的发生原因和证候特点，宜区分标本缓急，属虚属实，分而治之。

【Therapeutic principles】

The treatment should be given on the basis of different causes and symptoms.

【手法】

擦法、分推法、一指禅推法、滚法、按揉法、叩击法、拿法、抹法、扫散法、摩法。

【Manipulations】

Linear rubbing manipulation, pushing manipulation with two hands parting from each other, Yi Zhi Chan pushing, rolling manipulation, press-kneading manipulation, tapping manipulation, grasping manipulation, wiping manipulation, sweeping manipulation, circular rubbing manipulation.

【取穴】

头面部六阳经及督脉穴位、背俞穴和腹部任脉穴位。

【Selection of points】

Points on six yang meridians on the head and face, the Du meridian, the first lateral line of the foot solar bladder meridian on the back, and the Ren meridian in the abdomen.

【操作】

以头面部、腰背部和腹部内功推拿常规操作为主，然后随证施治，选择针对性的操作。

（1）头面部操作：自上而下推桥弓，先左后右，两侧交替进行。医者行一指禅“小∞字”和“大∞字”推法，反复分推3～5遍；继之指按、指揉印堂、神庭、攒竹、鱼腰、太阳、百会、四神聪等穴，每穴约1分钟；结合抹前额3～5遍；从前额发际处拿至风池穴处做

【Operations】

Operation is performed on head and face, waist and back and abdomen. Points selection for the treatment should be based on syndrome differentiation.

(1) Manipulation on the head and face: Push Bridge Arch from top to bottom, each time one side beginning at left one. Do ∞-manipulation (a tuina manipulation to exert constant force on the area to be treated with the tip or the palmar side of the thumb through active swing of the forearm) for 3 to 5 times. Press and knead Yintang (GV 29), Shenting (DU 24), Cuanzhu (BL 2), Yuyao (EX–HN 4), Temple (EX–HN 5), Baihui (DU 20) and Sishencong

五指拿法，反复3～5遍；行双手扫散法，约1分钟。

（2）腰背部操作：医者用滚法在患者背部、腰部操作，重点治疗心俞、厥阴俞、肝俞、胆俞、肾俞、命门等部位，时间约5分钟。捏脊，自上而下捏背部督脉脊骨皮，8～10遍。掌推督脉，自上而下掌推背部督脉，3～4遍。擦腰部肾俞、命门一线，以透热为度。

（3）胸腹部操作：术者站于受术者侧前方，以一手中指指腹着力于膻中穴，做轻柔缓和的环旋揉动。斜擦胁肋，术者站于受术者后方，以双掌在腋下胁肋部作斜向往返推擦。按揉腹部穴位，术者站于受术者右侧，以拇指按揉腹部关元、神阙、中脘等穴，重复数次。术者站于受术者右侧，一手掌紧贴于受术部位，而后做有节律的、顺时针方向的环形摩动。

(EX–HN 1) for 1 minute each; wipe the forehead for 3 to 5 times; grasp Fengchi (GB 20) with five fingers from the frontal hairline, repeating it 3 to 5 times. Do sweeping manipulation with two hands for about 1 minute.

(2) Manipulation on the waist and back: Do rolling manipulation with the proximal interphalangeal joints on the back and waist of the patients, with the focus on Xinshu (BL 15), Jueyinshu (BL 14), Ganshu (BL 18), Danshu (BL 19), Shenshu (BL 23) and Mingmen (DU 4) for about 5 minutes. Pinch the Du meridian along the spine for 8 to 10 times. Push the Du meridian with the palm for 3 to 4 times from top to bottom and rub the line between Shenshu (BL 23) and Mingmen (DU 4) to the penetration of heat.

(3) Manipulation on the chest and abdomen: Patients should stand when operating. Do circular rubbing manipulation on Danzhong (CV 17) of the patient gently and rub ribs. Press and knead the points on the abdomen with thumbs, with the focus on Guanyuan (RN 4), Shenque (RN 8) and Zhongwan (CV 12), repeating it for several times.

【辨证加减】

（1）肝阳上亢：头面部常规手法须加强应用，尤其是扫散法、推桥弓、按揉曲盆，并对胸、上腹、少腹加强平推。配合重拿风池穴2～3分钟，掐太冲、行间穴，各2～3分钟；摩揉肝俞、肾俞、涌泉穴，透热为度。

（2）痰浊壅盛：除头面扫散法外，还要推桥弓，加强胸及下肢部擦法。在擦胸部时配合按揉璇玑、天突，擦少腹时配合按揉水道、中极。一指禅推法结合指按、指揉丰隆、解溪穴，取泻法；推、擦足三

【Modification based on pattern identification】

(1) Hyperactivity of liver yang: Strengthen the manipulation for the head and face, especially sweeping manipulation, push Bridge Arch, press and knead Qupen (LI 11) ; strengthen flat-pushing manipulation in the upper chest and abdomen, lateral lower abdomen. Forcefully grasp Fengchi (GB 20) with strong force for 2 to 3 minutes, nip/pinch Taichong (LR 3) and Xingjian (LR 2) for 2 to 3 minutes respectively. Circular rub and knead Ganshu (BL 18), Shenshu (BL 23) and Yongquan (KI 1) to the penetration of heat.

(2) Obstruction of phlegm turbidity: Do sweeping manipulation on the head and face, push Bridge Arch and strengthen rub manipulation on chest and lower

里穴，摩中脘穴，取补法。

（3）阴虚阳亢：头面部的扫散法、推桥弓、拿风池做重点运用。如见心悸、失眠在头面部手法中尤以脑空穴为主，配合按揉心俞、神门穴。

（4）阴阳两虚：以头面操作为重点，即扫散法、推桥弓。如见行动气急，加强擦胸部及两胁；腰酸腿软、夜间多尿要加强腰部擦法，配合按揉肾俞、腰阳关。

limbs. When rub chest, press and knead Xuanji (CV 21), Tiantu (CV 22). When rub lower abdomen, press and knead Shuidao (ST 28) and Zhongji (CV 3). Do Yi Zhi Chan pushing, in the combination with pressing and kneading Fenglong (ST 40) and Jiexi (ST 41) with fingers in purgation method. Push and rub Zusanli (ST 36) and circularly rub Zhongwan (CV 12) in reinforcement method.

(3) Yin deficiency and yang hyperactivity: Do sweeping manipulation on head and face, with focus on pushing Bridge Arch and grasping Fengchi (GB 20). For patients with palpitations and insomnia, the manipulation should be focused on Naokong (GB 19) and press and knead Xinshu (BL 15) and Shenmen (HT 7).

(4) Deficiency of yin and yang: The manipulation should be focused on head and face, such as doing sweeping manipulation and pushing Bridge Arch. For patients who are out of breath when exercising, strengthen the linear rubbing manipulation on their chest and ribs; and for patients with aching back and legs and who have excessive urine at night, strengthen the linear rubbing manipulation on their waists, and press and knead Shenshu (BL 23) and Yaoyangguan (GV 3).

【功法处方】

练功是内功推拿治疗高血压的重要手段之一。患者须加强练习少林内功，可选择站裆势结合前怀中抱月、力劈华山等动作锻炼，也可选择坐裆势配合意念导引。每天早晚各锻炼1次，每次30分钟左右，以舒适为度。

【Exercise treatments】

Shaolin internal exercise is one of the most important methods to treat high blood pressure. Patients need to strengthen Shaolin Internal Exercise, taking standing stance combined with Huai Zhong Bao Yue (Embracing the Moon) and Li Pi Hua Shan (Splitting Hua Mountain with Vigorous Efforts). And they can also take sitting stance combined with guidance of the mind. Exercise once every morning and evening, about 30 minutes each time.

【注意事项】

（1）推拿疗法适用于1级和2级高血压病患者，必要时配合药物治疗。

【Attentions】

(1) Tuina therapy is suitable for the patients with grade 1 and grade 2 hypertension, and give drug treatment

（2）在推拿治疗高血压病时，手法要轻柔。

（3）高血压患者平时要节制饮食，减少盐的摄入量，忌食动物脂肪、内脏，防止体重超重，戒烟戒酒。生活要有规律，不宜过度疲劳和情绪激动，可在医生指导下进行适当的功法锻炼。

if necessary.

(2) The manipulation should be gentle and soft.

(3) Patients with hypertension should control their diet, reduce salt intake, avoid eating animal fat and viscera, prevent overweight, quit smoking and drinking. They should also remain a regular life and avoid excessive fatigue and intense emotion. And they can take appropriate exercise under the guidance of doctors.

五、肺痨

肺痨又称肺结核，以咳嗽、咯血、潮热、盗汗及身体逐渐消瘦等症为主要临床表现。是由结核菌引起的一种具有传染性的慢性消耗性疾病，可以分为原发性和继发性两大类，前者为人体第一次感染结核菌引起的病变，称为原发感染，多见于幼儿和少年。后者则是再次感染或者在原发感染的基础上，残留在病灶内当机体抵抗能力下降时，结核菌又可活跃、繁殖而致病，也称为内源性复发。肺痨临床可分为三期，即进展期、好转期和稳定期，其中进展期、好转期均属活动性，需要到传染病医院隔离治疗；稳定期仍有相关症状者可采用内功推拿治疗。肺痨是内功推拿早期治疗病种之一，李锡九等人曾患肺痨而受益于内功推拿。1959 年的《中医推拿学》教材，已将内功推拿治疗肺痨和肺胀列入其中。

Lung Tuberculosis

Lung tuberculosis, also known as Tuberculosis (TB), is an infectious chronic consumption disease caused by the bacterium mycobacterium tuberculosis (MTB). It has the classic symptoms of cough, hemoptysis, tidal fever, night sweats and weight loss. It can be classified as either primary tuberculosis or secondary tuberculosis. The former is a lesion caused by the first infection of the body with the tuberculosis bacterium and is called primary infection, mostly seen in young children and adolescents. In the latter case, the bacillus is re-infected or remains in the lesion parts based on primary infection, and when the body's resistance decreases, the bacilli can be active and multiply again. This is also called endogenous relapse. The clinical course of pulmonary tuberculosis can be divided into three stages, that is, progressive, improved, and stable, in which the progressive, improved stages are active and patients should be transferred to the infectious hospital for isolation; those who in the stable phase can be treated with internal tuina. Tuberculosis is one of the diseases to be treated by internal tuina in the early period. Li Xijiu's recovery from tuberculosis was one of the examples benefited from internal tuina. In 1959, the textbook *Chinese Tuina* (*Massage*) has included the tuina therapy for lung tuberculosis and lung distention.

【诊断要点】

有较密切的结核病接触史。起病可急可缓，多为低热（午后为著）、盗汗、乏力、纳差、消瘦、女性月经失调等。呼吸道症状有咳嗽、咳痰、咯血、胸痛、不同程度胸闷或呼吸困难。

（1）肺阴亏虚：干咳，咳声短促，或咯少量黏痰，或痰中带血丝或血点，血色鲜红，胸部隐隐闷痛，午后手足心热，皮肤干灼，口干咽燥，或有轻微盗汗。舌边尖红苔薄，脉细或细数。

（2）肺肾阴虚：可见咳嗽、痰中带血、食欲不振、倦怠消瘦等，或伴胸痛。舌红少苔或光剥，脉细数无力。

（3）肺脾两虚：可见咳嗽、痰中带血、食欲不振、倦怠消瘦等。舌质淡，苔薄白或白滑，脉细弱。

（4）阴阳两虚：咳逆喘息少气，咯痰色白，或夹血丝，血色暗淡，潮热，自汗，盗汗，声嘶或失音，面浮肢肿，心慌，唇紫，肢冷，形寒，或见五更泄泻，口舌生糜，大肉尽脱，男子滑精，女子经少、经闭。舌质淡或光嫩少津，脉微细而数，或虚大无力。

【Diagnoses】

A diagnosis of TB should be considered whether patients have close contact with confirmed cases. The onset can be acute and slow, and patients may have the symptoms of low-grade fever (late afternoon), night sweats, lack of strength, poor appetite, weight loss, and menstrual disturbances. Respiratory symptoms are cough, expectoration of phlegm and blood, chest pain, and oppression in the chest or dyspnea.

(1) Lung yin deficiency: Patients may have the symptoms of dry, short and quick cough, or cough with a small amount of mucous sputum, or sputum with little bright red blood or blood spots, pain in the chest, feverish sensations in palms and soles in the late afternoon, dry skin, slight night sweats, red tongue tip with thin tongue coating, thin or rapid pulse.

(2) Lung-kidney yin deficiency: Patients may have the symptoms of cough, sputum with blood, poor appetite, fatigue and emaciation or accompanied with pain in the chest, red tongue, sparse or peeled coating, thin, rapid and forceless pulse.

(3) Insufficiency of both lung and spleen: Patients may have the symptoms of cough, sputum with blood, poor appetite, fatigue and emaciation, pale tongue and white and thin or glossy tongue fur, thin and weak pulse.

(4) Deficiency of yin and yang: Patients may have the symptoms of cough with shortage of qi, white sputum or sputum with dark blood, tidal fever, spontaneous sweating, night sweats, light hoarseness or loss of voice, puffy face and swollen limbs, fluster, purple lips, cold extremities, physical cold. Patients may also have the symptoms of diarrhea before dawn, mouth and tongue sores, emaciation, spontaneous seminal emission of men, scanty menstruation or amenorrhea. Patients have pale or tender tongues with fluids scarcity, thin and rapid pulse or

weak and forceless pulse.

【治则】

"治之之法，一则杀其虫，以绝其根本；一则补虚，以复其真元。"抗痨杀虫，针对本病的特异病因进行治疗。内功推拿的主要作用是补虚培元，以培补肺气、健运中阳为主。在辨证施治的基础上，运用常规手法配合练功锻炼。旨在增强正气，以提高抗病能力，促进疾病的康复。

【Therapeutic principles】

"According to therapeutic principles, killing tubercle bacilli thoroughly is important. Then it is more important to make up for the deficiency to restore original qi." Treatment of TB uses antibiotics to kill the bacteria. The main function of internal tuina is to tonify deficiency and bank up the root, nurture and tonify lung qi, strengthen the transportation of middle yang. Based on the syndrome differentiation and treatment, combine routine manipulation with internal exercise. The aim is to strengthen healthy qi to resist disease and boost recovery.

【手法】

擦法、按揉法、拿法、棒击法。

【Manipulations】

Linear rubbing manipulation, press-kneading manipulation, grasping manipulation and stick-knocking manipulation.

【取穴】

中府、云门、大椎、肺俞、脊柱、肾俞、脑空、风池、桥弓、八髎。

【Selection of points】

Zhongfu (LU 1), Yunmen (LU 2), Dazhui (GV 14), Feishu (BL 13), Spinal Line[1], Naokong (GB 19), Fengchi (GB 20), Bridge Arch, Baliao (BL 31–34)

【操作】

以头面、躯干及上肢部常规手法操作为主，辅以棒击法常规操作。

【Operations】

The manipulation should be focused on head, face, trunk and upper limbs supplemented by stick-knocking manipulation.

【辨证加减】

（1）肺阴亏虚：应加强推桥弓穴，擦胸背，以温热为度；按揉中府、云门、大椎、肺俞等穴。

（2）肺肾阴虚：加强擦两胁及

【Modification based on pattern identification】

(1) Lung yin deficiency: Push Bridge Arch, scrub chest and back to the penetration of warmness, press Zhongfu (LU 1), Yunmen (LU 2), Dazhui (GV 14), Feishu (BL 13).

[1] Spinal Line: the arch from Yifeng (SJ 17) point to Quepen (ST 12) point.

少腹，横推肾俞，以温热为度；直擦脊柱两侧膀胱经，以透热为度；五指拿脑空穴、风池，推桥弓穴。

（3）肺脾两虚：加强擦腹及少腹，以温热为度；横擦肾俞、八髎，以透热为度。

（4）阴阳两虚：加强对胸背部操作，在胸背部可配合挡法，横擦大椎穴部，直擦脊柱两侧膀胱经，以透热为度。

(2) Lung-kidney yin deficiency: Scrub ribs and lateral lower abdomen, flat-push Shenshu (BL 23) to the penetration of warmness; rub bladder meridian on the two sides of vertebral column to the penetration of warmness; grasp Naokong (GB 19), Fengchi (GB 20) with five fingers and push Bridge Arch.

(3) Insufficiency of both lung and spleen: Scrub abdomen and lateral lower abdomen to the penetration of warmness; flat-scrub Shenshu (BL 23) and Baliao (BL 31–34) to the penetration of warmness.

(4) Dual deficiency of yin and yang: Strengthen the manipulation on the chest and back with warding manipulation, flat-scrub Dazhui (GV 14) and rub bladder meridian on the two sides of vertebral column to the penetration of warmness.

【功法处方】

一般在手法治疗 1 个疗程后可配合练习少林内功站裆式，适当选择前推八匹马、倒拉九头牛进行锻炼；第 2 疗程后可以配合马裆势、弓箭裆势，选择风摆荷叶、霸王举鼎等动作进行锻炼，锻炼时可配合出声发力。在练功稍休息后，再进行常规手法进行治疗。每天早晚各锻炼 1 次，每次 30 分钟左右，以略感疲劳为度。

【Exercise treatments】

After the first course of tuina therapy, patients can take standing stance combined with Qian Tui Ba Pi Ma (Pushing Eight Horses Forward) and Dao La Jiu Tou Niu (Pulling Nine Oxen Backward). And after the second course of tuina therapy, horse stance and bow stance can be better combined with the exercise Feng Bai He Ye (Wind Blowing Lotus Leaf) and Ba Wang Ju Ding (Hegemonic King Supporting Tripot). Speak out loudly when exercising. Have a rest first and then accept tuina manipulations. Exercise once every morning and evening, about 30 minutes each time, to feel slightly fatigue.

【注意事项】

（1）推拿治疗肺痨主要针对稳定期，进展期和好转期肺痨需要到专科医院进行隔离治疗。

（2）肺痨早期以药物治疗为主，加强休息，不宜做剧烈运动。稳定期加强推拿治疗和少林内功锻炼，

【Attentions】

(1) Tuina treatment of pulmonary tuberculosis is mainly aimed at the stable stage. At the progression and the improvement stage of pulmonary tuberculosis, patients need to go to specialized hospitals for isolation treatment.

(2) In the early stages of tuberculosis (TB), patients usually accept drug therapy. They should get enough

但亦需循序渐进，不可操之过急。

（3）肺痨属消耗性疾病，在治疗过程中需加强营养。

rest and avoid strenuous exercise. In the stable stages of tuberculosis (TB), they gradually accept tuina therapy and take Shaolin internal exercise.

(3) Tuberculosis (TB) is a consumption disease, and patients should ensure the abundant intake of nutrients.

六、哮喘

Asthma

哮喘是哮咳和喘息的简称，哮为喉中鸣息有声，喘为呼吸气促困难。目前全球哮喘患者约3亿人，中国哮喘患者约3 000万。哮喘是影响人们身心健康的重要疾病。治疗不及时、不规范，哮喘可能致命，而规范化治疗可使近80%的哮喘患者得到非常好的控制，工作、生活几乎不受影响。每年 5 月的第1个周二为世界哮喘日，旨在提醒公众对该疾病的认识，提高对哮喘的防治水平。推拿不仅可以缓解发作时的症状，而且通过手法治疗和功法锻炼扶正治疗，可以达到祛除夙根，控制复发的目的。

Asthma means croup and wheezing. Croup is a sound in the throat and wheezing is shortness of breath. The number of people with asthma is about 300 million globally, and about 30 million in China. Asthma is an important disease that affects people's physical and mental health. Asthma can be fatal if treatment is not timely and standardized. Standardized treatment allows nearly 80% of asthma patients to be very well controlled, with little or no impact on their work and life. World Asthma Day is celebrated every year on the 1st Tuesday of May to remind the public of the disease and to improve the prevention and treatment of asthma. Tuina not only relieves the symptoms of an asthma attack, but also helps to eliminate the root cause of the attack and control the recurrence of the disease through manipulations and exercise.

【诊断要点】

（1）风寒袭肺：喘息，呼吸困难，恶寒、发热，鼻流清涕。舌淡红苔薄白，脉浮紧。

（2）风热犯肺：气喘，咳嗽，痰黄黏稠，口干，便干，尿黄，或发热恶寒，或周身痛楚，头痛，或咽喉肿痛。舌红苔淡黄薄或黄。

（3）痰浊阻肺：喘息，咳嗽，痰多，咯出不爽，甚则喉中有痰鸣声，胸闷恶心，纳差口淡。舌苔白

【Diagnoses】

(1) Wind-cold attacking lung: Patients may have the symptoms of panting, dyspnea, aversion to cold, fever, runny nose with clear snivel, pale and red tongue and thin and white coating, floating and tight pulse.

(2) Wind-heat invading the lung: Patients may have the symptoms of panting, cough with thick yellow phlegm, dry mouth, dry stool, yellow urine, or fever and aversion to cold, or pantalgia and headache, or sore swollen throat and red tongue with thin and faint yellow or yellow coating.

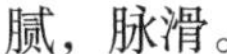

腻，脉滑。

（4）肺虚：咳嗽频发，动则呼吸促迫，吸短呼长，甚则张口抬肩。舌红苔白而滑，脉滑数。

（5）肾虚：动则喘急，呼多吸少，胸闷气促，心悸气短，夜间不能平卧，咳吐少量黏痰，面黄消瘦，腰酸痛，纳差，尿频。舌红苔薄黄，脉沉滑。

(3) Phlegm turbidity obstructing the lung: Patients may have the symptoms of panting, cough with profuse sputum, difficulty to cough sputum or cough with a phlegm sound in the throat, oppression in the chest and nausea, poor appetite, bland taste in the mouth, white and glossy tongue coating and slippery pulse.

(4) Lung deficiency: Patients may have the symptoms of frequent cough with rapid of breathing on exertion, short inhaling and long exhaling or even opening mouth and lifting shoulders, red tongue, white and slippery coating and rapid and slippery pulse.

(5) Kidney deficiency: Patients may have the symptoms of rapid of breathing on exertion, exhalation more than inhalation, oppression in the chest, hasty breathing, palpitations, shortness of breath, inability to lie flat at night, cough and spit scanty phlegm, sallow complexion and emaciation, soreness and pain of lumbus, poor appetite, frequent urination, red tongue and thin and yellow coating, sunken and slippery pulse.

【治则】

以宽胸理气，止咳平喘为原则。实证以祛邪为主，虚证以扶正为主。

【Therapeutic principles】

To soothe the chest and regulate qi and suppress cough and calm panting. Eliminate the pathogenic factors for excess pattern and reinforce the healthy qi for deficiency pattern.

【手法】

按揉法、擦法、推法、拿法、击法。

【Manipulations】

Press-kneading manipulation, scrubbing manipulation, pushing manipulation, grasping manipulation, tapping manipulation.

【取穴】

云门、大椎、命门、肩中俞、风门、璇玑、中府、囟门、膻中、内关、足三里等。

【Selection of points】

Yunmen (LU 2), Dazhui (GV 14), Mingmen (GV 4), Jianzhongshu (SI 15), Fengmen (BL 12), Xuanji (RN 21), Zhongfu (LU), Xinmen (GV 22), Danzhong (CV 17), Neiguan (PC 6), Zusanli (ST 36).

【操作】

按照头面、项部、躯干、上肢部的常规手法操作处理，加强重复头面部操作，震囟门、大椎、命门等穴。哮喘发作较甚者，先用按揉法在定喘、风门、肺俞、肩中俞、璇玑诸穴轻柔刺激，逐渐加大手法刺激量，以患者有明显的酸胀得气感为度，在哮喘缓解后再进行辨证施治。

【Operations】

The manipulation should be focused on head, face, neck, trunk and upper limbs. Do vibrating manipulation on Xinmen (GV 22), Dazhui (GV 14) and Mingmen (GV 4). If the asthma attack is very severe, do press-kneading manipulation on Dingchuan (EX–B 1), Fengmen (BL 12), Feishu (BL 13), Jianzhongshu (SI 15) and Xuanji (RN 21), generally adding strength to soreness and swelling.

【辨证加减】

（1）风寒袭肺：① 加强擦前胸的操作，擦前胸以透热为度。配合中指按揉璇玑、中府、云门、膻中穴。② 加强擦背部的操作，重点是大椎、定喘、肩中俞、风门、肺俞穴部，以透热为度，同时可以按揉上述诸穴。③ 直擦两侧膀胱经，以透热为度，配合提拿背部大筋。④ 加强对手三阴经的擦法，注意擦手太阴肺经，以透热为度。

（2）风热犯肺：① 加强手法对前胸的操作，擦前胸以温热为度，配合中指端螺纹按揉中府、云门、璇玑、膻中穴。② 加强手法对背部的操作，擦背部以大椎、定喘、肩中俞、风门、肺俞为重点，以温热为度。③ 加强对手三阴经的擦法，配合拿血海、曲池、合谷、尺泽穴。④ 擦两侧膀胱经，以温热为度。

（3）痰浊阻肺：① 加强手法对前胸的操作，擦前胸以透热为度。② 加强手法对穴位的刺激，按揉定喘、天突、膻中；按揉璇玑、尺泽、

【Modification based on pattern identification】

(1) Wind-cold attacking lung: ① strengthen the scrubbing manipulation on the chest to the penetration of heat. Press-knead Xuanji (CV 21), Zhongfu (LU 1), Yunmen (LU 2), Danzhong (CV 17) with the middle finger. ② strengthen the scrubbing manipulation or press-kneading manipulation on the back with a focus on Dazhui (GV 14), Dingchuan (EX–B 1), Jianzhongshu (SI 15), Fengmen (BL 12) and Feishu (BL 13) to the penetration of heat. ③ scrub the bladder meridian to the penetration of heat, and lift large sinews in the back. ④ strengthen the scrubbing manipulation on the three yin meridians of the hand, and pay attention to scrub lung meridian (LU) to the penetration of heat.

(2) Wind-heat invading the lung: ① strengthen the scrubbing manipulation on the chest to the penetration of warmness. Press-knead Zhongfu (LU), Yunmen (LU 2), Xuanji (CV 21) and Danzhong (CV 17) with the middle finger. ② strengthen the scrubbing manipulation on the back with a focus on Dazhui (GV 14), Dingchuan (EX–B 1), Jianzhongshu (SI 15), Fengmen (BL 12) and Feishu (BL 13) to the penetration of warmness. ③ strengthen the scrubbing manipulation on three yin meridians of the hand combined with the grasping manipulation on Xuehai (SP

内关、足三里、丰隆等穴，均以酸胀得气为宜。

（4）肺虚：① 加强手法对胸部的操作，擦法均宜透热为度。② 加强健补脾肾的手法，治本培元，擦脾俞、肾俞，以温热为度。

（5）肾虚：① 加强背部督脉及腰部的肾俞、命门的擦法，以补肾纳气，均以温热为度。② 按揉肾俞、肺俞、膏肓、命门，手法宜轻柔，均忌刺激太重。

10), Qvchi (LI 11), Hegu (LI 4) and Chize (LU 5). ④ srub the bladder meridian to the penetration of warmness.

(3) Phlegm turbidity obstructing the lung: ① strengthen the scrubbing manipulation on the chest to the penetration of warmness. ② strengthen the stimulation on points with manipulation, knead-press Dingchuan (EX–B 1), Tiantu (CV 22), Danzhong (CV 17); knead-press Xuanji (CV 21), Chize (LU 5), Neiguan (PC 6), Zusanli (ST 36), Fenglong (ST 40) to soreness and swelling.

(4) Lung deficiency: ① strengthen the scrubbing manipulation on the chest to the penetration of heat. ② scrub Pishu (BL 20), Shenshu (BL 23) to the penetration of warmness, to fortify the spleen and kidney and strengthen and consolidate body resistance.

(5) Kidney deficiency: ① strengthen the scrubbing manipulation of the governor vessel (GV) on the back and Shenshu (BL 23) and Mingmen (GV 4) on the waist to supplement the kidney to promote qi absorption to the penetration of warmness. ② knead Shenshu (BL 23), Feishu (BL 13) and Mingmen (GV 4). The manipulation should be soft and avoid over stimulation.

【功法处方】

内功推拿对本病治疗先以常规手法操作，结合辨证加减施治，通过1～2个疗程，病情缓解后，再指导患者练习站裆势，逐渐配合上肢动作，如前推八匹马、倒拉九头牛、风摆荷叶，以后逐渐加强马裆势、弓箭裆势的锻炼，并可配合双人锻炼法，锻炼时可配合出声发力。达到强身健体、扶正祛邪的目的，坚持长期锻炼。另外，可练习腹式呼吸法或做吐纳功，增加肺活量。每天早晚各锻炼1次，每次30分钟左右，以汗出或略感疲劳为度。

【Exercise treatments】

It is advisable for the patients to accept routine treatment first. After 1 to 2 courses of routine treatments, patients can take standing stance combined with movements of upper limbs, including Qian Tui Ba Pi Ma (Pushing Eight Horses Forward), Dao La Jiu Tou Niu (Pulling Nine Oxen Backward) and Feng Bai He Ye (Wind Blowing Lotus Leaf). Then patients can gradually take horse and bow stances combined with partner exercise. They can utter loud sounds when summoning up strengthen. Long-term exercise can help to strengthen the body and consolidate the constitution. In addition, practicing abdominal breathing or doing expiration and inspiration are conducive to improving lung capacity.

Exercise once every morning and evening, about 30 minutes each time, to sweat or feel slightly tired.

【注意事项】

（1）推拿适宜治疗慢性哮喘者，能提高呼吸道通气和局部抗病能力，加强药物的作用，达到久咳即止的效果。慢性咳嗽可参照本病治疗。

（2）在治疗过程中配合锻炼少林内功以扶正祛邪。

（3）季节交替时注意冷热，平时注意进行适当的户外活动。戒烟忌酒，忌食油腻、酸辣等刺激性食物。不宜接触有刺激性的气体和灰尘。

【Attentions】

(1) Tuina therapy is suitable for patients with chronic asthma and can improve their respiratory ventilation and local resistance to diseases, strengthen the effect of drugs, and relieve cough. Chronic cough can be referred to the treatment of this disease.

(2) During the treatment, do Shaolin internal exercise to reinforce the healthy qi and eliminate the pathogenic factors.

(3) Choose proper clothes during the changing of seasons and do some outdoor activities. Quit smoking and drinking, avoid eating greasy, sour and spicy food and keep away from irritant gas and dust.

七、肺胀

Lung Distension

肺胀是因咳嗽、哮喘等证，日久不愈，肺脾肾虚损，气道滞塞不利，出现以胸中胀满，痰涎壅盛，上气咳喘，动后尤显，甚则面色晦暗，唇舌发绀，颜面、四肢浮肿，病程缠绵，经久难愈为特征的疾病。肺气肿和慢阻肺可参照治疗。推拿防治肺胀不仅可以缓解胀满、咳喘等症状，而且可以通过功法锻炼扶正补虚，控制发作。

Lung distension is caused by long-time cough and asthma, deficiency of lung, spleen and kidneys, and airway obstruction. The symptoms are distention in the chest, excessive phlegm and saliva, cough especially after exercise, even dim complexion, paly and purple mouth and tongue, puffy face and four limbs. And the disease is lingering and hard to recover. Emphysema and chronic obstruction lung can refer to this treatment. Tuina therapy can not only relieve the symptoms of distention, panting and cough, but also be combined with the Shaolin internal exercise to reinforce the healthy qi and control its occurrence.

【诊断要点】

（1）有长期慢性咳喘的病史。

（2）以肿（胀）、喘、痰、咳、

【Diagnoses】

(1) The patients have a history of prolonged chronic panting and cough.

瘀为本病的证候特征，常因明显的外感而诱发或加重。其中，肿（胀）是指胸中胀满，并见四肢、颜面浮肿；喘是动则气短不续，吸少呼多，可闻及喘鸣音；痰为喘咳之时痰涎壅盛可闻痰喘；咳为长期反复发作咳嗽；瘀为唇舌紫绀，面色晦黯。

（3）有杵状指、唇甲紫绀及肺气肿的体征。

（4）X线片，可见肺容积增大，肺透亮度增强，肋骨平行间隙增宽，横膈活动度减弱，位置低平，心影缩小，常呈垂直性。肺功能检查示残气量增多，最大通气量降低，第1秒钟间肺活量降低，气体分布不均。

(2) The disease is characterized by swelling, panting, phlegm, cough and stasis, which are induced or aggravated by external pathogenic factors. Swelling refers to swelling in the chest and puffy face and four limbs; panting refers to short and intermittent breath when moving, and exhalation is more than inhalation with wheezing; phlegm refers to excessive phlegm and saliva when cough; cough refers to chronic cough; and stasis refers to paly and purple mouth and tongue and dull complexion.

(3) The patients have the signs of clubbed finger, paly and purple mouth and nails and emphysema.

(4) On radiographs, increased lung volume, enhanced lung lucency, widened parallel gaps of ribs, attenuated diaphragmatic mobility, low level of positioning, and reduced heart shadow, often vertically, are seen. Pulmonary function tests showed increased residual volume and decreased maximal ventilation. The interlobar vital capacity was reduced in the 1st second and the gas was unevenly distributed.

【治则】

扶正固本、宽胸理气，实证以祛痰为主、虚证以扶正为主。

【Therapeutic principles】

To strengthen and consolidate body resistance and soothe the chest and regulate qi. Dispel phlegm for excess pattern and reinforce the healthy qi for deficiency pattern.

【手法】

擦法、按法、揉法、拿法、点法、按揉法。

【Manipulations】

Linear rubbing manipulation, pressing manipulation, kneading manipulation, grasping manipulation, tapping manipulation and press-kneading manipulation.

【取穴】

天突、中府、云门、璇玑、膻中、神封、神藏、中脘、风门、定喘、肺俞、脾俞、肾俞、膏肓等。

【Selection of points】

Tiantu (CV 22), Zhongfu (LU 1), Yunmen (LU 2), Xuanji (CV 21), Danzhong (CV 17), Shenfeng (KI 23), Shencang (KI 25), Zhongwan (CV 12), Fengmen (BL 12), Dingchuan (EX–B 1), Feishu (BL 13), Pishu (BL 20), Shenshu (BL 23) and Gaohuang (BL 43).

【操作】

以胸背部为主的内功推拿常规操作。

（1）施术者站在受术者右边，右手横擦胸前，上下往返移动，紧擦慢移。

（2）施术者站在受术者右边，右手擦背部，从大椎穴开始，向下移至八髎，上下往返紧擦慢移；移动至受术者左边，用左手擦背部。

（3）左手擦胸前，上下往返操作，紧擦慢移。

（4）勾揉膻中、紫宫、神藏、神封、璇玑、华盖。

（5）擦左、右肺尖，勾揉中府、云门。

（6）擦两侧胁肋部，以透热为度。

（7）按揉风门、定喘、胞肓、膏肓、肺俞、脾俞、肾俞。

【Operations】

The routine manipulation should be focused on chest and back.

(1) Physicians should stand right of the patients, strongly flat-scrub the chest with the right hand up and down slowly.

(2) Physicians should stand right of the patients, strongly scrub chest with the right hand, from Dazhui (GV 14) to Baliao (BL 31–34) slowly. Then move to the left of the patient, scrubbing back with the left hand.

(3) Strongly and slowly scrub the chest with the left hand up and down.

(4) Knead Danzhong (CV 17), Zigong (CV 19), Shencang (KI 25), Shenfeng (KI 23), Xuanji (CV 21) and Huagai (CV 20).

(5) Scrub the lung apices on both sides, knead Zhongfu (LU 1) and Yunmen (LU 2).

(6) Scrub ribs on both sides to the penetration of heat.

(7) Knead-press Fengmen (BL 12), Dingchuan (EX–B 1), Baohuang (BL 53), Gaohuang (BL 43), Feishu (BL 13), Pishu (BL 20), and Shenshu (BL 23).

【功法处方】

练功是内功推拿治疗肺胀的重要手段之一。患者须加强练习少林内功，可选择站裆势结合风摆荷叶、顶天抱地等动作锻炼，锻炼时可配合出声发力。以后逐渐加强马裆势、弓箭裆势的锻炼，也可选择大裆势并配合意念导引。每天早晚各锻炼1次，每次30分钟左右，以汗出为度。

【Exercise treatments】

Patients need to strengthen Shaolin internal exercise, as it is one of the most important methods to treat lung distension. They can take standing stance combined with Feng Bai He Ye (Wind Blowing Lotus Leaf) and Ding Tian Bao Di (Supporting the Sky and Embracing the Earth) and uttering loud sounds. Then patients can gradually take horse and bow stances and splitting stance with hands backward combined with guidance of thought. Exercise once every morning and evening, about 30 minutes each time until sweating.

【注意事项】

（1）积极防治肺部疾病。本病乃由咳喘、哮病日久发展而成，故预防和及时治疗咳、喘、哮等病证，是本病预防的关键。

（2）饮食宜清淡，平时注意预防感冒，防止诱发因素。

（3）坚持锻炼，增强体质。患者可根据体质、病情与爱好，选择少林内功、六字诀、养生功等项目进行锻炼，以改善肺脏通气功能，提高抗病能力，防患于未然。可根据体力及病情选择，运动量宜由小到大，时间由短到长，避免剧烈运动。

【Attentions】

(1) It is advisable to prevent the occurrence of lung disease. This disease is developed from cough, panting and asthma for a long time. Therefore, prevention and timely treatment of cough, panting and asthma are the key to the prevention of this disease.

(2) Eat bland food and prevent colds.

(3) Do regular exercise and strengthen your body. Based on different constitutions, conditions and hobbies, patients can choose different exercises, including Shaolin internal exercise, six heeling sounds and exercise of nourishing life. The aim is to free qi in spleen and lungs, improve body resistance to diseases and take preventative measures. Avoid strenuous exercise and progressively extend exercise time and enlarge amount of exercise.

八、感冒

感冒，轻者俗称“伤风”，主要表现为鼻部症状，如喷嚏、鼻塞、流清水样鼻涕，也可表现为咳嗽、咽干、咽痒或灼热感等。发病同时或数小时后可有喷嚏、鼻塞、流清水样鼻涕等症状。2～3天后鼻涕变稠，常伴咽痛、流泪、味觉减退、呼吸不畅、声嘶等。一般无发热及全身症状，或仅有低热、不适、轻度畏寒、头痛。普通感冒是最常见的急性呼吸道感染性疾病，多呈自限性，但发生率较高。全年皆可发病，冬春季较多。一般数天即愈。病情较重，引起广泛流行者称为时行感冒。

Common Cold

Common cold, also known as wind attack, is a viral infectious disease of the upper respiratory tract that primarily affects the nose. Symptoms include sneezing, nasal congestion, runny nose, cough, throat dryness, itchy or scorching throat. After 2 to 3 days, the nasal discharge becomes thicker, often accompanied by sore throat, lacrimation, loss of taste, breathlessness and hoarseness. Generally, there is no fever or systemic symptoms, or only low fever, malaise, mild chills and headache. The common cold is the most common acute respiratory tract infection, mostly self-limiting, but with a high incidence. It can occur throughout the year but is more frequent in winter and spring. Patients can usually heal in a few days. The seasonal colds are usually more serious and contagious.

【诊断要点】

感冒初起，多见鼻塞、流涕、喷嚏、声重，或头痛、畏寒，或发热、咳嗽、喉痒或咽痛等。甚则恶寒高热、头痛、周身酸痛、疲乏等。根据病史、流行病学、鼻咽部的症状体征，结合周围血象和阴性胸部影像学检查可做出临床诊断，一般无须病因诊断。推拿防治感冒不仅可以缓解胀满、咳喘等症状，而且可以通过功法锻炼提高体质、扶正补虚，减少发作。

【Diagnoses】

At the beginning of common cold, patients may have the symptoms of nose congestion, runny nose, sneezing, hoarse voice, or headache, aversion to cold, or fever, cough, itchy throat and sore throat. Some may have the severe symptoms of aversion to cold, high fever, headache, aching pain of the whole body and fatigue. Clinical diagnosis can be made according to medical history, epidemiology, symptoms and signs of nasopharynx, combined with peripheral hemogram and negative chest imaging examination. And it is generally not possible to identify the virus type through symptoms. Tuina therapy can not only relieve cough, distention and fullness, but also improve body constitution, reinforce the healthy qi and tonify deficiency to prevent the occurrence of common cold.

【治则】

解表散邪，以对症治疗为主，必要时结合病因治疗。

【Therapeutic principles】

To release exterior and dissipate evil and suit the remedy to the case. If necessary, treat the underlying cause.

【手法】

一指禅推法、擦法、叩击法、推法、分推法、按法、揉法、拿法、抹法、扫散法。

【Manipulations】

Yi Zhi Chan pushing, linear rubbing manipulation, tapping manipulation, pushing manipulation, pushing manipulation with two hands parting from each other, pressing manipulation, kneading manipulation, grasping manipulation, wiping manipulation and sweeping manipulation.

【取穴】

头面部六阳经及督脉穴位，肺俞、定喘、大椎、背部膀胱经穴，上肢太阴经和阳明经穴。

【Selection of points】

Six yang meridians on the head and face, governor vessel (GV), Feishu (BL 13), Dingchuan (EX–B 1), Dazhui (GV 14), bladder meridian on the back, greater yin meridian on the upper body and yang brightness meridian.

【操作】

（1）患者坐位或仰卧位。医者行一指禅“小∞字”和“大∞字”推法，反复分推3～5遍；继之指按、指揉印堂、神庭、攒竹、鱼腰、太阳、百会、四神聪等穴，每穴约1分钟；结合抹前额3～5遍；从前额发际处拿至风池穴处做五指拿法，反复3～5遍。行双手扫散法，约1分钟。拿风池、拿肩井，汗出为度。

（2）按揉双侧肺俞、定喘穴，每侧1分钟；擦大椎，擦背部膀胱经（重点擦大杼至膈俞部位），以透热为度；拳背击大椎，以耐受为度。

（3）掌擦上肢手三阳经2～3分钟，结合按揉或拿揉尺泽、曲池、合谷、外关、鱼际穴，每穴0.5～1分钟。

【Operations】

(1) Patients sit or lie on the bed. Physicians do ∞-manipulation (a tuina manipulation to exert constant force on the area to be treated with the tip or the palmar side of the thumb through active swing of the forearm) for 3 to 5 times. Then press, and knead with fingers Yintang (EX–HN 3), Shenting (GV 24), Cuanzhu (BL 2), Yuyao (EX–HN 4), temple (EX–HN 5), Baihui (GV 20) and Sishencong (EX–HN 1) for 1 minutes respectively; wipe forehead for 3 to 5 times; do grasping manipulation with five fingers from forehead's hairline to Fengchi (GB 20) for 3 to 5 times. Do sweeping manipulation with two hands for about 1 minutes. Grasp Fengchi (GB 20) and Jianjing (GB 21) to sweat.

(2) Press and knead Feishu (BL 13) and Dingchuan (EX–B 1) for 1 minute each. Rub Dazhui (DU 14) and the bladder meridian to the penetration of heat (with a focus on Dashu to Geshu) and do knocking manipulation on Dazhui (DU 14) as hardly as patients can bear.

(3) Rub three yang meridian of upper limbs with the palms for 2 to 3 minutes, and press-knead or grasp-knead Chize (LU 5), Quchi (LI 11), Hegu (LI 4), Waiguan (SJ 5) and Yuji (LU 10) for 0.5 to 1 minute each.

【功法处方】

练功是内功推拿防治感冒的重要手段之一。在患者体力允许的情况下，可练习少林内功，选择站裆势结合前推八匹马、倒拉九头牛等动作锻炼，锻炼时可配合出声发力；以后逐渐加强马裆势、大裆势的锻炼，并可选择饿虎扑食、乌龙钻洞等动作进行锻炼。每天早晚各锻炼1次，每次30分钟左右，以汗出为度。

【Exercise treatments】

Patients can take Shaolin internal exercise, as it is one of the most important methods to prevent and treat common cold. If patients' physical strength permits, they can take standing stance combined with Qian Tui Ba Pi Ma (Pushing Eight Horses Forward) and Dao La Jiu Tou Niu (Pulling Nine Oxen Backward), combined with making loud sounds. Then patients can gradually take horse and splitting stance with hands backward combined with E Hu Pu Shi (Hunger Tiger Pouncing on its Prey) and Wu Long Zuan Dong (Black Dragon Crawling into Cave). Exercise once every morning and evening, about 30 minutes each time to sweat.

【注意事项】

（1）手法和功法能迅速减轻感冒的临床症状，缩短病程。平时应积极进行功法锻炼，提高防病能力，注意着衣随气温变化，降低易感性。

（2）病情较重或年老体弱者应卧床休息，多饮水，注意营养，进食易消化食物，保持室内空气通畅。

（3）有明确指征者，配合服用抗菌或抗病毒药物，不要盲目服用抗生素。

【Attentions】

(1) Manipulation and exercise can rapidly alleviate the clinical symptoms of common cold and reduce its duration. Patients should strengthen Shaolin Internal Exercise which can improve body resistance to disease and choose proper clothes according to the changing of temperature.

(2) Patients with severe condition and elderly patients should rest in bed, drink more water, get balanced nutrition, eat digestible food and keep air clean in the room.

(3) For patients with clear indicators, they should have antibacterial medicines or antiviral medicines and avoid abusing of antibiotics.

九、胃脘痛

胃脘痛又称胃痛，是指以上腹部经常发生疼痛为主症的一种消化道病症。历代文献中所称的“心痛”“心下痛”，多指胃痛。胃痛是临床上症状，多见于急慢性胃炎，胃、十二指肠溃疡病，胃神经症。

Abdominal Pain

Abdominal pain, also known as stomach pain, is an alimentary canal disease which usually happens in the epigastric region of the human body. The so-called “heart pain” and “pain under the heart” in ancient literatures are actually the abdominal pain. Abdominal pain is a common clinical symptom, mostly seen in acute and chronic gastritis, gastric and duodenal ulcer diseases, and gastric neurosis.

【诊断要点】

（1）寒邪停胃：胃凉暴痛，遇冷痛重，喜热饮食，口淡乏味。舌淡苔白，脉弦紧。

（2）饮食伤胃：暴饮暴食，胃饱胀痛，厌食拒按，嗳腐酸臭。舌苔厚腻，脉弦滑。

（3）肝气犯胃：胃脘胀痛，痛

【Diagnoses】

(1) Cold evil settling in the stomach: It is characterized by fulminant pain in the stomach due to cold, exacerbated by exposure to cold, desire for hot drinks and food, bland taste in the mouth, pale tongue and white tongue coating, wiry and tight pulse.

(2) Eating attacking the stomach: It is characterized by binge-eating, stomach distension, aversion to food,

窜胁背，嗳气痛轻，怒气痛重。舌边红、苔白，脉沉弦。

（4）脾胃虚寒：胃凉隐痛，喜热喜按，饮冷痛重，食少。舌淡齿痕苔薄白，脉沉细迟。

abdominal pain refusing to pressure, putrid belching and soar smelling, thick and slimy tongue fur and wiry and slippery pulse.

(3) Liver qi invading the stomach: It is characterized by distending pain in the stomach, pain in the hypochondrium and back, little pain with belching, and severe pain with angry mood. The margins of the tongue are red, white tongue coating, sunken and string-like pulse.

(4) Cold and deficiency of the spleen and stomach: It is characterized by little pain in the stomach due to cold, desire for warm and pressing, severe pain after having cold drinks, poor appetite, pale tongue with teeth marks, thin and white tongue coating, with deep, thready and slow pulse.

【治则】

散寒温中，消食导滞，疏肝理气，健脾止痛。

【Therapeutic principles】

To dissipate cold and warm the middle, promote digestion and remove food stagnation, soothe the liver and regulate qi, and fortify the spleen to relieve pain.

【手法】

擦法、按法、揉法、按揉法、点法、拿法、摩法、捏脊。

【Manipulations】

Linear rubbing manipulation, pressing manipulation, kneading manipulation, press-kneading manipulation, point-pressing manipulation, grasping manipulation, circular rubbing manipulation and pinch manipulation.

【取穴】

中脘、脾俞、胃俞、大椎、天枢、大肠俞、八髎、足三里、膻中、肝俞、胆俞、膈俞。

【Selection of points】

Zhongwan (CV 12), Pishu (BL 20), Weishu (BL 21), Dazhui (GV 14), Tianshu (ST 25), Dachangshu (BL 25), Baliao (BL 31–34), Zusanli (ST 36), Danzhong (CV 17), Ganshu (BL 18), Danshu (BL 19), Geshu (BL 17).

【操作】

疼痛剧烈者，先在背部脾俞、胃俞及附近的压痛点用轻重相继的按法或点法，待疼痛缓解后，再辨

【Operations】

For patients with severe pain, do pressing or point manipulation on Pishu (BL 20), Weishu (BL 21) and tender points softly and forcefully. After relieving pain, treatment

其证而治之。以胸腹部、背腰部及四肢部常规手法操作为主。

（1）医者于患者右侧，先用轻快的掌揉法胃脘部治疗；然后用四指摩法在中脘、气海、天枢等穴操作。

（2）医者于患者左侧，用按揉法，沿背部膀胱经自膈俞至三焦俞，往返操作5～10遍；然后用较重的按揉法于膈俞、肝俞、脾俞、胃俞、三焦俞穴操作，时间约5分钟。沿膀胱经循行部位施以擦法，透热为度。

（3）患者取坐势，按揉法结合提拿法在肩井、手三里、内关、合谷等穴做较强刺激地操作；然后搓肩臂和两胁，往返10～20遍；最后按揉足三里穴。

according to pattern identification. The manipulation should be mainly on the chest, abdomen, back, waist and four limbs.

(1) Physicians stand right of the patient, first softly press the stomach with palms and then do rubbing manipulation with four fingers on Zhongwan (CV 12), Qihai (CV 6) and Tianshu (ST 25).

(2) Physicians stand left of the patient, do press-kneading manipulation from the Geshu (BL 17) to Sanjiaoshu (BL 22) on the bladder meridian for 5 to 10 times, and then forcefully press and knead Geshu (BL 17), Ganshu (BL 18), Pishu (BL 20), Weishu (BL 21) and Sanjioashu (BL 22) for about 5 minutes. Do linear rubbing manipulation along the bladder meridian to the penetration of heat.

(3) With patients in the sitting stance, physicians do press-kneading manipulation and grasping manipulation on Jianjing (GB 21), Shousanli (LI 10), Neiguan (PC 6) and Hegu (LI 4). Then twist shoulders, back and both hypochondrium back and forth for 10 to 20 times. Finally, press and knead Zusanli (ST 36).

【辨证加减】

（1）寒邪停胃：宜散寒止痛。在常规手法的基础上，加强腹及两胁擦法；按揉中脘、脾俞、胃俞；以小鱼际横向擦大椎，直向擦两侧膀胱经，以透热为度。

（2）饮食伤胃：宜消食导滞。在常规手法操作时加强上腹及少腹擦法，按揉中脘、天枢，提拿天枢，摩腹。背部按揉脾俞、胃俞、大肠俞、八髎，下肢按足三里。

（3）肝气犯胃：宜疏肝理气。在常规手法操作时加强两胁及肝区的擦法，配按揉章门、期门；擦胸

【Treatment based on pattern identification】

(1) Cold evil settling in the stomach: It is advisable to dissipate cold to relieve pain. On the basis of routine treatment, strengthen the rubbing manipulation on abdomen and ribs. Press-knead Zhongwan (CV 12), Pishu (BL 20) and Weishu (BL 21), transversely rub Dazhui (DU 14) with hypothenar, vertically rub bladder meridian to the penetration of heat.

(2) Eating attacking the stomach: It is advisable to promote digestion and remove food stagnation. On the basis of routine treatment, strengthen the rubbing manipulation on the upper abdomen and lower abdomen. Press-knead Zhongwan (CV 12) and Tianshu (ST 25), lift Tianshu (ST 25) and rub the abdomen. For the back, press-

腹配合按揉中脘、膻中；在背部重点擦肝俞、胆俞、膈俞穴部。

（4）脾胃虚寒：宜温中散寒。在常规手法操作时，加强手法在上腹部及少腹部擦法，并配合中指按揉中脘、气海、关元。可以配合掌根揉中脘，手法徐徐下按，随后突然放松所按之掌，使患部感到局部温热。在背部捏脊可结合用小鱼际直擦两侧膀胱经及督脉经，以透热为度。在下肢可配合按揉足三里，以酸胀为度。

knead Pishu (BL 20), Weishu (BL 21), Dachangshu (BL 25), Baliao (BL 31–34) and press Zusanli (ST 36) on the lower limbs.

(3) Liver qi invading the stomach: It is advisable to soothe the liver and regulate qi. On the basis of routine treatment, strengthen the rubbing manipulation on ribs and liver areas. Press-knead Zhangmen (LR 13) and Qimen (LR 14) ; do the rubbing manipulation on the chest and abdomen combine with press-kneading Zhongwan (CV 12) and Danzhong (CV 17) ; rub the back with a focus on the Ganshu (BL 18), Danshu (BL 19) and Geshu (BL 17).

(4) Cold and deficiency of the spleen and stomach: It is advisable to dissipate cold and warm the middle. On the basis of routine treatment, strengthen the linear rubbing manipulation on the upper abdomen and lower abdomen and press-knead Zhongwan (CV 12), Qihai (CV 6) and Guanyuan (CV 4) with the middle finger. Knead Zhongwan (CV 12) with the heel of the hand, moving the hand downward slowly, then relax the hand and make patients feel warm. Pinch spine on the back and vertically rub the bladder meridian and the Du meridian with hypothenar to the penetration of heat. Press-knead Zusanli (ST 36) in the lower limbs to soreness and swelling.

【功法处方】

患者胃痛发作时可练习六字诀之“嘻”字诀，先大嘻三十遍，后细嘻十遍，中病即止，不可过量。胃痛缓解时可练习少林内功，选择站裆势结合摩腹或延年九转法锻炼，以后逐渐加强低裆势、悬裆势的锻炼，并可选择三起三落或海底捞月等动作进行锻炼，以耐受为度。胃脘痛表现虚实错杂，练功需要动静结合、消补并举。每天早晚各锻炼1

【Exercise treatments】

When the patient has an attack of stomach pain, he can first speak “Xi” loudly for 30 times, then speak softly for 10 times, until recover. Do not overdo it. When the stomach pain is relieved, do Shaolin internal exercise. Patients can choose standing stance combined with the circular rubbing manipulation on the abdomen or the exercise of nourishing life. Then gradually strengthen the lower stance and squatting-splitting stance with hands on the waist combined with the exercise of San Qi San Luo (Three Ups and Three Downs) or Hai Di Lao Yue

次，每次30分钟左右，以患者舒适为度。

(Scooping the Moon from Sea Bottom). Abdominal pain manifests a mixture of excess and deficiency, so the exercise requires both movement and stiffness, elimination and supplement. Exercise once in the morning and once in the evening, for about 30 minutes each time, to the extent that the patient is comfortable.

【注意事项】

（1）按时进餐，多食清淡，少食肥甘及各种生冷辛热及刺激性食物。戒烟忌酒。

（2）饮食定时定量，长期胃痛的患者每日三餐或加餐均应定时，间隔时间要合理。

（3）坚持锻炼，增强体质。可选择少林内功、延年九转法、养生功等进行锻炼，以改善胃肠功能，循序渐进，避免过于剧烈的运动。

【Attentions】

(1) Eat meals on time. Have a light diet and avoid eating greasy, sweet, cold, spicy and stimulating food. Quit smoking and avoid alcohol.

(2) Patients with chronic stomach pain should have three regular meals or extra meals daily with reasonable intervals.

(3) Adhere to exercise to enhance the body constitution. Patients can choose Shaolin internal exercise, the exercise of nourishing life and the exercise for life cultivation to improve gastrointestinal function. And patients should avoid overly strenuous exercise.

十、腹泻

腹泻又称泄泻，是指排便次数增多，粪便稀薄，甚至泻出如水样而言。本病一年四季均可发生，但以夏秋两季为多见。本证在《黄帝内经》称为泄，有“濡泻”“洞泄”“飧泄”“注泄”等名称。汉唐时代称为“下利”，宋代以后统称“泄泻”。亦有根据病因或病机而称为“署泄”“大肠泄”者，名称虽多，但都不离“泄泻”两字。按照发病缓急可分为急性泄泻和慢性泄泻。

Diarrhea

Diarrhea is characterized by increased frequency of bowel movements, loose stools, and watery stools. The disease can occur throughout the year but is more common in the summer and fall. The pattern is called diarrhea in *Yellow Emperor's Canon of Medicine*, and it has the name of Ruxie (watery diarrhea), Dongxie (torrential diarrhea), Sunxie (diarrhea with undigested food), and Zhuxie (outpoured diarrhea). In the Han and Tang Dynasties, it was called Xiali, and after the Song Dynasty, it was called diarrhea. And according to etiological factors and pathogenesis, it is called Shuxie (diarrhea caused by summer heat) and diarrhea. According to the urgency of onset, it can be divided into acute diarrhea and chronic diarrhea.

【诊断要点】

（1）湿邪侵袭：症见发病急骤，大便稀薄或夹黏液，每日数次或10余次，腹痛肠鸣，泻后痛止，肢体酸痛。苔黄腻或白腻，脉濡或滑数。

（2）伤食泄泻：发病突然，脘腹胀痛，泻下粪便臭如败卵，泻后则痛减，嗳腐吞酸。舌苔垢腻，脉滑数。

（3）肝气郁结：泄泻每因情绪波动时发作，平时感觉胸胁胀满，肠鸣腹痛，心烦不寐，嗳气纳少。舌苔淡红尖绛，脉弦。

（4）脾胃虚弱：大便时溏时泄，完谷不化，反复发作，稍食油腻后大便次数增多，甚则食入即泻，食欲不振，面色晄白。舌质淡苔薄，脉沉细或缓弱。

（5）肾虚泄泻：黎明前脐周腹痛，肠鸣辘辘有声，痛发即泻，泻后痛减，口渴，形寒肢冷，腰膝酸软。舌苔薄白，脉沉细。

【Diagnoses】

(1) Dampness attacking: The symptoms include rapid onset, thin stools or mucus, several times a day or more than 10 times a day, abdominal pain and bowel sounds, the pain stopping after diarrhea, and sore and painful limbs, yellow and greasy or white and greasy tongue fur, soft or slippery and rapid pulse.

(2) Food damage diarrhea: The symptoms include sudden onset, distended and painful abdomen, stink stools smelling like septic eggs, the pain which decreases after diarrhea, and belching and acid regurgitation, greasy and thick tongue coating, slippery and rapid pulse.

(3) Stagnation of liver qi: The diarrhea is caused by fluctuating emotions. The symptoms include swelling in the chest, bowel sounds, abdominal pain, vexation insomnia, burping, poor appetite, reddish tongue coating and wiry pulse.

(4) Spleen-stomach weakness: The symptoms include watery and loose stools, stools containing undigested food, increased stools after eating greasy food or immediate stools after eating, poor appetite, pale face, pale tongue, thin tongue fur, deep and thready pulse or slowdown and weak pulse.

(5) Diarrhea due to kidney deficiency: The symptoms include abdominal pain around the umbilicus before dawn, bowel sounds, diarrhea immediately after the onset of pain, pain decreasing after diarrhea, thirst, cold body and four limbs, and soreness and weakness of the waist and knees, thin and white tongue fur and deep and thready pulse.

【治则】

泄泻以祛湿健脾为总则，急性泄泻以祛湿止泻为主，慢性泄泻以健脾扶正为主。

【Therapeutic principles】

Dispelling dampness to fortify the spleen. Dispel dampness to stop diarrhea for acute diarrhea and reinforce the healthy qi to fortify the spleen for chronic diarrhea.

【手法】

按法、揉法、摩法、搓法、拿法、擦法。

【Manipulations】

Pressing manipulation, kneading manipulation, circular rubbing manipulation, twisting manipulation, grasping manipulation and linear rubbing manipulation.

【取穴】

气海、关元、中脘、天枢、脾俞、胃俞、肾俞、大肠俞、肩井、曲池、合谷、足三里等。

【Selection of points】

Qihai (CV 6), Guanyuan (CV 4), Zhongwan (CV 12), Tianshu (ST 25), Pishu (BL 20), Weishu (BL 21), Shenshu (BL 23), Dachangshu (BL 25), Jianjing (GB 21), Quchi (LI 11), Hegu (LI 4), Zusanli (ST 36).

【操作】

按照腹部、腰背部、四肢部的顺序实施内功推拿常规手法操作。

（1）患者取仰卧位，医者居于右侧，用沉着缓慢的一指禅推法、摩法，由中脘慢慢向下移动至气海、关元穴，往复数次；再指按揉中脘、天枢、气海。

（2）按揉脾俞、胃俞、大肠俞、上次髎穴约5分钟，以酸胀为度；擦大肠俞及八髎部，透热为度。

（3）患者取坐位，拿肩井、曲池、合谷，按揉足三里、三阴交等穴。

【Operations】

The manipulation should be focused on the abdomen, waist, back and four limbs.

(1) With the patient in supine position, physicians stand right side of the patient, do Yi Zhi Chan pushing and circular rubbing manipulation from Zhongwan (CV 12) to Qihai (RN 6) and Guanyuan (RN 4) back and forth for several times. Then press and knead Zhongwan (CV 12), Tianshu (ST 25) and Qihai (RN 6) with fingers.

(2) Press and knead Pishu (BL 20), Weishu (BL 21), Dachangshu (BL 25), for 5 minutes to soreness and swelling. Rub Dachangshu (BL 25) and Baliao (BL 31–34) to the penetration of heat.

(3) With the patient in sitting position, grasp Jianjing (GB 21), Quchi (LI 11), Hegu (LI 4), press and knead Zusanli (ST 36) and Sanyinjiao (SP 6).

【辨证加减】

（1）湿邪侵袭：加揉摩天枢、气海、关元，重按内关、足三里穴，加强擦八髎部。

（2）伤食泄泻：加摩脘腹部，顺时针方向进行15～20分钟，重按足三里，直擦大肠俞、八髎部。

【Modification based on pattern identification】

(1) Dampness attacking the body: Strengthen the kneading and rubbing manipulation on Tianshu (ST 25), Qihai (RN 6) and Guanyuan (RN 4), the pressing manipulation on Neiguan (PC 6) and Zusanli (ST 36), and the vertical scrubbing manipulation on Baliao (BL 31–34).

（3）肝气郁结：加推摩膻中、章门、期门，按揉肝胆俞、膈俞、行间、内关穴以酸胀为度，并擦两胁部以热为度。

（4）脾胃虚弱：用一指禅推法或摩法于中脘、天枢、气海、关元穴8分钟，接着再摩胃脘及下腹部各5分钟；坐位擦脾胃俞、肾俞、大肠俞，以透热为度。

（5）肾虚泄泻：加擦气海、关元穴部，直擦督脉，横擦肾俞、命门穴部，并逐渐下降到大肠俞、八髎穴部，以透热为度；按揉涌泉后再擦涌泉穴。若患者久病正气亏虚，加强擦背部膀胱经与督脉，按揉足三里，内关穴各半分钟，再配合捏脊8～10遍。

(2) Food damage diarrhea: Strengthen the rubbing manipulation on abdomen clockwise for 15 to 20 minutes, forcefully press Zusanli (ST 36), and vertically scrubbing Dachangshu (BL 25) and Baliao (BL 31–34).

(3) Stagnation of liver qi: Strengthen the pushing manipulation on Danzhong (CV 17), Zhangmen (LR 13) and Qimen (LR 14), press and knead Ganshu (BL 18), Danshu (BL 19), Geshu (BL 17), Xingjian (LR 2), Neiguan (PC 6) to soreness and swelling, and scrub both hypochondrium to heat.

(4) Spleen-stomach weakness: Do Yi Zhi Chan pushing or circular rubbing manipulation on Zhongwan (CV 12), Tianshu (ST 25), Qihai (RN 6) and Guanyuan (RN 4) for 8 minutes, the circular rubbing manipulation on the stomach and lower abdomen for 5 minutes each, and patients should sit when receiving the linear rubbing manipulation on Pishu (BL 20), Weishu (BL 21) and Dachangshu (BL 25) to the penetration of heat.

(5) Diarrhea due to kidney deficiency: Strengthen the linear rubbing manipulation on Qihai (RN 6) and Guanyuan (RN 4), and vertically rub the Du meridian, transversely rub Shenshu (BL 23), Mingmen (DU 4), Dachangshu (BL 25) and Baliao (BL 31–34) to the penetration of heat. Press and knead Yongquan (KI 1), and then rub it. For patients suffering the disease for a long time resulting inthe deficiency of healthy qi, strengthen the linear rubbing manipulation on the bladder meridian and the Du meridian on the back, press and knead Zusanli (ST 36) and Neiguan (PC 6) for half a minute each and then pinch the spine for 8 to 10 times.

【功法处方】

慢性腹泻可练习少林内功，选择站裆势结合摩腹或延年九转法锻炼，以后逐渐加强低裆势、马裆势的锻炼，并可选择三起三落或海底

【Exercise treatments】

Patients with chronic diarrhea can choose standing stance combined with circular rubbing manipulation on the abdomen or the exercise of nourishing life. And then strengthen the exercise of lower stance and horse stance

捞月等动作进行锻炼，以耐受为度。每天早晚各锻炼1次，每次30分钟左右，以患者舒适为度。

and and choose the exercise of San Qi San Luo (Three Ups and Three Downs) or Hai Di Lao Yue (Scooping the Moon from Sea Bottom). Exercise once in the morning and evening, 30 minutes each.

【注意事项】

（1）注意饮食、饮水卫生。

（2）急性腹泻患者随时注意病情变化，必要时应中西医结合治疗，慢性腹泻者注意腹部保暖，避免零食冷饮及油腻食物。

（3）出现高热及明显脱水、酸中毒患者，应在高热减退、水电介质平衡后再采用推拿治疗。

【Attentions】

(1) Pay attention to keep the diet and drinking water clean.

(2) Patients with acute diarrhea should be alert to the changes of their own condition, and if necessary, accept both TCM and western treatment. Patients with chronic diarrhea should keep their abdomen warm and avoid eating snacks, cold drinks and greasy food.

(3) Patients with hyperthermia, dehydration and acidosis should be treated with tuina therapy after the hyperthermia has subsided and the hydropower mediators have been balanced.

十一、便秘

Constipation

便秘是指大便秘结不通，排便时间延长，或欲大便而艰涩不畅的一种病证。便秘的一般症状是排便困难，经常三五日或六七日才能大便一次。有部分患者大便次数正常，但粪质干燥，坚硬难排；或少数患者时有便意，大便并不干燥，但排出艰难。而另一部分患者由于便秘导致腑气不通，浊气不降，往往有头痛头晕，腹中胀满，甚则出现疼痛，可伴有脘闷嗳气、食欲减退、睡眠不安、心烦易怒等症。长期便秘，会引起痔疮、肛裂。本证多见于各种急慢性疾病中。本节所论便秘，是以排便异常为主要症状者。

Constipation is a condition in which the bowels are constipated with prolonged defecation time or difficulty to pass stool. The general symptom of constipation is difficulty in passing stool, often only once every three to five days or six to seven days. Some patients have a normal frequency of stools, but the stool is dry and hard to pass; or a few patients have the intention to pass stool, and the stool is not dry, but it is difficult to pass. And some patients have headache and dizziness, fullness in the abdomen, and even pain due to constipation, which can be accompanied by distention in the abdomen and stuffy belching, loss of appetite, sleep disturbance, irritability and other symptoms. Long-term constipation can cause hemorrhoids and anal fissures. Constipation is mostly seen in various acute and chronic diseases. The constipation discussed in this section

由于其他疾病而兼见大便秘结者，不在论述范围。

is mainly focused on the constipation as the main symptom in patients.

【诊断要点】

（1）热秘：大便干结，小便短赤，面红身热，或兼有腹胀腹痛，口干口臭。舌红苔黄或黄燥，脉滑数。

（2）气秘：大便秘结，欲便不得，嗳气频作，胸胁痞满，甚则腹中胀痛，纳食减少。舌苔薄腻，脉弦。

（3）虚秘：① 气虚便秘：虽有便意，临厕努挣乏力，挣则汗出短气，便后疲乏，大便并不干硬，面色晄白。舌淡苔薄，脉虚。② 血虚便秘：大便秘结，面色少华，头晕目眩，心悸，唇色淡。舌淡，脉细涩。

（4）冷秘：大便艰涩，排出困难，小便清长，面色㿠白，四肢不温，喜热恶冷，腹中冷痛，或腰脊酸冷。舌淡苔白，脉沉迟。

【Diagnoses】

(1) Heat constipation: It is characterized by dry defecation, short and red urine, red face and feverish body, abdominal distention and pain, dry mouth and bad breath, red tongue and yellow or yellow and dry tongue fur and slippery and rapid pulse.

(2) Qi constipation: It is characterized by constipation, inability to pass stool, frequent belching, fullness in the chest, or even distension and pain in the abdomen, and reduced appetite, thin and greasy tongue coating and wiry pulse.

(3) Deficiency constipation: ① Qi deficiency and constipation is manifested as inability to pass stool, fatigue after passing stool, pale face, light tongue and thin tongue fur and weak pulse. ②Blood deficiency and constipation is manifested as constipation, less florid face, dizziness, palpitations, pale lips, light tongue, thin and hesitant pulse.

(4) Cold constipation: It is characterized by difficulty to pass stool, clear and long urine, pale complexion, cold extremities, desire to heat and aversion to cold, coldness and pain in the abdomen, or soreness and coldness of the lumbar spine, light tongue, white tongue coating and deep and slow pulse.

【治则】

推拿对便秘的治疗原则是和肠通便，但是还需进一步审证求因，辨证论治。

【Therapeutic principles】

Therapeutic principles are to harmonize the stomach and unblock defecation. However, it is necessary to further examine the cause and identify the evidence for treatment based on syndrome differentiation.

【手法】

按法、揉法、摩法、擦法、分推法、一指禅推法、搓法、提拿法。

【Manipulations】

Pressing manipulation, kneading manipulation, circular rubbing manipulation, rubbing manipulation, pushing manipulation with two hands parting from each other, Yi Zhi Chan pushing, palm-twisting manipulation and lifting manipulation.

【取穴】

中脘、关元、天枢、大横、脾俞、胃俞、肝俞、肾俞、大肠俞、八髎、长强、足三里、支沟等。

【Selection of points】

Zhongwan (CV 12), Guanyuan (CV 4), Tianshu (ST 25), Daheng (SP 15), Pishu (BL 20), Weishu (BL 21), Ganshu (BL 18), Shenshu (BL 23), Dachangshu (BL 25), Baliao (BL 31–34), Changqiang (DU 1), Zusanli (ST 36) and Zhigou (SJ 6)

【操作】

按照腹部、腰背部、四肢部的顺序实施内功推拿常规手法操作，然后再随证施治，进行针对性治疗。

（1）患者取仰卧位，医者居于患者右侧，摩脘腹部，顺时针方向进行15～20分钟摩法，使热量深透至腹部，增强肠胃的蠕动；在中脘、天枢、关元、大横穴用轻快的一指禅推法，然后搓揉腹部，分推腹部。

（2）再取俯卧位，按揉患者背部脾俞、胃俞、肝俞、大肠俞等穴；直擦大肠俞、八髎穴部；用指按法按肾俞、长强，然后自上而下掌推督脉。

（3）患者取坐位，拇指按揉支沟、足三里等穴。

【Operations】

According to the order of the abdomen, waist and back, the limbs of the internal tuina routine operation, and then apply targeted treatment according to the symptom.

(1) With the patient in a supine position, the physician stands on the patient's right side. Circularly rub the abdomen for 15 to 20 minutes in a clockwise direction to make the abdomen warm, with the purpose of enhancing bowel movement. Do the Yi Zhi Chan pushing on Zhongwan (CV 12), Tianshu (ST 25), Guanyuan (CV 4) and Daheng (SP 15). Then press and knead the abdomen and do parting-pushing manipulation on the abdomen.

(2) With the patient in a prone position, the physician presses and kneads Pishu (BL 20), Weishu (BL 21), Ganshu (BL 18) and Dachangshu (BL 25) ; rubs Dachangshu (BL 25) and Baliao (BL 31–34) directly. Press Shenshu (BL 23) and Changqiang (DU 1) and push Du meridian with the palm from the top down.

(3) With the patient in a sitting position, the physician presses and kneads Zhigou (SJ 6) and Zusanli (ST 36) with thumbs.

【辨证加减】

（1）热秘：重用直擦八髎穴部，以透热为度；按揉足三里、大肠俞，

【Modification based on pattern identification】

(1) Heat constipation: Vertically rub Baliao (BL 31–34) to the penetration of heat. Press and knead Zusanli

以酸胀为度。

（2）气秘：加摩膻中、章门、期门穴，按揉膈俞、肝俞，均以酸胀为度；擦两肋及腹部气海、关元、大横；重用直擦腰骶八髎穴部。

（3）虚秘：横擦胸上部、背部及腰骶部，均以透热为度；重用按揉足三里、支沟穴，以酸胀为度。

（4）寒秘：横擦脘腹部和腰骶部，以透热为度；直擦背部督脉，以透热为度。

(ST 36) and Dachangshu (BL 25) to soreness and swelling.

(2) Qi constipation: Circularly rub Danzhong (RN 17), Zhangmen (LR 13) and Qimen (LR 14), press and knead Geshu (BL 17) and Ganshu (BL 18) to soreness and swelling; linearly rub two ribs and Qihai (RN 6), Guanyuan (RN 4) and Daheng (SP 15) ; directly rub Baliao (BL 31–34) with strong force.

(3) Deficiency constipation: Linearly rub upper thorax, back and lumbosacral regions to the penetration of heat; heavily press and knead Zusanli (ST 36) and Zhigou (SJ 6) to soreness and swelling.

(4) Cold constipation: Linearly rub the abdomen and lumbosacral regions to the penetration of heat; vertically rub Du meridian on the back to the penetration of heat.

【功法处方】

练功是内功推拿治疗便秘的重要手段之一。患者须加强练习少林内功，可选择站裆势结合顺水推舟、海底捞月等动作锻炼，也可选择低裆势或坐裆势配合意念导引法。每天早晚各锻炼1次，每次30分钟左右，以患者舒适为度。

【Exercise treatments】

Shaolin internal exercise is one of the important effective methods to treat constipation. Patients can take the standing stance with Shun Shui Tui Zhou (Pushing Boat along Water-Flowing) and Hai Di Lao Yue (Scooping the Moon from Sea Bottom). Or they can choose lower stance or sitting stance with the guidance of thought. Exercise once in the morning and once in the evening, 30 minutes each.

【注意事项】

（1）养成每天按时排便的习惯。

（2）避免食物过于精细，适当进食富含植物性纤维的食物，如蔬菜、水果。

（3）可每天自行按摩腹部，刺激肠蠕动，或练习腹式呼吸，提高肠蠕动力量。

【Attentions】

(1) Develop a good habit of having a bowel movement on a daily basis.

(2) Avoid too fine food and eat food rich in plant fiber, such as vegetables and fruits.

(3) Massage your abdomen daily to stimulate bowel movement or practice abdominal breathing to improve bowel movement strength.

十二、消渴

消渴泛指以多饮、多食、多尿、形体消瘦，或尿有甜味为特征的疾病。本病在《黄帝内经》中称为“消瘅”。口渴引饮为上消；善食易饥为中消；饮一溲一为下消，统称消渴。与现代医学中糖尿病的临床表现相似。空腹血糖≥7.0 mmol/L，和（或）餐后2小时血糖≥11.1 mmol/L即可确诊。推拿干预消渴以对症处理为主，对糖尿病并发症的预防有积极作用。

Wasting and Thirst

Wasting and thirst refers to a group of disorders characterized by polydipsia, polyphagia and polyuria, emaciation and sweet urination. In *Yellow Emperor's Canon of Medicine,* it is called “Xiaodan”. Wasting of the upper jiao (Diaphragm wasting) is characterized by excessive thirst and excessive drinking. Wasting of the middle jiao (spleen/stomach wasting) is characterized by increased appetite but rapid hunger after eating food. Wasting of the lower jiao (kidney wasting) is characterized by excessive drinking and profuse urination. It is similar to the clinical presentation of diabetes in modern medicine. Fasting blood glucose ≥ 7.0 mmol/L, and/or 2 hours postprandial blood glucose ≥ 11.1 mmol/L can confirm the diagnosis. Tuina treatment for wasting and thirst are based on different symptoms, and it has a positive effect on the prevention of diabetic complications.

【诊断要点】

（1）燥热伤肺：烦渴多饮，口干咽燥，多食易饥，小便量多，大便干结。舌质红，苔薄黄，脉数。

（2）胃燥津伤：消谷善饥，大便秘结，口干欲饮，形体消瘦。舌红苔黄，脉滑有力。

（3）肝肾阴虚：尿频量多，浑如脂膏，头晕目眩，耳鸣，视物模糊，口干唇燥，失眠心烦。舌红无苔，脉细、弦数。

（4）阴阳两虚：尿频，饮一溲一，色混如膏。面色黧黑，耳轮枯焦，腰膝酸软，消瘦显著，阳痿或月经不调，畏寒面浮。舌淡苔白，脉沉细、无力。

【Diagnoses】

(1) Dryness and heat damage the lung: It is characterized by thirst and excessive drinking, dry mouth and throat, excessive eating and easy to feel hungry, excessive urination and dry stools, red tongue, thin and yellow tongue coating and rapid pulse.

(2) Stomach dryness due to loss of fluids: It is characterized by fast digestion with rapid hunger, constipation, dry mouth and desire to drink, emaciation, red tongue, yellow tongue and slippery and strong pulse.

(3) Yin deficiency of the liver and the kidney: It is characterized by frequent and excessive urination like mixed grease, dizziness, tinnitus, blurred vision, dry mouth and lips, insomnia and distress, red tongue without coating and thready, wiry and rapid pulse.

(4) Dual deficiency of yin and yang: It is characterized

by frequent urination, like mixed grease, sallow face, withered and scorched ears, soreness and weakness of the waist and knees, emaciation, impotence or irregular menstruation, fear of cold and floating face, light tongue, white tongue coating, deep, thready and weak pulse.

【治则】

清热育阳，生津止渴。

【Therapeutic principles】

Clear heat and nourish yang, generate fluids and relieve thirst.

【手法】

一指禅推法、擦法、拿法、按法、揉法、点按法、拍法、搓法、抖法等。

【Manipulations】

Yi Zhi Chan pushing, linear rubbing manipulation, grasping manipulation, pressing manipulation, kneading manipulation, point-pressing manipulation, patting manipulation, palm-twisting manipulation and shaking manipulation.

【取穴】

以手太阴、手阳明、足阳明、足少阴经腧穴为主。取肺俞、肝俞、胆俞、脾俞、胃俞、肾俞、期门、章门、中脘、神阙、三阴交、足三里、血海等穴。

【Selection of points】

Feishu (BL 13), Ganshu (BL 18), Danshu (BL 19), Pishu (BL 20), Weishu (BL 21), Shenshu (BL 23), Qimen (LR 14), Zhangmen (LR 13), Zhongwan (CV 12), Shenque (RN 8), Sanyinjiao (SP 6), Zusanli (ST 36) and Xuehai (SP 10) and other points on the lung meridian, the large intestine meridian, the stomach meridian and the kidney meridian.

【操作】

俯卧位：先用一指禅推法于背脊部，自大椎穴开始，沿两侧足太阳膀胱经循行路线，由上而下推至腰骶部，上下往返操作治疗3～5遍；继之用掌揉法沿膀胱经走行，后按揉肺俞、肝俞、胆俞、脾俞、胃俞、肾俞诸穴反复操作按揉3～5分钟；再用掌擦法于督脉和膀胱经，以脾俞为主，斜擦两侧肾俞，均以

【Operations】

Prone position: First, use the Yi Zhi Chan pushing on the dorsal spine, starting from Dazhui (DU 14) following the route of the bladder meridian on both sides to the lumbosacral region and repeat it for 3 to 5 times. Then, do kneading manipulation with the palm along the bladder meridian and press and knead Feishu (BL 13), Ganshu (BL 18), Danshu (BL 19), Pishu (BL 20), Weishu (BL 21) and Shenshu (BL 23) for 3 to 5 minutes. Do kneading manipulation with the palm on the Du meridian and

热透入里为佳；在背脊部运用掌拍法，自大椎穴开始逐次拍打至腰骶部，上下往返操作3～5遍；再拿揉肩井穴5～7次。

bladder meridian, with the focus on Pishu (BL 20) and rub Shenshu (BL 23) on the two sides to the penetration of heat. Then pat the back with the palm from Dazhui (DU 14) to lumbosacral region and repeat it for 3 to 5 times; and then grasp and knead Jianjing (GB 21) for 5 to 7 times.

十三、中风后遗症

Sequelae of Wind Stroke

中风后遗症是指患者出现一侧肢体瘫痪、口眼歪斜、舌强语涩等症状，大多为中风（脑血管意外）引起的后遗症。本书介绍的是中风引起的以半身不遂为主的后遗症。半身不遂患者大部分有高血压病史，发病以老年人为多见。由于肢体功能的丧失，患者健康受到严重威胁。推拿治疗对促进肢体功能的康复，具有一定的临床效果，且以早期治疗为宜。

Sequelae of wind stroke are sequelae mostly caused by stroke (cerebrovascular accident), which has symptoms as paralysis of one side of the limb, distorted mouth and eyes, stiff tongue with difficulty in speaking. This book describes the sequelae of hemiplegia caused by stroke. Most patients with hemiplegia have a history of hypertension, and the onset is more common in the elderly. Due to the loss of limb function, the patient's health is at serious risk. Tuina treatment is clinically effective in promoting the rehabilitation of limb functions, and early treatment is generally preferable.

【诊断要点】

中风后遗症以单侧上下肢瘫痪无力，口眼歪斜，舌强语涩等为主症。初期，患者肢体软弱无力，知觉迟钝或稍有强硬，活动功能受限，以后逐渐趋于强直挛急，患侧肢体姿势常发生改变和畸形等。

口眼歪斜：口角及鼻唇沟歪向健侧，两腮鼓起漏气，但能做皱额蹙眉和闭眼等动作。

半身不遂：患侧肢体肌张力增高，关节挛缩畸形，感觉略减退，活动功能基本丧失，患侧上肢的肱二头肌、肱三头肌腱反射亢进，下肢膝腱和跟腱反射均为亢进、健侧

【Diagnoses】

Sequelae of wind stroke is characterized by unilateral paralysis of extremities, distorted mouth and eyes, and stiff tongue with difficulty in speaking. In the initial stage, the patient's limbs are weak, bradyesthesia or slightly stiff with limited in movement, and then gradually become tonic and contractile, and the posture of the affected limbs are often changed and deformed.

The corners of the mouth and the nasolabial folds are skewed to the healthy side, the cheeks are bulging and leaking, but the patient can make movements such as frowning and closing the eyes.

Hemiplegia, which is characterized by increased muscle tone, joint contracture and deformity, slightly decreased sensation, and the loss of basic movement

正常。CT或MRI检查可确诊为出血栓塞性脑病。

本病以早期以药物或手术治疗为主，中风后2周适宜推拿治疗。

function. The biceps and triceps tendon reflexes of the affected upper limb are hyperactive, and the knee and Achilles tendon reflexes of the lower limb are hyperactive, while the healthy side is normal. The diagnosis of hemorrhagic embolic encephalopathy can be confirmed by CT or MRI.

The disease is mainly treated by medication or surgery in the early stage, and massage therapy is appropriate to be applied 2 weeks later after stroke.

【治则】

平肝熄风、行气活血、舒筋通络、滑利关节是本病的治疗原则。

【Therapeutic principles】

To sooth the liver and extinguish the wind, circulate qi and blood, promote tendons and unblock collaterals and lubricate joints.

【手法】

㨰法、一指禅推法、按法、揉法、拿法、摇法、捻法、配合患肢关节的被动运动。

【Manipulations】

Rolling manipulation with the proximal interphalangeal joints, Yi Zhi Chan pushing, pressing manipulation, kneading manipulation, grasping manipulation, rotating manipulation, finger-twisting manipulation and passive movement of joints of the patients.

【取穴】

大椎、肩井、曲池、手三里、合谷、居髎、环跳、殷门、承扶、委中、承山、昆仑、血海、足三里、阳陵泉、风市、梁丘、肾俞、大肠俞、命门等穴。

【Selection of points】

Dazhui (DU 14), Jianjing (GB 21), Quchi (LI 11), Shousanli (LI 10), Hegu (LI 4), Juliao (GB 29), Huantiao (GB 30), Yinmen (BL 37), Chengfu (BL 36), Weizhong (BL 40), Chengshan (BL 57), Kunlun (BL 60), Xuehai (SP 10), Zusanli (ST 36), Yanglingquan (GB 34), Fengshi (GB 31), Liangqiu (ST 34), Shenyu (BL 23), Dachangshu (BL 25) and Mingmen (DU 4).

【操作】

先行内功推拿常规套路操作。然后选取俯卧或仰卧位针对性手法操作治疗。

（1）俯卧位：㨰背部脊柱两侧，

【Operations】

First apply the routine operation and then choose targeted manipulation treatment.

(1) Prone position: Rolling both sides of the back spine, together with the passive movement of lumbar

同时配合腰后伸被动运动；㨰臀部及下肢后侧及跟腱配合髋外展被动运动；按揉大椎、膈俞、肾俞、命门、大肠俞、环跳、委中、承山诸穴以酸胀为度；擦腰骶部以热为度。

（2）仰卧位：㨰大腿前侧、小腿前外侧至足背部；并被动屈曲患侧膝关节，按揉伏兔、梁丘、两膝眼、足三里、丘墟、解溪、太冲诸穴，以酸胀为度；拿委中、承山、昆仑、太溪部以有酸胀麻的感应为佳。

（3）坐位：㨰肩井和肩关节周围到上肢掌指部，在㨰肩前缘时结合肩关节上举、外展的被动运动，㨰腕部时结合腕关节屈伸被动运动；按揉肩内陵穴以酸为度；拿曲池、合谷穴以酸胀为度；摇掌指关节，捻指关节，搓肩部及上肢。按揉下关、颊车、地仓、人中、承浆等穴；拿两侧风池、肩井穴结束。

posterior extension, roll the hip and the posterior side of the lower limb and the Achilles tendon accompanied with passive hip abduction. Press and knead Dazhui (DU 14), Geshu (BL 17), Shenshu (BL 23), Mingmen (DU 4), Dachangshu (BL 25), Huantiao (GB 30), Weizhong (BL 40), Chengshan (BL 57) to soreness and swelling. Rub the lumbosacral area to heat.

(2) Supine position: Roll the anterior thigh, anterolateral calf to the back of the foot and passively flex the affected knee joint. Press and knead Fu Tu (ST 32), Liangqiu (ST 34), Liangxiyan (EX–LE 5), Zusanli (ST 36), Qiuxu (GB 40), Jiexi (ST 41) and Taichong (LR 3) to soreness and swelling. Grasp Weizhong (BL 40), Chengshan (BL 57), Kunlun (BL 60), Taixi (KI 3) to soreness and swelling.

(3) Sitting position: Roll Jianjing (GB 21) and around the shoulder joint to the palm and fingers. Roll the front edge of the shoulder in combination with passive movements of shoulder joint elevation and abduction and roll the wrist in combination with passive movements of wrist joint flexion and extension. Press and knead Jianneiling point to the degree of soreness, take the Quchi (LI 11) and Hegu (LI 4) to the degree of soreness and swelling. Shake the metacarpal and finger joints, twist the finger joints, and rub the shoulder and upper limbs. Press and knead Xiaguan (ST 7), Jiache (ST 6), Dicang (ST 4), Renzhong (DU 26) and Chengjiang (RN 24), grasp Fengchi (GB 20) and Jianjing (GB 21).

【功法处方】

练功是中风后遗症功能康复的重要手段之一。患者可选择锻炼少林内功站裆势结合倒拉九头牛、凤凰展翅等动作，并可配合双人锻炼法。若患者站立困难，可由医师或家属帮助进行，先训练手指或足趾

【Exercise treatments】

Shaolin internal exercise is one of the important effective methods to treat post-stroke sequelae. Patients can choose Dao La Jiu Tou Niu (Pulling Nine Oxen Backward) and Feng Huang Zhan Chi (Chinese Phoenix Spreading its Wings) combined with exercise in pairs with standing stance. If the patient has difficulty in standing, the

的运动，再训练膝、肘关节及肩、髋关节。每天早晚各锻炼1次，每次30分钟左右，以患者能耐受为度。

physician or family members can help him/her to train the fingers or toes first, then the knees, elbows, shoulders and hip joints. Exercise once in the morning and once in the evening, for 30 minutes each time.

【注意事项】

（1）中风后遗症疗程较长，医患双方都要有耐心。手法治疗和功法训练循序渐进，不可操之过急，以免引发意外。

（2）卧床不起的患者应注意经常翻身，预防褥疮的发生。

（3）注意情绪和生活饮食的调摄，防止再中风。

【Attentions】

(1) Post-stroke sequelae have a long course of treatment, and both doctors and patients should have patience. The intensity of manipulation and exercise treatment should be added slowly to avoid accidents.

(2) Patients who are bedridden should be turned frequently to prevent the occurrence of bed sores.

(3) Take care of emotions and diet to prevent another stroke.

十四、颈椎病

Cervical Spondylosis

颈椎病又称颈椎综合征，是一种中年以上年龄的慢性疾病，近年有年轻化的趋势。颈椎病是由于损伤或颈椎及其椎间盘、椎周筋肉退变引起的脊柱平衡失调，刺激颈部血管、交感神经、脊神经根和脊髓等，产生颈、肩、背、上肢、头、胸、部疼痛及其他伴随症状，甚至合并肢体功能丧失等。推拿能较好地改善症状，对于颈椎病有较好的治疗作用。

Cervical spondylosis, also known as cervical spine syndrome, is a chronic disease of middle age and older, with a trend toward younger age in recent years. Cervical spine or cervical spondylosis is a disorder of spinal balance caused by injury or degeneration of the cervical spine, its intervertebral discs and peri-vertebral muscles, which stimulates the blood vessels, sympathetic nerves, spinal nerve roots and spinal cord in the neck. This can lead to pain in the neck, shoulders, back, upper limbs, head, chest, and other symptoms, and even loss of limb function. Tuina can improve the symptoms and has a good treatment effect on cervical spondylosis.

【诊断要点】

颈椎病的临床症状复杂多变，以颈项、肩臂、肩胛上背、上胸壁及上肢疼痛或麻痛为最常见。患者往往因颈部过劳、扭伤或寒冷刺激

【Diagnoses】

The symptoms of cervical spondylosis are complex and variable, with pain or numbness in the neck, shoulders and arms, upper back of the scapula, upper chest wall and upper limbs being the most common. The disease is often

使症状加剧而诱发。临床症状的产生随病变在颈椎的平面及范围而有差异。

（1）分型

1）颈型：颈椎各椎间关节及周围筋肉损伤，导致颈肩背局部酸胀、疼痛、僵硬，不能做点头、仰头及头颈部旋转活动，呈斜颈姿势。患者回头时，颈部与躯干需共同旋转。

2）神经根型：颈丛和臂丛神经受压，造成颈项、肩胛上背、上胸壁、肩臂和手部放射性麻木、疼痛无力和肌肉萎缩，感觉异常。患者睡眠时，喜取伤肢在上的屈肘侧卧位。

3）椎动脉型：颈椎关节退变，增生而压迫椎动脉，致使椎动脉、脊髓前动脉、脊髓后动脉供血不足，造成头晕、耳鸣、记忆力减退、猝倒（猝倒后因颈部位置改变，而立即清醒，并可起来走路）。颈部侧弯及后伸到一定位置，则出现头晕加重，甚至猝倒。

4）脊髓型：颈部脊髓因受压而缺血、变性，导致脊髓传导障碍。造成四肢无力，走路不稳，瘫痪，大小便障碍等。

5）交感神经型：颈交感神经受压，造成心率异常、假性心绞痛、胸闷、顽固性头痛、眼痛、视物模糊、眼窝发胀、流泪、肢体发凉、指端红肿、出汗障碍等综合征（即霍纳尔征）。

6）混合型：临床上同时存在上述两型或两型以上症状、体征者，

triggered by symptoms exacerbated by neck overwork, sprain or cold stimulation. The clinical symptoms vary according to the plane and extent of the lesion in the cervical spine.

(1) Classification

1) Cervical type: Injury to the intervertebral joints and surrounding muscles of the cervical spine, resulting in localized soreness, pain and stiffness of the neck, shoulders and back, and inability to nod, tilt the head and rotate the head and neck, and has an oblique neck posture. When the patient turns back, the neck and trunk need to rotate together.

2) Nerve root type: Compression of the cervical plexus and brachial plexus nerves causing radiated numbness, pain, weakness, muscle atrophy and abnormal sensation in the neck, upper scapular back, upper chest wall, shoulders, arms and hands. The patient prefers to sleep in a lateral position with the injured limb on top bent.

3) Vertebral artery type: Cervical joint degeneration, hyperplasia and compression of the vertebral artery, resulting in insufficient blood supply to the vertebral artery, anterior spinal cord artery and posterior spinal cord artery, resulting in dizziness, tinnitus, memory loss, sudden collapse (after sudden collapse, the neck position changes and the person wakes up immediately and walks). If the neck is laterally bent and posteriorly extended to a certain position, patients will fell intense dizziness and even hit the floor.

4) Spinal cord type: Ischemia and degeneration of the cervical spinal cord due to compression, resulting in spinal cord conduction disorders. This causes limb weakness, unstable walking, paralysis, and difficulty in urine and stools.

5) Sympathetic type: Cervical sympathetic nerve compression, resulting in abnormal heart rate, pseudo-angina, chest tightness, intractable headache, eye pain,

即可诊断为混合型颈椎病。

（2）相应检查

1）检查颈项活动幅度是否正常。医师立于患者背后，一手安抚患者肩部，另一手扶其头部，将头颈部前屈、后伸、侧弯及旋转活动。注意其活动在何角度出现肢体放射痛，或沿何神经分布区放射。并注意其他症状的出现，有助于确定颈椎病的类型。

2）触诊时医师立于患者后方，一手扶其头部。另一手拇指由上而下逐个触摸颈椎棘突，可发现：①患椎棘突偏离脊柱中心轴线；②患椎后方项韧带剥离、钝厚、压痛或有索条状硬物；③多数患者向棘突偏歪侧转头受限或有僵硬感；④患椎平面棘突旁开一横指处可有压痛，并沿一定的神经分布区放射至伤侧上肢。

3）注意伤侧肢体有无发凉、肌萎缩与肌力、肌张力等情况。

4）椎间孔压缩试验阳性、闭气缩肛试验阳性、臂丛神经牵拉试验阳性，对神经根型和椎动脉型颈椎病的诊断具有临床意义。

5）神经协同检查应注意颈神经分布区的痛觉、触觉、温度觉有无改变，肱二头肌、三头肌腱反射有否减弱或消失，并注意下肢腱反射情况及有无病理反射。

6）为了协助或明确诊断，一般须拍正、侧、斜位X线片。重点观察颈椎生理曲线、钩椎关节、关节突间关节、椎间开、椎间隙、棘突顺列、椎体缘等变化情况。必要时

blurred vision, swelling of the eye sockets, tearing, coldness of the limbs, redness and swelling of the fingertips, sweating disorder and other syndromes (i.e. Hornar's sign).

6) Mixed type: If the above two or more types of symptoms and signs exist at the same time, it can be diagnosed as mixed type cervical spondylosis.

(2) Corresponding inspection

1) Check for the normal movement of the neck. The physician stands behind the patient, with one hand on the patient's shoulder, and the other hand on the patient's head, make the patient's head and neck do forward flexion, back extension, lateral bending and rotation activities. Note the angle at which the limb radiates pain, or along which nerve distribution area. The presence of other symptoms can help determine the type of cervical spondylosis.

2) During palpation, the physician stands behind the patient and holds his or her head with one hand. The thumb of the other hand touches the cervical spine from top to bottom one by one. ① deviation of the affected spinous process from the central axis of the spine; ② peeling, dull thickness, pressure pain or rigidity of the cords of the posterior collateral ligaments of the affected vertebrae; ③ most patients have limited head rotation or stiffness on the skewed side of the spinous process; ④ there may be pressure pain at a transverse finger opening next to the spinous process of the affected vertebra. The pressure pain can be found at the transverse finger of the spinous process in the affected plane and radiates to the injured upper limb along a certain nerve distribution area.

3) Note the presence of coldness, muscle atrophy and muscle strength, and muscle tone in the injured limb.

4) Positive intervertebral foramen compression test, positive closed-air retraction test, and positive brachial plexus nerve pull test have clinical significance in the diagnosis of neurogenic and pushing chakra type cervical

可进行CT、MRI等检查。

spondylosis.

5) The synergistic neurological examination should pay attention to the changes in pain, touch and temperature sensation in the cervical nerve distribution area and see whether the biceps and triceps tendon reflexes are weakened or absent. And attention should also be paid to the tendon reflexes of the lower extremities and the presence of pathological reflexes.

6) To assist or clarify the diagnosis, frontal, lateral and oblique X-rays are generally required. Focus on the physiological curve of the cervical spine, the changes in the hook vertebral joint, interarticular joint, intervertebral opening, vertebral space, spinous process paralleling, vertebral body margin, etc. If necessary, CT, MRI and other examinations can be performed.

【治则】

舒筋活血，理筋整复。刺激性手法与调整类手法并重，颈项部操作与循经手法刺激相结合，以颈项部操作为主的原则。

【Therapeutic principles】

To relax tendons and circulate blood and manipulate tendons and relocate joints. Give equal importance to stimulating manipulation and adjusting manipulation, combined the manipulation on the neck with the manipulation along the meridian, with the focus on the manipulation on the neck.

【手法】

选用一指禅推法、㨰法、推法、拿法、按揉法、拔伸法，拨法、分推法、合推法和颈椎调整手法等。

【Manipulations】

Yi Zhi Chan pushing, rolling manipulation with the proximal interphalangeal joints, pushing manipulation, grasping manipulation, pressing-kneading manipulation, pulling-stretching manipulation, pulling manipulation, pushing manipulation with two hands parting from each other, pushing manipulation with two hands meeting with each other, cervical spine adjustment manipulation.

【取穴】

取穴以风池、颈夹脊、肩井、天宗、肩中俞、肩外俞、天鼎、缺

【Selection of points】

Fengchi (GB 20), Jiaji (EX–B 2), Jianjing (GB 21), Tianzong (SI 11), Jianzhongshu (SI 15), Jianwaishu (SI

盆、手三里、阿是穴等为主。以颈项部、枕后部、肩胛部、横突后结节和胸椎夹脊等部位为重点。

14), Tianding (LI 17), Quepen (ST 12), Shousanli (LI 10), Ashi points, with the focus on points on the neck, posterior occipital region, scapula, posterior transverse process nodule and thoracic spine.

【操作】

按照颈项部、上背部、上肢部的顺序实施内功推拿常规操作，然后根据分型随证施治，选择针对性的操作。

推拿操作常规：由松解手法、颈椎调整手法和整理手法三部分组成。松解手法宜在逐步放松的情况下用轻缓柔和的刺激性手法，如一指禅推法、㨰法、拇指按揉法在颈项肩背部操作，刺激关键穴位及部位，并在手法刺激的同时，轻巧地小幅度被动运动头颈部。当患者颈肩背部肌肉逐渐放松之后，宜在颈椎拔伸状态下小幅度旋摇颈椎，以调整颈椎微小错移。整理手法主要采用拿法刺激两侧风池穴、两侧颈椎诸夹脊穴及两侧肩井穴，双掌从肩井向两侧分推，以枕、项部的合法结束。

（1）神经根型：常规操作基础上再以轻柔手法沿放射性神经痛路线循经推拿，小幅度持续拔伸颈椎2～3次，每次1分钟，以进一步消除神经痛；用拇指与示指相对捏住治疗部位，稍用力，做对称的快速捻动手指；然后用夹住患指，从指根部至指端，做急速的勒法。

（2）椎动脉型：在常规操作的基础上加强风池、风府等穴位的手法，再以手法轻柔地分抹患者两颞

【Operations】

The manipulation should be focused on the neck, upper back and limbs.

Routine manipulation: relaxation manipulation, cervical spine adjustment manipulation and finishing manipulation. The relaxation manipulation should be combined with gentle and stimulating manipulation, such as Yi Zhi Chan pushing, rolling manipulation, and thumb press-kneading manipulation, to operate on the back of the neck, shoulders and back. The patient's head and neck should be stimulated with key acupuncture points and areas, and the head and neck should be moved gently and passively while the patient is being stimulated. After the muscles in the back of the shoulders and neck are gradually relaxed, it is advisable to rotate the cervical vertebrae in the state of cervical extension and extraction to adjust the small misshift of the cervical vertebrae. The finishing manipulation is to stimulate the Fengchi (GB 20) on both sides, the cervical spine points on both sides and Jianjing (GB 21) on both sides. Do parting-pushing manipulation with the palms from Jianjing (GB 21) to both sides, ending with the legal occiput and collar.

(1) Nerve root type: On the basis of the conventional operation, gentle techniques are used to follow the route of radioactive neuralgia and push and stretch the cervical vertebrae along the meridians, with small amplitude and continuous. The cervical spine is extracted and stretched 2 to 3 times for 1 minute each time to further eliminate the neuralgia; the treatment area is pinched with the thumb and index finger opposite each other and then, the affected finger is held, and a sharp strangulation is performed from

及前额，以消除头面部症状。

（3）交感神经型：在常规操作的基础上以轻巧的手法在颈前气管两侧循序推移，使痉挛椎前肌群放松；然后根据患者临床症状，采用针对性的手法操作。

the root to the end of the finger.

(2) Vertebral artery type: On the basis of the conventional operation, the techniques of Fengchi (GB 20) and Fengfu (GV 16) acupuncture points were strengthened, and then the techniques were gently divided and wiped on patient's two temporal and forehead areas to eliminate head and facial symptoms.

(3) Sympathetic nerve type: Based on the conventional operation, a gentle technique is used to push on both sides of the anterior cervical trachea in a sequential manner to make the spastic vertebral anterior muscles are relaxed. Then, according to the patient's clinical symptoms, a targeted manipulation is applied.

【功法处方】

患者可选择少林内功站裆势结合乌龙钻洞、顶天抱地等动作锻炼，也可选择易筋经的九鬼拔马刀势。每天早晚各锻炼1次，每次30分钟左右，以汗出或舒适为度。

【Exercise treatments】

Patients can choose standing stance combined with the exercise of Wu Long Zuan Dong (Black Dragon Crawling into Cave) and Ding Tian Bao Di (Supporting the Sky and Embracing the Earth). Exercise once in the morning and once in the evening, 30 minutes each time to sweat or feel comfortable.

【注意事项】

（1）颈椎病患者平时宜贯彻"仰头抬臂，协调平衡"的原则，以锻炼颈部后伸肌群，平衡长期低头位而引起的颈部应力和稳定平衡失调。

（2）注意纠正平时的不良习惯姿势，肩颈部的保暖和用枕的合理性，立足于预防。

（3）推拿治疗颈椎病务必选择适应证型，注意手法安全性，避免推拿意外。

【Attentions】

(1) Patients with cervical spondylosis should usually conform to the principle of "tilting the head and raising the arms, coordinating and balancing" to exercise the posterior extension muscles of the neck and moderate the stress and stable imbalance of the neck caused by long-term low head position.

(2) Pay attention to the correction of the bad habits posture, keep the shoulders and neck warm, and use the suitable pillow for prevention of the disease.

(3) It is important to choose the appropriate type of tuina treatment for cervical spondylosis, pay attention to the safety of the manipulation, and avoid accidents.

十五、胸胁屏伤

Pain in the Chest When Breathing

胸胁屏伤又称岔气，是指由于身体姿势不当时用力引起胸胁部气机壅滞，出现以胸部板紧掣痛、胸闷不舒为主要症状的一种病症。胸廓由全部胸椎、胸骨和12对肋脊柱关节和韧带连结而成。在正常的呼吸运动中，胸廓中各关节活动范围较小，随着呼吸运动而活动。若胸壁肌肉受到牵拉或挤压，而产生痉挛或撕裂伤，会刺激肋间神经，引起疼痛。

Pain in the chest when breathing, also known side stitch, is a condition in which the stagnation of qi in the chest caused by drawing on strength in improper body posture. The main symptoms are tightness, pain and oppression in the chest. The thorax consists of all thoracic vertebrae, sternums and 12 pairs of rib spinal joints and ligaments. During normal respiratory movements, the joints in the thorax have a small range of motion and move with the respiratory movement. If the muscles of the chest wall are stretched or squeezed, resulting in spasm or laceration, the intercostal nerves will be stimulated, causing pain.

【诊断要点】

（1）外伤史：一般均有明显外伤史，伤后出现疼痛，多呈窜痛，疼痛区域模糊，范围较广，深呼吸及咳嗽时疼痛加重，疼痛有时牵扯背部，并可伴有胸闷不适等症状。

（2）体征及检查：胸壁无明显压痛，患者呼吸运动减小，呼吸浅促，不敢咳嗽，动作缓慢。如胸壁肌损伤，损伤部位可有肿胀、压痛明显。

（3）X线检查：由于胸椎后关节错位乃解剖位置上的细微变化，故X线片常不易显示。但X线检查可除外胸椎结核、肿瘤、骨折、类风湿等疾病。

【Diagnoses】

(1) History of trauma: There is usually a history of significant trauma and pain after the injury. Most of the pains are flickering, with a vague and widespread pain area. The pain increases with deep breathing and coughing, sometimes involving the back, and may be accompanied by oppression in the chest and other symptoms.

(2) Signs and examinations: There is no obvious pressure pain in the chest wall. The patient's respiratory movement has reduced with short and rapid breathing with slow movement and avoids coughing. And if the chest wall muscle is injured, there may be obvious swelling and pressure pain at the injury site.

(3) X-ray examination: Because posterior thoracic joint misalignment is a subtle change in anatomic position, it is often not easily revealed on X-ray. However, X-rays can exclude diseases such as thoracic spine tuberculosis, tumors, fractures, rheumatoid diseases, etc.

【治则】

活血化瘀，理气止痛。

【Therapeutic principles】

Circulating blood to reslove stasis, regulating qi to

relieve pain.

【手法】

擦法、按揉法、拿法等。

【Manipulations】

Linear rubbing manipulation, pressing-kneading manipulation and grasping manipulation.

【取穴】

章门、期门、阿是穴等。

【Selection of points】

Zhang Men (LR 13), Qi Men (LA 14) and Ashi points.

【操作】

按照前胸部、后背部及上肢部的常规套路操作，然后选择下述方法采用局部治疗。

（1）擦胸、背胁肋部，以患侧局部为主；按揉章门、期门、压痛点，以行气止痛。

（2）用鱼际擦胁部，小鱼际直向擦背部，以冬青膏辅之，以透热为度。

（3）局部配合热敷。

【Operations】

Follow the routine treatment of the front chest, back and upper limbs, then select the following methods for local treatment.

(1) Rub the chest and dorsal hypochondrium with a focus on the affected side, press and knead Zhang Men (LR 13), Qi Men (LA 14) and press points, to circulate qi and alleviate pain.

(2) Rub the ribs with thenar, vertically rub the back with hypothenar with holly ointment to the penetration of heat.

(3) Do hot compresses.

【功法处方】

患者可选择锻炼少林内功站坐裆势，逐渐配合上肢动作，如凤凰展翅、风摆荷叶等，锻炼时可配合出声发力。以后逐渐加强马裆势、弓箭裆势的锻炼，并可配合双人锻炼法。每天早晚各锻炼1次，每次30分钟左右，以汗出或舒适为度。

【Exercise treatments】

Patients can choose standing and sitting stances combined with the movement of upper limbs, as Feng Huang Zhan Chi (Chinese Phoenix Spreading its Wings) and Feng Bai He Ye (Wind Blowing Lotus Leaf). Speak loudly when exercising. Then increase the exercise of horse stance and bow stance combined with exercise in pairs. Exercise once in the morning and once in the evening, for 30 minutes each time.

【注意事项】

（1）需注意排除胸膜炎、肿瘤及其他骨关节病，需要先明确诊断。

（2）治疗期间注意保暖和休息，

【Attentions】

(1) Care needs to be taken to rule out pleurisy, tumors and other osteoarthropathies, which require a clear diagnosis first.

避免负重和劳累。

（3）卧硬板床。

(2) Keep warm and rest during treatment, avoid weight bearing and straining.

(3) Sleeping on a hard board bed.

十六、腰肌劳损

Lumbar Strain

腰肌劳损是指腰骶部肌肉、筋膜以及韧带等软组织的慢性损伤，导致局部无菌性炎症，从而引起腰臀部一侧或两侧的弥漫性疼痛。本病又称腰臀肌筋膜炎或功能性腰痛，中医学称为肾虚腰痛，是慢性腰腿痛中常见的疾病之一。

Lumbar strain is a chronic injury to the lumbosacral muscles, fascia, and soft tissues such as ligaments, resulting in local sterile inflammation that causes diffuse pain on one or both sides of the lumbar hip. This disease is also known as lumbar gluteal myofasciitis or functional lumbago, and in Chinese medicine is called as kidney deficiency lumbago. It is one of the common diseases of chronic low back pain.

【诊断要点】

（1）症状：长期反复发作的腰背部酸痛不适，或钝性胀痛，腰部重着板紧如负重物，时轻时重，缠绵不愈。充分休息、加强保暖、适当活动或改变体位姿势可使症状减轻，劳累或遇阴雨天气，受风寒湿影响则症状加重。腰部活动基本正常，一般无明显障碍，但有时有牵掣不适感。不能久坐久站，不能胜任弯腰工作，弯腰稍久，便直腰困难，常喜双手捶击腰背部。急性发作时，诸症明显加重，可有明显的肌痉挛，甚至出现腰脊柱侧弯，下肢牵掣作痛等症状。

（2）体征：腰背部压痛范围较广泛，压痛点多在竖脊肌、腰椎横突及髂嵴后缘等部位。肌痉挛：触诊时腰部肌肉紧张痉挛，或有硬结及肥厚感。

【Diagnoses】

(1) Symptoms: It is characterized by long-term recurrent episodes of low back pain, or dull pain, lumbar heavy plate tight as a heavy load, sometimes light, sometimes heavy. Have a good rest and keep warm. Do some activities or change postures can alleviate the symptoms. But excessive fatigue or rainy days will aggravate the symptoms. The lumbar performance is basically normal, generally there are no obvious obstacles but pulling discomfort. The patient is unable to sit, bend and stand for a long time, or do bending work. And the patients will find it difficult to straighten his waist, so he likes to pound his waist and back with hands. In acute attacks, the symptoms will aggravate with obvious muscle spasm, and even scoliosis of the lumbar spine and painful pulling of the lower limbs.

(2) Physical signs: The pressure pain in the low back is widespread, with pressure points mostly in the erector spinae, the transverse process of the lumbar spine and the posterior border of the iliac crest. Muscle Spasm: Tension

（3）X 线检查：少数患者可有先天性畸形或骨质增生，余无异常发现。

and spasm of the lumbar muscles on palpation, or a feeling of hardness and hypertrophy.

(3) X-ray examination: Few patients may have congenital malformations or osteophytes.

【治则】

舒筋活血，温经通络。

【Therapeutic principles】

Relaxing tendons to circulate blood, warming meridians to unblock collaterals.

【手法】

擦法、㨰法、按法、揉法、推法、拿法、点法、拨法、搓法、背法等。

【Manipulations】

Linear rubbing manipulation, rolling manipulation with the proximal interphalangeal joints, pressing manipulation, kneading manipulation, pushing manipulation, grasping manipulation, point-pressing manipulation, plucking manipulation, palm-twisting manipulation and back-carrying manipulation.

【取穴】

肾俞、腰阳关、大肠俞、八髎、秩边、委中、承山。

【Selection of points】

Shenshu (BL 23), Yaoyangguan (GV 3), Dachangshu (BL 25), Baliao (BL 31–34), Zhibian (BL 54), Weizhong (BL 40) and Chengshan (BL 57).

【操作】

按照腰背部、下肢部的顺序实施内功推拿常规套路的操作。然后再选择以下针对性的治疗。

（1）松解手法：患者俯卧位，医者站于一侧，先用㨰、按揉法沿两侧膀胱经由上而下往返施术3～5遍，用力由轻到重；然后用双手拇指按揉肾俞、腰阳关、大肠俞、八髎等穴，以酸胀为度，并配合腰部后伸被动运动数次。

（2）解痉止痛法：医者用点压、弹拨手法施术于痛点及肌痉挛处，反复3～5遍，以达到提高痛阈、松

【Operations】

According to the routine order of waist and back, lower limbs. Then select the following targeted treatments.

(1) Relaxing manipulation: With the patient in prone position and the practitioner standing on one side, first roll and press the bladder meridian along both sides from top to bottom and back again. Apply 3 to 5 times with light to heavy pressure. Then press and knead Shenshu (BL 23), Yaoyangguan (GV 3), Dachangyu (BL 25) and Baliao (BL 31–34) to soreness and swelling combined with several times of passively posterior movement of back.

(2) Alleviate spasm and pain: Do point-pressing manipulation and plucking manipulation on the pain point and the muscle spasm for 3 to 5 times, with the purpose to

解粘连、解痉止痛的目的。

（3）调整关节紊乱：患者侧卧位，医者面向患者站立，施腰部斜扳法，左右各 1 次，再取仰卧位，双下肢屈膝屈髋，医者抱住患者双膝做腰骶旋转，顺、逆时针各 8 ～ 10 次，然后做抱膝滚腰 16 ～ 20 次。亦可采用背法操作以调整腰骶关节。

（4）整理手法：患者俯卧位，医者先分别用㨰法、揉法在腰臀及大腿后外侧依次施术，往返3 ～ 5 遍，并点按秩边、委中、承山等穴；然后用小鱼际直擦腰背两侧膀胱经，横擦腰骶部，以透热为度；最后用五指并拢，腕部放松，有节律地叩打腰背及下肢膀胱经部位。用力宜由轻到重，以患者能忍受为度。

alleviate spasm and pain.

(3) Adjustment of joint disorders: The patient was lying on his side, the doctor stood facing the patient and applied obliquely pulling manipulation on lumbar vertebrae method, one time on each of side. Then the patient takes the supine position, bending knees and hips, and the doctor holds the patient's knees and does lumbosacral rotation, clockwise and counterclockwise 8 to 10 times each, and then bow the knees and roll the waist for 16 to 20 times. The back method can also be used to adjust the lumbosacral joints.

(4) Finishing manipulation: With the patient in prone position, the practitioner first applies the rolling and kneading manipulations on the waist and buttocks for 3 to 5 times in turn. Then, the practitioner point-presses Zhibian (BL 54), Weizhong (BL 40) and Chengshan (BL 57) and rubs the bladder meridian on both sides of the waist and back with hypothenar, and transversely rubs the lumbosacral area to the penetration of heat. Finally, with the five fingers together and the wrist relaxed, tap rhythmically on the bladder meridians of the waist and back and lower limbs. And the force should be within the tolerance of the patient.

【功法处方】

练功是内功推拿治疗腰肌劳损的重要手段之一。患者可选择少林内功站裆势结合前推八匹马、倒拉九头牛等动作锻炼，以后逐渐加强马裆势、弓箭裆势的锻炼，并可配合双人锻炼法。每天早晚各锻炼 1 次，每次 30 分钟左右，以汗出或略感疲劳为度。也可进行仰卧位拱桥式锻炼、俯卧位的飞燕式锻炼，早晚各 1 次，每次各做 20 ～ 30 遍。有利于腰背肌力的恢复。

【Exercise treatments】

Shaolin internal exercise is one of the important effective methods to treat lumbar strain. Patients can choose standing stance combined with the exercise of Qian Tui Ba Pi Ma (Pushing Eight Horses Forward) and Dao La Jiu Tou Niu (Pulling Nine Oxen Backward). Then gradually strengthen the exercise of horse stance and bow stance combined with exercise in pairs. Exercise once in the morning and once in the evening, for 30 minutes each time. Patients can also choose the Arch-bridge-like exercise and Flying-swallow-like exercise once in the morning and once in the evening, for 20 to 30 times each time. They do good for the recovery of the waist and back.

【注意事项】

（1）在日常生活和工作中，纠正不良姿势，经常变换体位，勿使过度疲劳。

（2）注意休息和局部保暖，节制房事。

（3）平日加强腰背肌肉锻炼，适当参加户外活动或功法锻炼。

【Attentions】

(1) In daily life and work, correct postures, change positions frequently. Do not make excessive fatigue.

(2) Take care of rest and local warmth, and abstain from sexual intercourse.

(3) Strengthen the muscle exercise of the lower back and participate in outdoor activities or exercises as appropriate.